T0417921

YOGA AND MEDITATION

Past and Present Evidence

YOGA AND MEDITATION

Past and Present Evidence

Edited by
Sachi Nandan Mohanty, PhD
Rabindra Kumar Pradhan, PhD
Sugyanta Priyadarshini, PhD

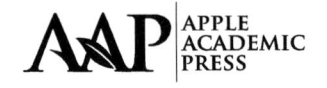

APPLE ACADEMIC PRESS

First edition published 2025

Apple Academic Press Inc.
1265 Goldenrod Circle, NE,
Palm Bay, FL 32905 USA

760 Laurentian Drive, Unit 19,
Burlington, ON L7N 0A4, CANADA

CRC Press
2385 NW Executive Center Drive,
Suite 320, Boca Raton FL 33431

4 Park Square, Milton Park,
Abingdon, Oxon, OX14 4RN UK

Library and Archives Canada Cataloguing in Publication

Title: Yoga and meditation : past and present evidence / edited by Sachi Nandan Mohanty, PhD, Rabindra Kumar Pradhan, PhD, Sugyanta Priyadarshini, PhD.
Other titles: Yoga and meditation (Palm Bay, Fla.)
Names: Mohanty, Sachi Nandan, editor | Pradhan, Rabindra Kumar, editor | Priyadarshini, Sugyanta, editor.
Description: First edition. | Includes bibliographical references and index.
Identifiers: Canadiana (print) 20240465040 | Canadiana (ebook) 20240465121 | ISBN 9781774918340 (hardcover) | ISBN 9781774918357 (softcover) | ISBN 9781003568308 (ebook)
Subjects: LCSH: Yoga—Therapeutic use. | LCSH: Yoga—Health aspects.
Classification: LCC RM727.Y64 Y54 2025 | DDC 615.8/24—dc23

Library of Congress Cataloging-in-Publication Data

CIP data on file with US Library of Congress

ISBN: 978-1-77491-834-0 (hbk)
ISBN: 978-1-77491-835-7 (pbk)
ISBN: 978-1-00356-830-8 (ebk)

About the Editors

Sachi Nandan Mohanty, PhD (FIE.FIETE, EAI)
Professor, VIT-AP University, Andhra Pradesh, India

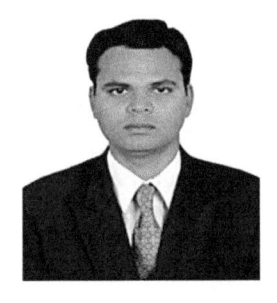

Sachi Nandan Mohanty, PhD, has been recognized on the list of Top 2% World Scientists Ranking by Stanford University and Elsevier for the years 2022 and 2023. He received his postdoctoral degree from the Indian Institute of Technology Kanpur, India, in the year 2019 and PhD from the same university in the 2015, with a MHRD scholarship from the Government of India. He has authored/edited 52 books, published by IEEE, Wiley, Springer, Wiley, CRC Press, Nova Science Publishers, and DeGruyter. His research areas include data mining, big data analysis, cognitive science, fuzzy decision making, brain-computer interface, cognition, and computational intelligence. Prof. Mohanty has received four best paper awards during his PhD from an international conference in Beijing, China, and the other at International Conference on Soft Computing Applications, organized by IIT Rookee in the year 2013. He has awarded a best thesis award first prize by the Computer Society of India in the year 2015. He has guided nine PhD scholars and 23 postgraduate students. He has published 120 papers in international journals of repute. He has received many international and national awards from the Government of India Department of Science and Technology, along with SERB funding for international travel for presenting research papers. He has received many awards and fellowships during his career, including election as a fellow of the Institute of Engineers, Ambassador European Alliance Innovation (EAI) Springer, and senior member of the IEEE Computer Society Hyderabad chapter. He also received the Prof. Ganesh Mishra Memorial Award on the 61st Annual Technical Session and 19th Prof. Bhubaneswar Behera Lecturer on 23-24th June 2020 from The Institution of Engineers (India) Odisha State Center, Bhubaneswar.

He is a member of professional bodies like IETE, CSI, IE, IEEE (Hyderabad section). He also a reviewer for the Journal of Robotics and

Autonomous Systems (Elsevier), Computational and Structural Biotechnology Journal (Elsevier), Artificial Intelligence Review (Springer), and Spatial Information Research (Springer). He is leading as general chair of two international conferences such as ICISML and AIHC and is editor in chief of the international journal EAI Endorsed Transactions on Intelligent Systems and Machine. Dr. Mohanty has gone for academic assignments to USA, Paris, Slovakia, Singapore, Abu Dhabi, Dubai, Malaysia, and Germany for delivering keynote talks and chairing sessions of international conferences with travel support from the Department of Science & Technology, Government of India, New Delhi, India.

He is a member of professional bodies like IETE, CSI, IE, IEEE (Hyderabad section). He also the reviewer of Journal of Robotics and Autonomous Systems (Elsevier), Computational and Structural Biotechnology Journal (Elsevier), Artificial Intelligence Review (Springer), Spatial Information Research (Springer). He is leading as General chair of 2 international conferences such as ICISML, AIHC and editor in chief of international journal Intelligent System and Machine learning Application. Dr. Mohanty has gone for academic assignment to USA, Paris, Slovakia, Singapore, Abu Dhabi, Dubai, Malaysia, and Germany for delivering Key note talk and chair the sessions in international conferences with travel support from Department of Science & Technology, Government of India, New Delhi, India.

Rabindra Kumar Pradhan, PhD
Full Professor, Psychology and Human Resources, Department of Humanities and Social Sciences, Indian Institute of Technology, Kharagpur, India

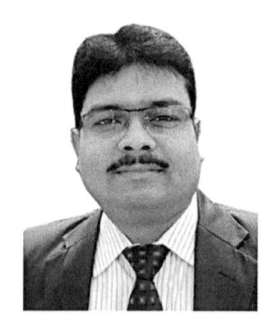

Rabindra Kumar Pradhan, PhD, is currently working as a Full Professor of Psychology and Human Resources in the Department of Humanities and Social Sciences at the Indian Institute of Technology Kharagpur, India. With more than 22 years of experience in research and teaching, Prof. Pradhan has worked in various aspects of psychology and human resources. He has served as a guest faculty and adjunct faculty at IIM Indore, IIM Kozhikode, and many other institutes and universities. He has successfully completed over 20 major research projects sponsored by various agencies of the Government of India and other international agencies. Under his supervision, 12 PhD research theses and over 35 master-level dissertations have been awarded. He has authored five books, more than 25 book chapters, and over 80 research papers in peer-reviewed journals of international repute. His academic works have been published in journals and books by publishers such as Routledge, Emerald, Inderscience, Sage, Springer, Taylor & Francis, CRC Press, Apple Academic Press, Lambert Academic Publishing, and Pearson Education, among others. His current research interests include spirituality at work, psychological capital, emotional intelligence, yoga, resilience, happiness, and well-being. Prof. Pradhan has conducted training sessions for thousands of executives at different levels in various organizations, including the Indian Army, Navy & Air Force personnel, teachers, managers, and professionals from NGOs and other service sectors. He is a member of the International Association of Applied Psychology, Academy of Management, National Academy of Psychology (India), Indian Academy of Applied Psychology, and other prestigious organizations. Prof. Pradhan has received several awards, including the ISTD Best Trainer Award, Best Teacher Award in HRD, and Best Research Paper Award at ICOM, among others.

Sugyanta Priyadarshini, PhD
Assistant Professor, Department of Humanities, Kalinga Institute of Industrial Technology (KIIT), Deemed to be University, Bhubaneswar, Odisha, India

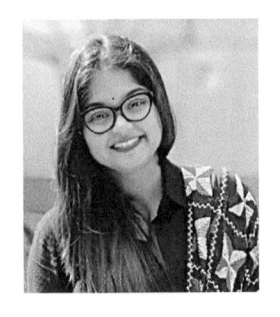

Sugyanta Priyadarshini, PhD, is an Assistant Professor in the Department of Economics and Commerce, Kalinga Institute of Industrial Technology (KIIT), Deemed to be University, Bhubaneswar, Odisha, India. Dr. Sugyanta earned her doctoral degree (PhD) in 2021 and was a university topper and gold medalist in her master's examination in 2016. She has successfully published approximately 20 research articles and book chapters in journals and books of high repute. She has participated in more than 30 international/national conferences and has been a moderator for several workshops and seminars. Presently, she is guiding two doctoral candidates. Her research areas are gender economics, artificial intelligence in social issues, and behavioral economics. She has successfully received three research grants from the Indian Council of Social Science Research (ICSSR) (one major and two minor projects) as Project Director and Project Coordinator.

Recently, she has revealed her interest in spiritual interventions by participating in a national conference on "spiritualism: a potential key for stress management." She is a regular reviewer for several journals, such as Human Rights Review (Springer), Lancet Regional Health Southeast Asia (Lancet Group), Technology, Knowledge and Learning (Springer) Asian Journal of Women's Studies (Taylor and Francis), International Journal of Qualitative Methods (Sage Publishing), Gender in Management (Emerald), and Management in Environment Quality (Emerald). Additionally, she has remained the awardee of the best paper at the 22nd Pattaya International Conference on Economics, Education and Humanities and Social Sciences (PEEHSS-19), best paper at the International Conference on Education 4.0 (IMHRC 2020), and best paper award at the M.S. Gore Centenary Conference 2021 by Tata Institute of Social Sciences (TISS), Mumbai 2021. She is currently an active member of Odisha Economic Association (OEA).

Contents

Contributors .... *xi*

Preface .... *xv*

1. **Yoga: Legacy Illuminates the Future** 1
   Antriksh and Ambika Warrier

2. **Impact of Yoga on Social Life and Humanity** 19
   Yogita Bisht and Pawan Singh Mehra

3. **Well-Being and Quality of Life Through Yoga: Rethinking Our Notions of Happiness** 31
   Richa Chopra, Shashank Shekhar Tripathi, Rahul Sanal, and Kashinath G. Metri

4. **Effect of Yoga and Meditation on "Quality of Life": Comparison among People Who Practice and Those Who Don't** 61
   Mousumi Sethy, Pallabi Mishra, Puspita Bharati Samantaray, and Rituparna Mitra

5. **Mental Component Study to Ensure Sustainable Health Through Quality of Life of Participants in Challenging Situations of the 21st Century** 79
   Rohit Rastogi, Tribhuvan Mishra, Vaishnavi Mishra, Saransh Chauhan, Rohan Tyagi, and Utkarsh Pratap Shahi

6. **Female Adolescents are a Step Ahead of Male Adolescents in Decision-Making via Yoga-Cultivated Attentiveness: Pedagogy Interventions in Indian Settings** 113
   Sugyanta Priyadarshini, Sarthak Dash, Sukanya Priyadarshini, and Nisrutha Dulla

7. **Impact of Yoga and Meditation with Mudras in Building Quality of Life** 135
   Sheelu Sagar, Rohit Rastogi, Ishwar V. Basavaraddi, and Vikas Garg

8. **Managing Polycystic Ovarian Syndrome Through Suryanamaskar** 159
   Yashvi Panjrath, Anjalee, and Vijendra Nath Pathak

9. **Statistically Examining the Effect of Herbal and Spiritual
    Environment on Various Dimensions of Adolescents'
    Fitness Post-COVID Effects**...175
    Rohit Rastogi, Mamta Saxena, Pranav Sharma, Yati Varshney,
    Vaibhav Aggarwal, and Richa Singh

10. **Statistical Surveillance on Effect of Ayurvedic Herbs on
    Improvement in Brain Power of Children**..233
    Rohit Rastogi, Mamta Saxena, Charu Tripathi, Yati Varshney,
    Rayush Jain, and Prabhinav Mishra

11. **Yoga as a Protective Factor for Arresting Cognitive Impairment
    and Promoting Well-Being Among Institutionalized Seniors**.............271
    Eshva Shah and Urmi Nanda Biswas

12. **Yoga and Mindfulness: A Positive Health Framework**.......................297
    Kailash Jandu and Rabindra Kumar Pradhan

13. **Yoga for the Management of Diabetes**...315
    Ravi Shanker Datti

Index...*329*

Contributors

Vaibhav Aggarwal
Department of Electronics and Communication Engineering, ABES Engineering College, Ghaziabad, Uttar Pradesh, India

Anjalee
Department of Psychology, Gurukula Kangari University, Haridwar, Uttarakhand, India

Antriksh
Practitioner Marma Chikitsa, Acupuncture (Registered with MCA), Adyant Health, India

Ishwar V. Basavaraddi
Morarji Desai National Institute of Yoga, Ministry of AYUSH, New Delhi, India

Yogita Bisht
Department of Kayachikitsa, GS Ayurveda Medical College and Hospital, Pilkhuwa, Uttar Pradesh, India

Urmi Nanda Biswas
Department of Psychology, Faculty of Arts, Delhi University

Saransh Chauhan
Student, Department of CSE, ABES Engineering College, Ghaziabad, Uttar Pradesh, India

Richa Chopra
Center of Excellence for Indian Knowledge Systems, Indian Institute of Technology (IIT), Kharagpur, West Bengal, India

Sarthak Dash
School of Humanities, KIIT Deemed to be University, Bhubaneswar, Odisha, India

Ravi Shanker Datti
Assistant Professor, Department of Applied Psychology, GITAM School of Gandhian Studies, GITAM (Deemed to be University), Visakhapatnam, Andhra Pradesh, India

Nisrutha Dulla
School of Humanities, KIIT Deemed to be University, Bhubaneswar, Odisha, India

Vikas Garg
Amity Business School, Amity University, Noida, Uttar Pradesh, India

Rayush Jain
Student, Department of CSE, ABES Engineering College, Ghaziabad, Uttar Pradesh, India

Kailash Jandu
Scientist-B, DRDO, 14 Services Selection Board, Selection Centre East, Prayagraj, Uttar Pradesh, India

Pawan Singh Mehra
Department of Computer Science Engineering, Delhi Technological University, New Delhi, India

Kashinath G. Metri
Department of Yoga, Central University of Rajasthan, Ajmer, Rajasthan, India

Pallabi Mishra
Assistant Professor, Department of Business Administration, Utkal University, Bhubaneswar, Odisha, India

Prabhinav Mishra
Student, Department of CSE, ABES Engineering College, Ghaziabad, Uttar Pradesh, India

Tribhuvan Mishra
Student, Department of CSE, ABES Engineering College, Ghaziabad, Uttar Pradesh, India

Vaishnavi Mishra
Student, Department of CSE, ABES Engineering College, Ghaziabad, Uttar Pradesh, India

Rituparna Mitra
Post-Graduate in Psychology, Department of Psychology, Utkal University, India

Yashvi Panjrath
Department of Psychology, School of Social Science and Language, Lovely Professional University, Punjab, India

Vijendra Nath Pathak
Department of Psychology, School of Social Science and Language, Lovely Professional University, Punjab, India

Rabindra Kumar Pradhan
Professor, Department of Humanities and Social Sciences, Indian Institute of Technology, Kharagpur, West Medinipur, West Bengal, India

Sugyanta Priyadarshini
School of Humanities, KIIT Deemed to be University, Bhubaneswar, Odisha, India

Sukanya Priyadarshini
Berhampur University, Odisha, India

Rohit Rastogi
Associate Professor, Department of Computer Science and Engineering, ABES Engineering College, Ghaziabad, Uttar Pradesh, India

Sheelu Sagar
Amity International Business School, Amity University, Noida, Uttar Pradesh, India

Puspita Bharati Samantaray
Post-Graduate in Psychology, Department of Psychology, Utkal University, India

Rahul Sanal
Freelancer, Sanal Kumar Foundation, Thiruvananthapuram, India

Mamta Saxena
Ex-DG, MoS-PI, Government of India, New Delhi, India

Mousumi Sethy
Assistant Professor, Department of Psychology, Utkal University, Bhubaneswar, Odisha, India

Eshva Shah
Ahmedabad University, Ahmedabad

Utkarsh Pratap Shahi
Student, Department of CSE, ABES Engineering College, Ghaziabad, Uttar Pradesh, India

Pranav Sharma
Dayalbagh Educational Institute, Agra, Uttar Pradesh, India

Richa Singh
Ramjas College, Delhi University, India

Charu Tripathi
BAMS, MD(Ayu.) CMO, MCD, Delhi, India

Shashank Shekhar Tripathi
Pragyan Ritam Yog Aranya Nyas (PRYAN) Ashram, Udaipur, Rajasthan, India

Rohan Tyagi
Student, Department of CSE, ABES Engineering College, Ghaziabad, Uttar Pradesh, India

Yati Varshney
Student, Department of Computer Science and Engineering, ABES Engineering College, Ghaziabad, Uttar Pradesh, India

Ambika Warrier
Founder, RCI Registered Rehabilitation Counsellor, Psychotherapist, Aananda Center for Counselling, India

Preface

This book provides a holistic insight into the perennial bliss of yoga on body, mind, and spirit. This book isn't just a manual of the yogic postures for a body of any shape and size; it also highlights the ways to achieve optimum mental and spiritual health. Collectively, it gives an idea about how physical, mental, spiritual, and social health can be improved by practicing yoga diligently. The book highlights the simple fact that there is more to yoga than just the poses. It gives you a glimpse of the beneficial effects of yoga on improving certain medical conditions and uplifting the quality of life.

With an amalgamation of multiple chapters, this book is an important resource of knowledge for all yoga practitioners and believers. Each chapter of the book provides a succinct introduction to the benefits of yoga in different spheres.

The book begins with an introductory chapter on the benefits of practicing yoga on social life and humanity. Further, the second chapter of the book elucidates the robust impact of yoga on socio-emotional development, focusing on notions of happiness. It emphasizes the benefits of yoga in cultivating mindfulness, managing stress and anxiety, developing positive psychology, and bringing oneness of body, mind, and spirit. Further, the third book chapter attempts to draw an analogy between yoga and happiness for both yoga practitioners and non-practitioners. It tries to establish the relation between a person's well-being, quality of life, and cultivating happiness by practicing yoga. Moreover, the book also makes an effort to emphasize certain yogic postures that focus on the science of happiness, developing sustainable health, and enhancing the level of happiness in life.

Additionally, the book focuses on the improvement of the quality of life by practicing yoga especially for female and male adolescents via yoga-cultivated attentiveness pedagogy interventions. One chapter explains the role of yoga in improving memory and mental health, boosting immunity, lowering the symptoms of stress and anxiety, and improving sleep quality with yogic mudras and surya namaskar. It draws a picture of the long-term benefits of yoga and the ways in which yoga has catapulted the lives of people in every aspect. The comparison between yoga practitioners and non-practitioners brings a strong contrast in the dimensions of happiness level, mental balance, stress management, and medical conditions. This chapter provides sheer motivation to start practicing yoga.

The book further goes on to present a chapter titled, Mental Component Study to Ensure Sustainable Health through Quality of Life of Participants in Challenging Situations of the 21st Century. It emphasizes how yogic practices affect the quality of life of people and improve their health standards.

The book has an interesting chapter on how female adolescents are a step ahead of male adolescents in decision-making via yoga-cultivated attentiveness pedagogy interventions in Indian settings. This also brings to light the benefits of incorporating yoga in schools to improve attentiveness, enhance the ability to focus on work and stay on task, ameliorate socio-emotional quotient in learning, enhance ways to instill positive coping mechanisms to counteract stress, and lastly, to provide methodologies to enhance self-control.

Moreover, the book also covers the use of mudras or hand postures to channelize inner energy and recharge the energy levels within. More often, the use of mudras is overlooked. Hence, one chapter guides on ways in which benefits of yoga can be maximized by practicing yoga mudras. It also emphasizes the different ways in which deepening the practice of mudras can act as a medium to bring significant changes, like controlling mood swings, clearing the mind, adding clarity in life, and sharpening focus.

The book also has a chapter on the role of Surya Namaskar in controlling a common hormonal problem in many women, which is polycystic ovarian syndrome (PCOS). This book chapter explains the steps of doing a perfect Surya Namaskar and also its role in maintaining lipid profile, reducing fat, and regulating the menstrual cycle. The book presents a statistical examination of the effect of herbal and spiritual environment on various dimensions of adolescents' fitness in the post-Covid scenario. It gives an idea about the significant improvement in the spirituality quotient amongst the adolescents by herbal and spiritual environment. The book also has a unique chapter that presents a statistical surveillance on the effect of Ayurvedic herbs on the improvement in the brainpower of children.

This book provides encompassing knowledge on the multiple benefits of practicing yoga in all age groups. It is an ideal book for yoga lovers, with simple and lucid language for better reading and understanding. With many interesting and dynamic chapters of timeless lessons, comparisons, and deep analysis, this book goes beyond the physical benefits of yoga and will inspire readers to explore different dimensions of yoga.

CHAPTER 1

Yoga: Legacy Illuminates the Future

ANTRIKSH[1] and AMBIKA WARRIER[2]

[1]Founder, Practitioner Marma Chikitsa, Acupuncture (Registered with MCA), Adyant Health, India

[2]Founder, RCI Registered Rehabilitation Counsellor, Psychotherapist, Aananda Center for Counselling, India

ABSTRACT

Yoga is a system of liberation from the cycles. The health benefits are consequential to fundamental reformation as part of the yogic process. It is meant for those prepared to dissociate from the patterns of life and realize the true nature of existence. This chapter extrapolates the foundation and purpose of a yogic life. In this chapter, we have made an effort to exemplify the concepts of *Vayus*, *Doshas*, and *Naḍis*, as their complete understanding is only possible through the experiential process of Yoga. However, we are hopeful that these cognitive concepts have the potential to illuminate the path to discovery of a life we never thought possible. The collective effort of like-minded individuals can help bring back the *Bharatiya parampara* to the mainstream and not be addressed as 'alternate systems.'

1.1 WHAT IS YOGA?

योगश्चित्तवृत्तिनिरोधः (Anand, Chandla, & Dogra, 2018) The Yoga Sutras of *Patanjali* is perhaps the most well-preserved documentation that explicates the method and purpose of Yoga. Purpose precedes pursuance, and

Yoga and Meditation: Past and Present Evidence. Sachi Nandan Mohanty, Rabindra Kumar Pradhan, & Sugyanta Priyadarshini (Eds.)

it's explicitly expressed in the *Samadhi Pada* (first chapter): *Yogaś citta vṛitti nirodhaḥ*. In modern vernacular: The restraint of the modifications of the mind is *Yoga*. The hallmark of the sutras is that their purpose is the consequence of the preparation and not what one strives for. It is not a struggle for attainment, but a process of liberation. It's a journey from perception to observation.

1.2   THE LEGACY

Yoga is a journey of many paths; we can call them 'schools' depending on the source of transcendence of knowledge. The *Srimad Bhagavad Gita* offers *Trimarga*, the three-forked path to liberation comprising *Jnana, Karma*, and *Bhakti* forms of Yoga (Charaka, & Valiathan, 2023). Traditionally, Yoga is practiced as *Ashtanga, Hatha, Jnana, Karma, Kriya, Bhakti*, and besides these, variations and adaptations exist. The origin of Yoga as a system is an intricate foray into antiquity with contrasting chronological narratives. However, knowledge holds value when contextualized to time, place, and operator; hence Yoga assumes multiple forms, with one purpose: Liberation. For simplicity, we shall focus on the Yoga Sutras of *Patanjali* for its structure, archival veracity, and pragmatism. The deliberation that follows from here is a humble attempt at capturing the spirit of these yogic formulations, for the intellectual pre-eminence of Maharishi *Patanjali* is unparalleled. Fundamentally, the Yogic process is beyond academic deliberations; any act to confine the process to intellectual comprehension will severely dilute its purpose and intent. It's a path and an experience to surpass the bounds of intellect; hence it cannot be understood by the very tool it's designed to transcend. This chapter offers a window to the path; to walk the path, one has to open the doors.

1.3   THE YOGIC PROCESS

Yoga is a method of unification through separation, like all processes, carried out in stages. These stages are explicated through four chapters: *Samadhi, Sadhana, Vibhuti, Kaivalya*. The process continues through 8 stages, hence the name Aṣtanga Yoga (eight limbs of Yoga). Before we proceed, it's important to acquaint ourselves with terminology that forms the rest of the discussion:

- **Prakṛti:** Matter, which exhibits three *Gunas* (attributes): *Sattva* (active calmness), *Rajas* (action), *Tamas* (inertia).
- **Puruṣa:** Universal consciousness, the witness of all that exists (*Prakriti*). "Know that *Prakriti* and *Purusha* are beginningless, and their modifications and their qualities originate, manifest, from *Prakritī*" (B.G. 13.19).
- **Manas:** The orchestrator of action and the coordinator of senses. It's part of the collective called *Antahkarna.* The mind function is simply to collect and carry impressions and present them to the *Buddhi* (Gheranda & Saraswati, 2012). Gita elaborates the gunas of *Manas* as the 11th sense whose function is thinking and doubting (sankalpa and vikalpa) (B.G. 13.06).
- **Buddhi:** This is the finest state of existence of Matter, and goes on becoming grosser and grosser, until it becomes this universe (Gupta & Ojha, 2018). The knowledge derived from *Buddhi* becomes intelligence. Since *Buddhi* is an evolute of *Prakriti* (but made sentient by the presence of *Purusha*), studying itself as different forms of *Prakriti*, hence is binding. The Seer thus seeks liberation by identifying himself with *Purusha.*
- **Prāṇa:** This is not the breath. But that which causes the motion of breath (Gupta & Ojha, 2019). The foundation of life is flow, blood, nerve impulse, emotions, thoughts, flow to give symptoms of presence of life. Any stagnation shows symptoms we call 'disease.' Death is the cessation of flow of *Prana. Prana* is action, movement, the precursor to any process of transformation.
- **Yogi:** One who has attained *sthita prajña* (steady intellect) and is *samādhi-stha* (situated in trance) [*B.G. 02.54*]. The final limb of *Ashtanga* Yoga culminates in the state of *Samādhi*, where "one is established in his own essential and fundamental nature."
- **Ċitta:** It's the source of consciousness in a living being. In itself, it's the reflection of the universal consciousness, *Puruṣa.*
- **Mahābhūtas:** These are the evolutes of *Prakriti* and correspond to the denser aspects of existence. All matter is a unique combination of these 5 *Mahābhūtas.*

Maharṣi *Patanjali* exhibits an uncanny disposition to deliberately dilute any pleasure a reader might draw from reading; hence, the Yoga *sutras* seldom find recommendations from avid readers. The *Yogasutra* is the beginning of a journey at a stage in life when all worldly distractions have become uninspiring and a yearning spawn to seek beyond the ordinary (it's not about age, but time in life). The first chapter is just two words; अथ योगानुशासनम् (Now, Yoga). The purpose is not amusement, but to end the cycles of life.

Yoga as a journey begins with breaking down predispositions with *Yama*, subsequently establishing new order as *Niyama*, which helps our body and mind to become established in one place with Asana (it is literally one posture called *sthira sukham* asana *m*), which paves the way for the breath to flow in *Pranayama*, so we can draw our consciousness inwards as *Pratyahara*, and hold our focus in singularity in *Dharna*. Meditation ensues as a consequence in the form of *Dhyana*, eventually becoming a witness to reality in *Samadhi*.

1.4   DYNAMICS OF YOGA

How does the Yogic process function? Prior to that, we may want to know, perhaps, why we would want to walk that path. Swami Vivekananda explicates that "he (a *yogi*) sees that he has been coming and going so many times (following the cycles of life), determined that this time he will be free, that he will no more come and go, and be the slave of Nature." But before we leave, we can truly say "Blessed am I that I was born, how wonderful this body (and Mind) really is" (Iyengar, 2014).

Now, we may delve into the dynamics of the yogic process, and it begins with *Prāṇa*. Often understood as breath or oxygen, *Prāṇa* is not the breath. But that which causes the motion of breath. *Prāṇa* is *Vayu*, the second *Mahabhuta* formed out of the evolution of *Prakriti* (the *Mahābhūtas* themselves contribute to a larger classification, known as *Dravyas*, or anything that has a guna and karma). All processes including chemical, nuclear, to cell division, involve activity, which beginning of something, where potential transitions into action is *Vayu*, without this fundamental attribute (*guna*) of *Prakriti*, there is no transformation, everything remains stalled. The transformation a cell undergoes, as it splits infinitesimally to create the form we identify as human, is a consequence of the flow of *Prana*, how it flows, determines the attributes and qualities of that human, or the *guna* and *karma*. This aspect is beautifully explicated by *Maharshi Suśruta* in *Suśruta Samhita* as he writes:

"When the woman conceives, the developing fetus blocks the channel carrying menstrual blood, causing the cessation of menstrual flow. As the obstruction progresses, there is pressure for the upward movement of blood, which results in upward movement of placenta; further upward movement causes the engorgement of breasts…

Channels in the body are opened up by *vaata* in partnership with pitta; entering into the fleshy mass, *vaata* separates individual muscles; it forms blood vessels and ligaments by mild heating of the fatty component of the fats; it creates a chamber or cavity by remaining stagnant in one place… This pattern is followed throughout fetal development, when *vaata* in the company of fire cuts and enlarges channels in all directions– up, down, and around" (Iyengar, 2014).

This brings us closer to life. A curiosity that spans human history, a yearning to explore what differentiates the living from the inanimate. Maharshi Charaka explicates life as "शरीर इन्द्रिये सत्व आत्मा संयोग धारी जीवितम इति आयु" or the "conjunction of body, senses, mind, and *atma*, is life" (C.S. Su. 1.42). *Bhagavad Gita* illuminates *Atma* as *avikāryaḥ* or unchanging [B.G. 2.25]. As *Prakriti* is always modifying or changing, *atma* is not an evolute of *Prakriti*; hence, it cannot be understood and studied as matter. This is an exclusive cosmic arrangement where life engages with matter and transforms it (a phenomenon already explained by Charaka above). This also sheds light on the inexplicable origins of diseases where physical evaluations fall short of an explanation.

In essence, Ayurveda as an *upa-veda* is seminal to the exclusivity of matter-life engagement. A phenomenon systematically formulated in 3 humors: *Vata, Pitta,* and *Kapha* to explain the *Prakriti* of the body, and *Gunas; Sattva, Rajas, Tamas,* explaining the state of mind. These states of mind are not exclusive to human behavior but are the three basic attributes of *Prakriti* itself. Each element of *Prakriti* will exhibit the prominence of one or two of these attributes. Since the mind is a finer evolute of *Prakriti* compared to the body, it readily exhibits those subtle qualities and can also become influenced by them. The body, however, is gross and exhibits the denser combinations of *Mahābhūtās* (*see* Figure 1.4). The body corresponds to the *Aṇamaya kosha* (accumulated through consumption), followed by *Pranayama kosha* (the causative body), *Manomaya kosha* (where emotions catalyze experiences: *Manas*), *Vijñanamaya kosha* (wisdom nurtured through intellect), and *Ananda maya kosha* (liberated from *Manas* and *indriyas*). Developments and disturbances in a *Kosha* can influence the others (Figure 1.1).

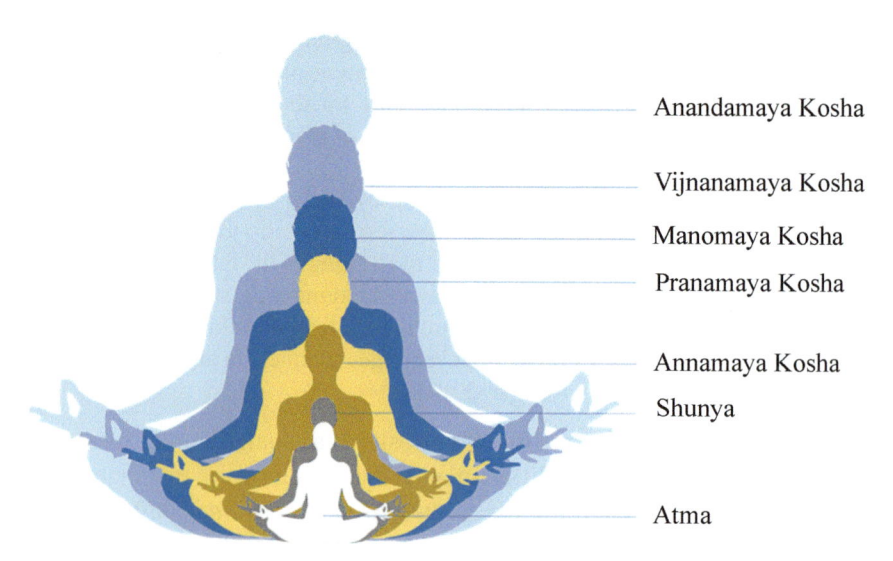

Anandamaya Kosha

Vijnanamaya Kosha

Manomaya Kosha

Pranamaya Kosha

Annamaya Kosha

Shunya

Atma

FIGURE 1.1 The *Kosha*.
Source: Own work.

Wisdom has its own eminence, as its failure is known as *Prājñā-aparādh*, a condition where the mind is no longer restrained, manifesting in erroneous decisions, leading to unfavorable consequences (explored in section: The future with Yoga and beyond). This is the primary reason for a variety of psychological disorders, which are disturbances of *Manomaya kosha*. Similarly, chronic physical diseases are often known to affect the emotional state (Sushruta & Valiathan, 2007). Here we can see *Aṇamaya kosha* affecting the *Manomaya Kosha*. However, *Manomaya kosha* can also affect *Annamaya Kosha*. *Manas* is deeply integrated with the physical body since it directly engages with sense organs and action organs. Inexplicable body aches, diseases, and disorders are often a result of disturbances in the *Manas* and are usually dealt with as psychological disorders (this can be looked at as psychosomatic issues). *Manas* is also the regulator and preserver of the body; hence, *vikrutis* or disturbances of *Manas* will have a consequential influence on the body. We can clearly see how matter (body) is influenced in the presence of life. Today, we infer it through body chemistry and imaging; as humans, we experience it, but as yogis, we can witness the transformation of *Prakriti* (Matter) and its innumerable forms.

Since we are coursing through the evolutionary process of *Prakriti* (*see* Figure 1.4), the *Mahābhūtās* demand their own conceptual hearing.

Prakriti is an organizational framework of material existence, hierarchically arranged from the finest to the grossest. The finest creation is *Buddhi* (often approximated as intellect, however that is an oversimplification as Sanskrit terms are densely packed with layers of meanings and experiential wisdom. Hence, intellect may be exclusive to human beings, but *Buddhi* is a cosmic phenomenon). *Akash, Vayu, Agni, Jal, Prithvi* connote different attributes and qualities of Matter. These are often misappropriated through symbolic representations. *Akash* does not mean Space; similarly, *Prithvi* does not mean Earth. The *Mahābhūtās* combine in varied proportions to form different forms of matter. Let us explore these in detail (Figures 1.2 and 1.3):

1. ***Aakash***: It's possibility, that which allows activity to take place. Think of this as your fist. When all fingers are closed to form a fist, the uniqueness and qualities of each finger are diluted. For each finger to exhibit its quality, they need to be allowed before they can carry out an action. This is *Aakash*. The possibility of activity. This also limits unrestrained activity.

2. ***Vayu***: This is activity. The beginning of something, where potential transitions into action. Wherever there is activity, irrespective of its scale, is *Vayu*.

3. ***Agni***: It is transformation. All active processes are mechanisms of transformation.

4. ***Jal***: This is the first order binding force, weaker, but allows refined activity.

5. ***Prithvi***: This is second order binding force, stronger, resists change. This is also the sum total of all the *Mahābhūtās*.

Vaata or *Prāṇa*, governs life, and Yoga is the process of governing the flow of *Prana*, so it invigorates, illuminates, and distills various aspects of our physical, intellectual, emotional, sensorial, and spiritual existence. That is the process one undergoes in *Prāṇāyāma*. *Prana*, which appears to be abiding, is also the medium of liberation. *Citta* is the engine that draws in *Prana* (Iyengar, 2014), first nourishing the preservatory processes, followed by thought and will. We may see this in practice: when ill, thought becomes an effort (which otherwise flows effortlessly, rather unnecessarily); in case the severity of illness advances, the perception of reality may be distorted (understood as hallucinations), consciousness may be lost, completely crippling the thought mechanism, and at last the survival processes may be affected. *Prana* flows in pathways called *Naḍis* (Lad, 2016). The *Naḍis*

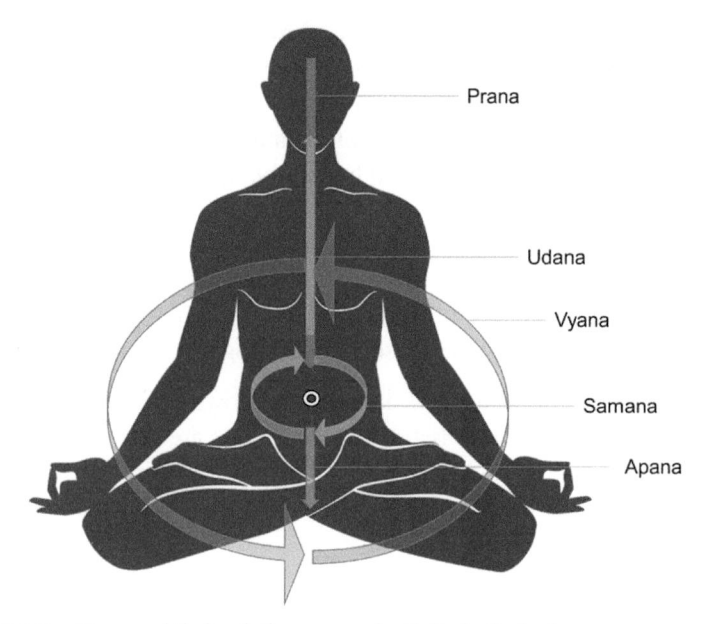

FIGURE 1.2 *Vayus* and their relative space of activity in the body.

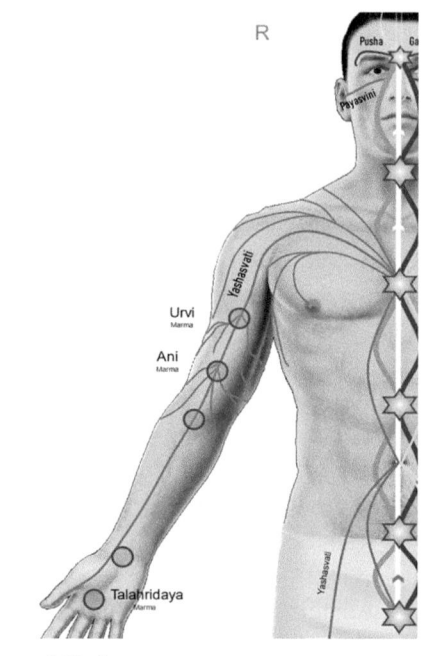

FIGURE 1.3 *Marma* and *Nadis*.

originate from *Kanda*, a region approximately 4 fingers below the navel. *Nadis* are neither nerve, artery, nor vein as they originate in regions different from the location of *Kanda*. In *Marma Chikitsa*, *Prana* nourishes the centers of *Prana* first, known as *sadyah Prana Hara Marmani* (Patil, 2019). These are *Brahmarandharā, Shivarandharā, Sthapani, Ṣankha, Hṛidaya, Nābhi, Gūda, Basti*. *Prana* is then carried out with the help of *vayus* through the *Nadis* to the rest of the body. *Marma* are located at the site of distribution of *Prana* from the primary *Pranavaha srotas* (*Nadis* carrying *Prana*). The tributaries that emanate from the *Nadis* thus nourish the nearby regions. For example, *Ani* and *Urvi Marma* are located on the *Yashasvati Nadi* on the left upper arm. Injury or blockage of any of these *Marma sthalas* (locations) can lead to dysfunction or paralysis of the arm or impaired sensory or motor function. *Talahridaya Marma*, as can be seen in the image, represents the anatomical, emotional, and energetic function of the Heart. Stimulation of this *Marma* enhances the flow of *Prana* in the body, balances the emotional response, and brings about a sense of stability in the body and the mind.

As we have understood, all functions are a result of the flow of *Prana* or *Vayu*, and the extensive network of *Nadis*, and *Marma* sthalas are fundamental to the functions of the body. The yogic practices influence the *Vayu*s, consequently altering the functions of the body and the state of the mind. To illustrate this aspect, the 5 fundamental *Vayus* are: *Prana, Apana, Udana, Vyana,* and *Samana. Udana Vayu* is a purgatory action anywhere in the body and mind. So, activities like defecation, menstruation, delivery, urination, ejaculation, sweating, nails, hair, and expulsion of emotional accumulations are functions of *Udana*. Disruption in the flow of *Udana* may result in symptoms like dysmenorrhea, amenorrhea, dysuria, urinary incontinence, diarrhea, constipation, hair loss, brittle nails, oily or dry skin, inability to let go (emotions), worry, anxiousness, fibroids in the uterus, etc. Yogic *asanas* like *Sarvangasana, Halasana, Matsyasana* help rectify the vitiation of *Udana Vayu*. As a consequence, the blood and body chemistry and physiology change to reflect the restored function of *vayu*. This is why ailments known and unknown can be treated through yogic practices since they fundamentally change who we are.

However, health is an intermediary step in the yogic process. The purpose is not merely to alleviate migraines, lose weight, or cure cancer, but liberation from the cycles of many forms: habits, predispositions, identities, instincts, temper, emotional outbursts, birth, and death. The health benefits we witness during the journey are effects of the transformations happening at all levels of existence.

1.5   MENDING THE FLAW

Instinctively, happiness is what we seek, and in its absence, sadness follows. A cycle we know well enough. The same can be said for everything sought after in life. For most, this is life, and with life it ends, only to begin with another. We seek what we see, but do we see enough? Take a look at Figure 1.4. Here you are, arriving in an unfamiliar city (holding the red umbrella). Surrounded by people, you seek to cross the road. Not sure how large the crowd is, you decide to follow. But the crowd has no direction, and the one in front may not head towards your destination. Yet, you follow, not sure if it's the same you saw moments earlier, until you discover the unpleasant feeling of being stranded. Tiredness dawns upon you as you ask yourself, "Where am I?" Each person here is a thought, multitudes crisscrossing the pathways of your mind, obscuring what lies beyond. When the destination is unknown, distraction takes the wheel. For many, this is life, and some seek to change it, for them, there is Yoga.

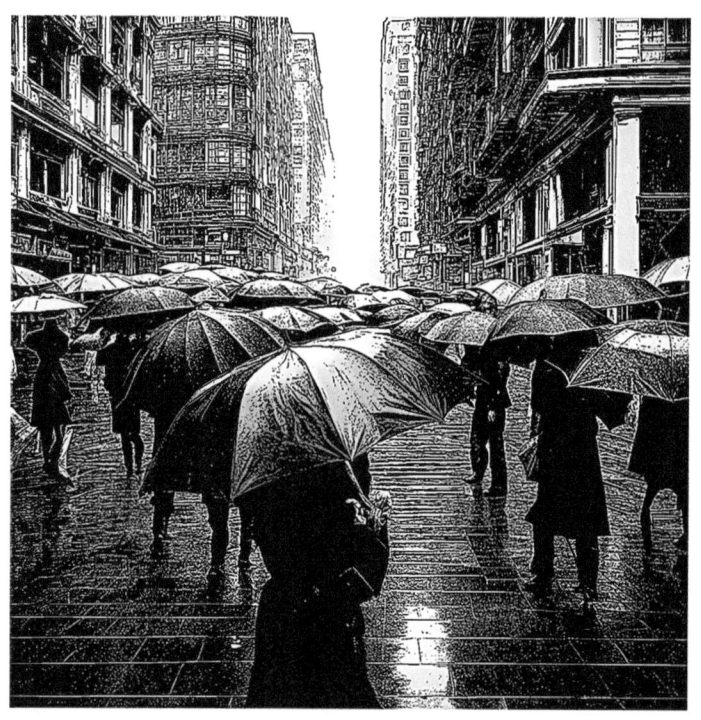

FIGURE 1.4   Thoughts obscuring the truth.

Source: Own work

These thoughts are ripples generated by the impressions gathered from the external world (Prabhupada, 2019). We merely see the reflections of our own thoughts. This phenomenon is similar to holding a mirror against another. Each mirror is reflecting the reflection of another, infinitely. The image has form, but none is real. This is the nature of *Prakriti*, its forms are multitudes, but none represent the true nature of *Prakriti*, and the mind with its associative behavior identifies with the forms, which are many. Yoga is a method to bypass the mind, so the vision of a world beyond forms is thus revealed. Figure 1.5 is likely to help us with the phenomenon:

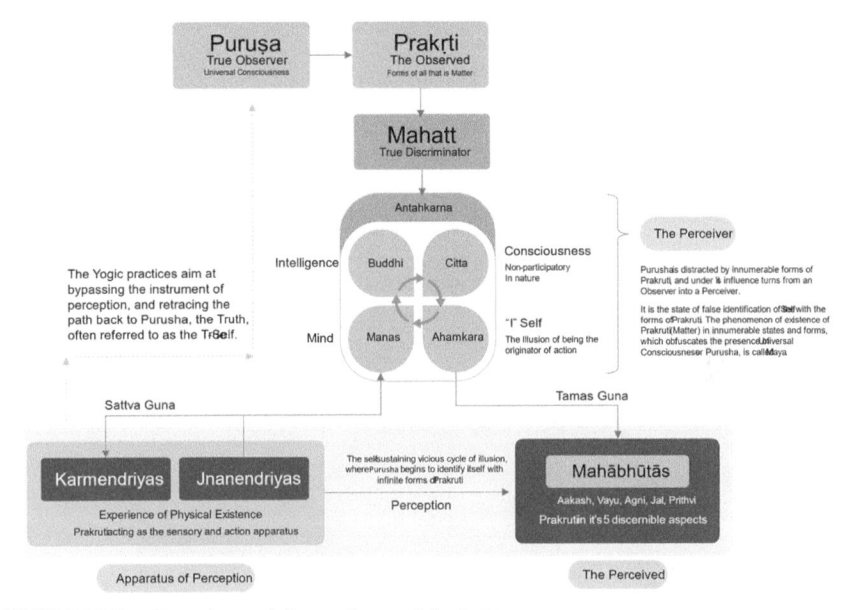

FIGURE 1.5   *Purusha*, and the evolutes of *Prakriti*.

Source: Own work.

Prakriti is the 'reality' as we know it. *Purusha* is real consciousness that pervades everything. It is through this that we become aware of many aspects of this cosmos. All matter is *Prakriti*, as all matter follows the same set of laws that we are aware of. In the yogic system, matter exhibits three gunas, or attributes: *Sattva*, *Rajas*, and *Tamas* arranged in order of activity, with *Sattva* being the highest, but it is also the most 'structured,' 'systematic,' and 'controlled.' This is how the mind is measured, with *Sattvik* being the purest, and *Tamasic* being the least. As matter becomes gross, its inertia increases; hence, the densest forms of *Prakriti* are the 5 *Mahābhūtās*, with *Aakasa* being the least and *Prithvi* being the most. The sense organs or Jnanendriyas respond to the qualities of these *Mahābhūtās*, so they are also 5. But the sense organs are composed of the *Mahābhūtās* themselves. This is where 'reality' is orchestrated, and the mind is tricked. Here *Prakriti* becomes both the observer and the observed, looking at itself. Hence the mind is unable to see beyond the forms of the world, and to be able to look beyond, mind needs to be circumvented, so the *Purusha* can witness its true identity (Figure 1.6).

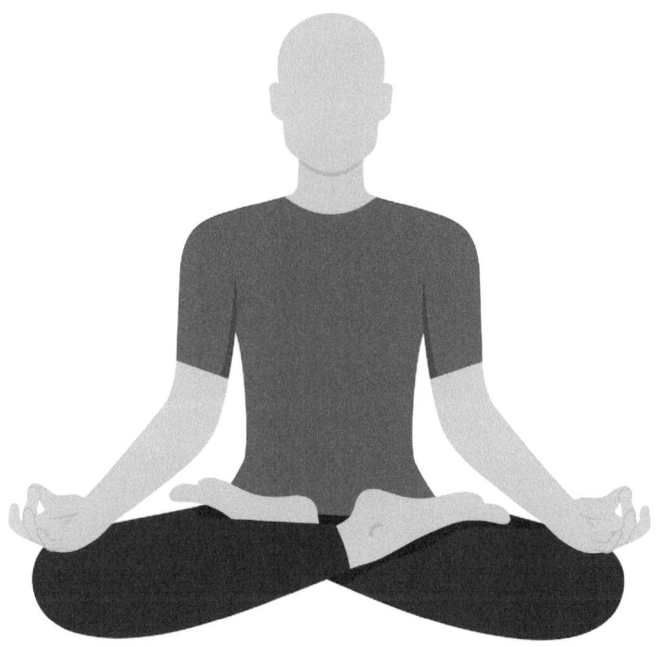

FIGURE 1.6   A yogi in *Siddha Asana*.

Source: Vecteezy.com. https://www.vecteezy.com/vector-art/47587386-abstract-bald-man-sitting-in-lotus-pose-meditating-male-isolated-on-white-background-international-yoga-day-illustration

1.6   A WORD ON ASANAS

There are 8,400,000 Asanas described by Lord Shiva, the knowledge of which is lost, and 84 *asanas* continue to be practiced till this day. Yet *Maharshi Patanjali* defines one *asana*, the '*sthirasukhamaasana m*,' that posture which one can hold steadily and with comfort. There are 8,400,000 *yonis* or species, and each asana corresponds to each [G.S. p. 167]. Suggesting, a posture is unique and natural to step into for each creature. Thus, *asana* is that physical state where the being is in its natural state. Hence, the names of *asanas* are frequently found to be derived from forms of *Prakriti* in their natural states. For example; *Garbha Pind*asana, *Garudasana, Kurmasana, Makarasana, Mandukasana, Padmasana, Simhasana*.

Since the past few decades, the word *asana* has become synonymous with Yoga. *Asanas* are one path to achieve union with the higher consciousness or Yoga, and hence asanas too have their importance and should be seen as something much higher than an exercise regime.

An *asana* is a posture beyond the physical. It's the synchronization of the body and the mind resulting in an equilibrium of movement and resistance. We all know that the mind controls the body. In *asana*, the mind becomes aware of the body. This helps in becoming aware of the subtle processes and movements enhancing our understanding of our natural state of balance. This is the only way we can recognize the stress that disturbs the mind and the body before we can decide to eliminate them.

The *asanas* or poses have research-based evidence that they help by releasing the blockages and tension at a physical, mental, and emotional level thus opening the energy channels and allowing the *Prana* to flow freely. It has been found that Yoga has an immediate quieting effect on the HPA axis response to stress and anxiety. The practice of asanas helps increase brain GABA levels which are otherwise reduced in anxiety and mood disorders (Vivekananda, 2021).

Asanas can be categorized into six types (Vivekananda, 2021):

1. **Sitting *Asanas*:** These *asanas* remove stiffness and tension in the upper part of the body and relax the mind and nervous system, thus helping the organs function optimally.
2. **Twists:** The organs in the abdominal area are rejuvenated with easy blood flow. These asanas make the spine agile, improving the blood flow to the nervous system and aiding in energy flow.
3. **Forward Bends:** Improve blood flow to the brain, thus reducing stress, fatigue, and strengthening the paraspinal muscles.
4. **Inversions:** Aid in blood flow to the vital organs of the body.
5. **Back Bends:** Stabilize the central nervous system. Beneficial for people with depression.
6. **Reclining:** These are asanas that are performed to conclude the Yoga sessions as they relax the body and strengthen the joints.

When an asana is performed, the focus is on a particular part of the body, and that part becomes the "brain" of the pose (Vivekananda, 2021).

Various *asanas* target the body's different systems, including the immunological, reproductive, hormonal, digestive, and respiratory ones. In order to facilitate healing, the combination and sequencing of asanas are essential (Vivekananda, 2021).

1.7   THE FUTURE WITH YOGA AND BEYOND

A species more aware of its choices in life, responsibilities, engagements, and necessities, enhanced sensitivity towards life, irrespective of its form. This is an eventuality if the yogic path becomes the way of life. A revisit to the image illustrated above exemplifies that 'intellect' or 'intelligence' is one of the many faculties of human awareness, the other being the *Manas* (often translated as the Mind) which engages with senses to interpret reality. Above all, it's the *Ċitta*, a direct descendent of the *Purusha*, which is the source of consciousness. Only in the human form can we direct the intellect to disengage from the *Manas* and realize our true nature. The yogic pathway requires patience and the willingness to unlearn; this is where an endeavor into the system of *Marma* can bridge the distance. It's a swift-acting system of regulating the flow of *Prana* that primarily influences the *Aṇṇamaya* and *Manōmaya Koshas* or the Body and the Mind. Since our association with the physical is more convincing, the effects are observed more readily. *Marma sthalas* (locations) like *Brahmarandhra, Shivarandhra, Ajñya (Sthapani), Talahridaya* are known to calm the mind and are also used in treating the symptoms associated with ADHD (Saraswati, 2008). The understanding of the role of intellect is essential to our path of liberation. The capacity of intellect (*Buddhi* or *dhi)* is to preserve knowledge, rational thinking, and the ability to make decisions (Satchidanand, 2020). The main function of *Buddhi* is firmness, contentment, and resolution. *Manas*, on the contrary, being engaged with the senses, is easily distracted by infinite modifications of *Prakriti* or the physical world. It's clear that the failure of the function of *Buddhi* will reflect upon our decisions, wisdom, actions, and eventually, life. This failure of intellect is known as *Prājñā-aparādh*. In Ayurveda (C.S. S.S), *Dhidhrutismrutivibrashtta* corresponds to the failure of intellect. It is the *vibhransha* or vitiation of *Dhee* (intellect), *Dhṛiti* (restraint of the *Manas*), and *Smṛiti* (memory). This is also the reason why psychological disorders exist. Consider the image. A person decides to hold his hand on the burning flame and begins to writhe in pain, seeking help. With a burning candle still held in the other hand, he desperately seeks treatment. Our wisdom indicates that this is an act of foolishness. Why would a person inflict such pain? More importantly, why would he not withdraw his hand when he felt the pain to begin with? Furthermore, can a person be treated while the flame is still alight beneath the hand? Did the candle cause the damage? It all began with the failure of intellect, where we failed to perceive the consequences of the supposed action. This is the way we inflict mental and emotional trauma upon ourselves, and since we cannot see the error in judgment, damage continues until the catastrophe has become a physical ailment. Yet, we cannot see the source that caused the ailment. The *Samkhya Karika* explains that *Buddhi* in its purest *Sattvik* form exhibits the qualities of *Dharma* (righteous behavior), *Jñana* (true knowledge*), Vairagya* (non-attachment), and *Aishwarya* (auspicious attainments) (Turner & Kelly, 2000). However, in its *Tamasik* state, it reflects the opposite qualities. This also gives insight into human behavior as the person becomes attached, physically or emotionally, he is not able to see the true nature of things and becomes susceptible to *Ajñāna*, which is nothing, but ignorance disguised as knowledge (Figure 1.7).

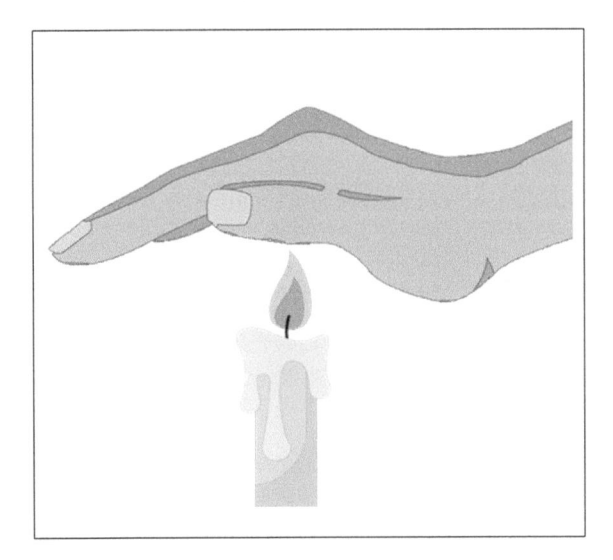

FIGURE 1.7   The burning candle model.
Source: Own work.

Maharṣi Gheranda, with his seminal work on Yoga, the *Gheranda Samhita*, postulates that there is no force greater than Yoga, "*Nasti Yogaat-param balam*" (Vivekananda, 2021). Yoga is a pure experience, and no combination of words does any justice to the Yogic experience of life. A yogic way of life is a conscious choice of being aware of each breath, and to utilize it in the most effective way possible, where each act complements our progression. And this is how the legacy of Yoga illuminates our future.

KEYWORDS

- **Chakra**
- **Indian healing systems**
- **meditation**
- **Naḍis**
- **Vayus**
- **Yoga**

REFERENCES

Anand, P., Chandla, S. S., & Dogra, R. (2018). Effect of yogic asanas on anxiety and general well-being of nursing students. *International Journal of Health Sciences and Research, 8*(5), 23–27.

Charaka, & Valiathan, M. S. (2023). *Legacy of Charaka.* University Press, India.

Gheranda, M., & Saraswati, N. (2012). *Gheranda Samhita.* Yoga Publications Trust, Bihar, India.

Gupta, S., & Ojha, N. (2018). Role of Shirodhara in the management of attention deficit hyperactivity disorder (ADHD) in children. *IJCRT, 6*(2), 557–559.

Gupta, S., & Ojha, N. (2019). Role of Ayurveda therapy in attention deficit hyperactivity disorder in children. p. 37. *International Journal of Emerging Technologies and Innovative Research, 6*(2), 35–43 (www.jetir.org | UGC and issn Approved), ISSN:2349–5162, February-2019.

Iyengar, B. K. S. (2014). *B.K.S. Iyengar Yoga: The Path to Holistic Health* (pp. 64–65, 263). Dorling Kindersley Limited, Great Britain.

Lad, V. (2016). *Marma Points of Ayurveda: The Energy Pathways for Healing Body, Mind & Consciousness with A Comparison to Traditional Chinese Medicine.* Ayurvedic Press, UK.

Patil, A. (2019). The concept of Pragyaparadh with respect to the factors that cause lifestyle disorders. *International Ayurvedic Medical Journal, 7*(1), 111–114.

Prabhupada, S. (2019). *Bhagavad Gita as it is*. Bhaktivedanta book trust, India. Referenced to Jnana yoga (B.G. 06.08), Bhakti yoga (B.G. 12.22), Karma yoga (B.G. 05.03).

Saraswati, N. S. (2008). *Samkhya Darshan*. Yoga publication trust, Bihar, India.

Satchidanand, S. (2020). *The Yoga Sutras of Patanjali* (pp. 3–4). Integral Yoga Publications, Virginia, USA.

Sharma, S. (2014). *Yogic Nadis (The Subtle Flow of Vibration)*. Chaukhambha Orientalia, Delhi.

Sushruta, M., & Valiathan, M. S. (2007). *The Legacy of Sushruta* (Chapter 4: The development of fetus). Universities Press, India.

Turner, J., & Kelly, B. (2000). Emotional dimensions of chronic disease. *Western Journal of Medicine, 172*(2), 124–128.

Vivekananda, S. (2021). *The Yoga Sutras of Patanjali* (pp. 11, 39, 73, 96, 97). Srishti Publishers & Distributors, India.

CHAPTER 2

Impact of Yoga on Social Life and Humanity

YOGITA BISHT[1] and PAWAN SINGH MEHRA[2]

[1]*Department of Kayachikitsa, GS Ayurveda Medical College and Hospital, Pilkhuwa, Uttar Pradesh, India*

[2]*Department of Computer Science Engineering, Delhi Technological University, New Delhi, India*

ABSTRACT

The young generation faces mental turmoil in this fast-growing, busy, hectic life with job insecurity, financial insecurity, and mismanaged lifestyle. There is pressure to perform on a professional front, and no one wants to figure out their daily routine, eating schedule, and physical fitness routine. In this race, we lose our overall development by neglecting our physical or mental health and social well-being. Because of all this, society faces many problems like drug addiction, depression, terrorism, etc. With the practice of Yoga, this social distress or havoc can be well managed by giving strength to the body and evoking spirituality. This work briefly describes Yoga theoretically and scientifically to prove its positive impact on social life and humanity.

2.1 INTRODUCTION

Yoga is the science that establishes the harmony of self with the systems of body and surroundings, thus bringing about positive physical and mental

Yoga and Meditation: Past and Present Evidence. Sachi Nandan Mohanty, Rabindra Kumar Pradhan, & Sugyanta Priyadarshini (Eds.)

changes. Henceforth, it helps to maintain homeostasis, where the body's internal environment remains relatively stable so a person can easily withstand imbalances in the surroundings, whether physical or mental. Yoga has its roots in Indian Philosophy. Except for a few Ayurvedic books, *Patanjali* Yoga-*Darshan* remains the main source of Yoga literature. The word "Yoga" means "unite or integrate." Here the union is of the body with the soul or with God. According to the *Patanjali Yoga sutra*, cessation of mental modifications due to Mind, intellect, and ego are Yoga (Vivekananda, 2021). Remaining unbounded with happiness and miseries of the world is Yoga. According to Swami Aravinda, the role of Yoga is also about personality development on the physical, mental, emotional, spiritual, and intellectual levels (Rao, 2011). In other words, we can say that Yoga is the union of the body with the psychological and spiritual aspects of the human body and the environment in which he lives. Now, when we talk about humans and their environment, the role of human relations, Society, and mental health comes into play. According to WHO, health is a state of complete physical, mental, social, and spiritual wellbeing. Social wellbeing is equally important for a healthy state according to this definition (Park, 2021; World Health Organization (WHO), 2022). It is a matter of misfortune that today, with a rapidly improving standard of living, we are harvesting a tragic crop of explosive, violent, and anti-social youth. It is rightly said that economic planning becomes meaningless if it disregards moral values, democracy becomes a mockery if it ignores the rhythm of education, and education becomes a farce if it deviates from the aim of character formation. There is an urgent need to turn the searchlight towards ourselves to achieve reforms from within in the first place.

2.2 SOCIAL LIFE

A society is a group of persons united by modes of behavior or certain relations that separate them from others. There is a close relationship between individuals and society. Essentially, "society" is the regularities and ground rules of anti-human behavior. These rules and regulations are extremely important to understand how people interact and act with one another. There is no existence of society without individuals, and society exists to aid people. The lives of human beings and society almost go side by side. Human beings are biologically and psychologically equipped to live in groups. For human life to thrive and continue, society has become vital. One of the profound problems of social philosophy is the relationship between society and individuals. As it involves the question of moral values, it is more theoretical than sociological. Man depends on society. A societal force called "culture" surrounds an individual living in society. In society, one has to obey norms, inhabit status, and become a participant in groups. The relationship between man and society is based on the fact that one grows with the help of the other. So, the two are mutually dependent. Though precise information about society's exact origin is still unknown, it is believed that man has lived in society for centuries.

According to Aristotle, "Man is a social animal by nature." He is supposed to be either a beast or God if he lives away from society. In other words, he cannot survive without society. Man requires to live in society for his welfare and existence. Man feels the necessity of society in almost every part of his life. It would be impossible to develop his language, personality, culture, and character without society. The core of the fact is that man has always been related to some society, without which he cannot exist. Society provides security and fulfills all his needs. Every human is born, lives, grows, and takes his last breath in society. Both are closely interrelated, interconnected, and interdependent. Hence, there exist a lot of close relationships between man and society. Man is a social animal mainly because of the following three reasons (Hossain & Ali, 2014):

- By nature;
- Necessity; and
- For mental and intellectual development.

Being social means living in groups or associating with people in a normal or friendly manner. A good social life is also important for a healthy mind and positive thinking. According to "Psychology Today," a person's social life includes various connections they form with others, such as family, friends, colleagues, and community members (Psychology Today, 2022). Having good relationships makes people happy. Happy people lead a better and longer life. Without a positive social surrounding, both minds and bodies can fall prey to many disorders. Ayurveda also believes in a link between physical and mental health. A diseased state of the body can affect the mind, and the mind with anxiety, depression, etc., can affect various systems in the body.

Today, man is not at peace with himself, nature, and society. This mental turbulence, aggressiveness, and loss of peace in mind have given birth to many lifestyle disorders, especially in youths. The youth in any society are like the backbone. The other age groups depend on them, and the youth also determine the future of society. Due to many reasons like social inactivity, improper diet, poor lifestyle, and various criminal activities going around, the youth are suffering the most. Now the time has come when people have started realizing that they need to move towards a deeper understanding of how to live, how and what to eat, exercise, and have the right attitude towards life. So, it is here that Yoga seems to be a remedy to most of the problems of this century, especially for a healthy mental and social life (Figure 2.1).

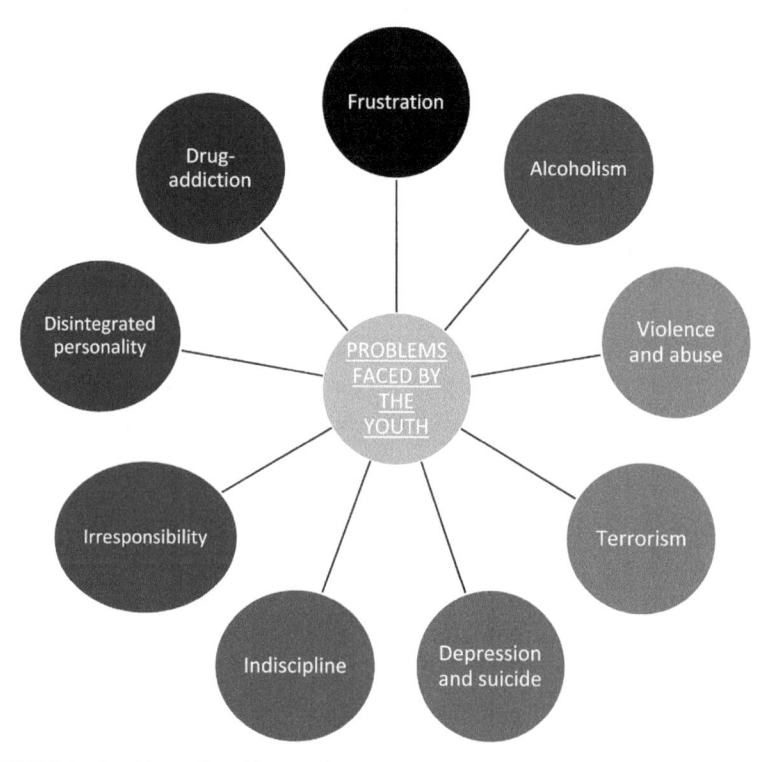

FIGURE 2.1 Problems faced by youth.

2.3   ORIGIN OF YOGA (1700–500 B.C.)

The Yogic practices are believed to have commenced at the very beginning of civilization, long before the first belief systems or religions took birth. The science of Yoga originated. In the yogic history, the first teacher and the first yogi is Lord Shiva. The description of Yoga is obtainable in Harappan civilization, Vedic and Upanishadic legacy, *Darshanas*, classics of Ramayana and Mahabharat, Buddhist, and Jain civilizations, theistic traditions of *Shaivas*, *Vaishnavas*, and *Tantric* customs. In South Asian tradition, there is a description of an ancient form of Yoga. This type of yogic practice was observed under the direct supervision of the *Guru*. It was given special importance and was inbuilt into their rituals. It is important to note that the highest position was given to the Sun during the Vedic period. After being influenced by this practice, the practice of 'Surya namaskara' may have been developed later. *Pranayama* was also a part of routine customary.

After the pre-Vedic era, the then-existing Yoga practices, their meaning, and associated knowledge were organized by Sage Maharshi Patanjali in a systematic way through his Yoga Sutras. Besides covering various aspects of Yoga, Patanjali's Yoga sutra is mainly identified with the eight-fold path of Yoga. Many other sages and Yoga Teachers contributed significantly to the field's conservation and advancement through their well-documented texts and practices. The description of Yoga can also be found in four *Vedas* as *Rig-Veda*, *Yajur-Veda*, *Sama-Veda*, and *Atharva Veda*. Also, evidence that survived in the *Vedas* is scarce and indirect. Nonetheless, the existence of accomplished yogis in Vedic times cannot be doubted. Thus, Vedic Yoga is determined as a foundation of Yoga. A master of Vedic Yoga was recognized as a "Rishi" in Sanskrit.

The most productive and noticeable period in the history and growth of Yoga is the period between 500 BC and 800 A.D. During this time, interpretations of Sage Vyasa on Yoga Sutras and *Bhagavad-Gita*, etc., were written. Also, India's great spiritual teachers, Mahavir and Buddha, enlightened the world with their teachings in this period only. The theory of *Pancha mahavrata* (Five great oaths) – by Mahavir and Ashta-Magga (eight-fold path) by Buddha can be regarded as an initial form of *Yoga sadhana*. We find its more obvious description in *Bhagavad-Gita*, which has richly demonstrated the notion of *Gyan Yoga*, *Bhakti Yoga*, and *Karma Yoga*, which are still the utmost illustration of human insight. Even now, people find serenity and accord by following the teachings in *Bhagavad-Gita*.

Between 800 A.D. and 1700 A.D. has been acknowledged for the pearls of wisdom of three eminent *Acharyas*: Adi Shankaracharya,

Ramanujacharya, and Madhavacharya. Some of the great *Natha* Yogis of *Hatha* Yoga who promoted and propagated the *Hatha* Yoga practices are Matsyendranatha, Gorakshanatha, Swatmaram Suri, Gheranda, and Shrinivasa Bhatt (Basavaraddi, 2015). Between 1700 and 1900 A.D., Yogacharyas who contributed to the development of Raj Yoga are Ramakrishna Paramhansa, Maharshi Ramana, Paramhansa Yogananda, Vivekananda, etc. In conclusion, Vedic Yoga strives to surpass the limitations of the mind. Therefore, Vedic Yoga is considered a way to link with the unseen world and revolves around a sacrifice of the self for the ultimate goal of union with God by practicing *Tapas*, *Asana*, and *Samadhi*.

2.3.1   TYPES OF YOGA (RAO, 2011)

2.3.1.1   GYAN YOGA

Atma-gyan is called *Gyan* Yoga. The person devoid of desire, hatred, anger, and passion becomes *Param-atma* (superior being/soul) by gaining self-knowledge.

2.3.1.2   BHAKTI YOGA

Inner love towards God, which leads to liberation. According to *Devi Bhagavata*, love is compared to uninterrupted thought towards God.

2.3.1.3   KARMA YOGA

Duties should be performed without expecting fruit, and one should take success and failure equally. This balance is also Yoga.

2.3.1.4   MANTRA YOGA

It involves chanting hymns that contain mystical sounds with or without meaning. Each hymn has a certain vibration which produces an effect that calms the mind.

2.3.1.5 LAYA YOGA

Meditating over the ultimate soul while walking, sitting, sleeping, and eating are *Laya* Yoga.

2.3.1.6 KUNDALINI YOGA

Kundalini is divine cosmic energy generally residing at the base of the spinal cord. This energy can be awakened through yogic practices. This is known as *Kundalini* Yoga.

2.3.1.7 HATHA YOGA

With the help of gross body control of mental modifications through the practice of *Pranayama*, *asana*, etc., by a strong person is called *Hatha* Yoga. It gives importance to strengthening the body. It is a preliminary process so that the person can withstand higher energy levels. First, there is the involvement of the physique, the breath, the thoughts, and ultimately the inner self.

2.3.1.8 RAJ YOGA

It involves gaining victory over unhappiness and mental modifications. Also, there is a description of *Ashtanga* Yoga, i.e., 8 limbs or 8 steps of Yoga. The eight limbs or branches are depicted in Figure 2.2.

Through all these steps, one can control the Mind and get a healthy body.

2.4 NEED OF YOGA

2.4.1 YOGA AND QUALITY OF LIFE

Currently, the workplace and home are filled with many factors that bring about stress and aggression, leading to many psychological and psycho-somatic disorders like Diabetes Mellitus, Hypertension, hormonal imbal-ances, infertility, insomnia, etc.

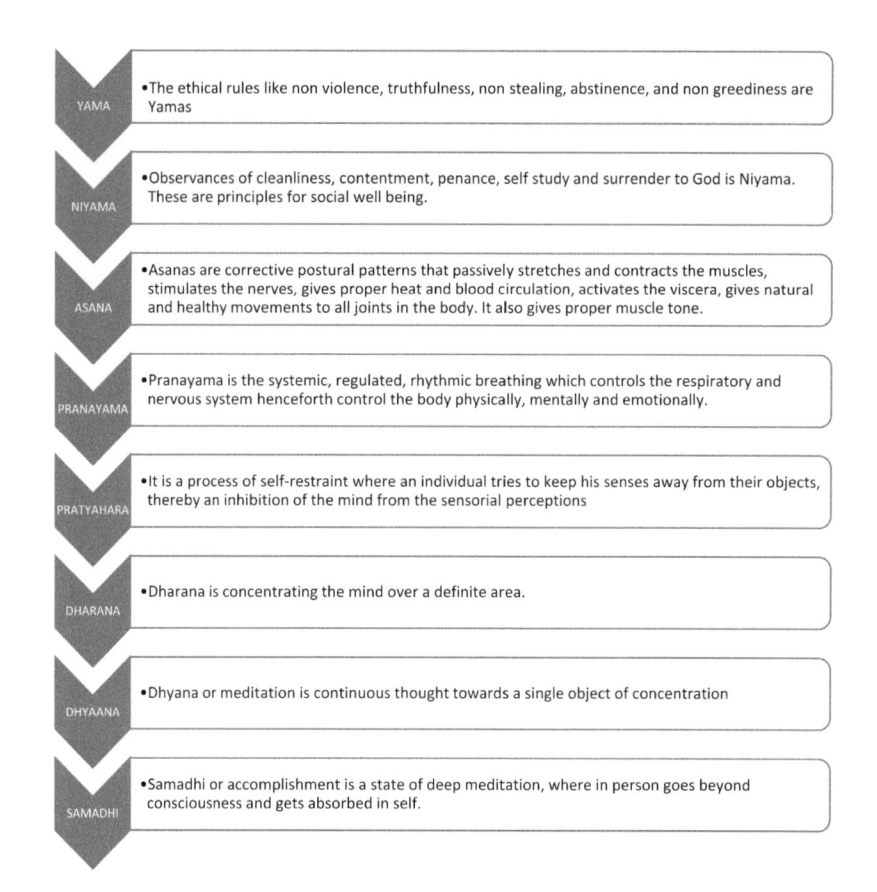

FIGURE 2.2   Eight limbs of yoga.

Swami Vivekananda has mentioned that physical power becomes brutal and blind if not transformed into mental and moral energy. Man needs mental training along with that of his physique to become a perfect being. In today's rat race, from early morning traffic rush to coping with work competition, tension, and the pressure of becoming the best, the only thing that comes to our mind as the best possible answer for standing up to these situations is Yoga. In recent years, many research articles have been published in national and international journals concluding the usefulness of Yoga. In a study of Yoga's effects on health by Naragatti (2020), the effect of Yoga on domains of the quality of life of healthy volunteers was measured. The study showed a noteworthy improvement in the Yoga group on all four domains of the QOL scale (by WHO): physical health, psychological, social relationship, and environmental. It was established that the quality of life improved with this simple practice of regular Yoga. Another study by Woodyard (2011) showed that Yoga helps increase the body's flexibility and muscular strength. It also improves respiratory and cardiovascular functions, aids in recovery from addiction, eases stress, anxiety, depression, and chronic pain, improves sleep, and enhances overall wellness. In another study, "Yoga and mental health: a review" by Shroff & Asgharpour (2017), in their meta-analysis emphasized that Yoga improves complete symptom scores for anxiety and depression by about 40% both by itself and as an add-on treatment across several RCTs using different Yoga practices in different study populations. Also, it produced no reported harmful side effects.

2.4.2   YOGA AND REHABILITATION

Besides the role of Yoga practice in preventing and treating disease, it has several applications in rehabilitation too. Rehabilitation means restoring a person's normal healthy life. It aims at enhancing and restoring abilities that are needed for daily routine. The disability can be physical, psychological, and social. Yoga has helped persons with many diseases return to health; examples are already mentioned.

Regarding psychological rehabilitation, Yoga has helped establish the psychological function and mental balance in persons with depression, anxiety, posttraumatic stress disorder and even certain psychiatric disorders. Yoga can help people in jail like criminals and offenders, those from the slums or economically weak class, children in detention homes, and older people living in convalescent homes. Social rehabilitation includes assistance provided to such people for returning to society or finding new ways of living (Telles, Kozasa, Bernardi, & Cohen, 2013).

2.4.3   YOGA AND POSITIVE PSYCHOLOGY

Researchers have now proven a strong connection between Yoga and positive psychology. However, in the Vedic era, Yoga originated with a spiritual focus. The withdrawal of sense organs from worldly objects is Yoga. As already discussed, *Yama* and *Niyama* are concerned with social behavior. The practice of *Yama* and *Niyama* is necessary to achieve *Samadhi*. In other words, these steps pave the path for cleansing the mind from negativity like anxiety, stress, depression, low self-esteem, criticism, pessimism, and insecurity. Such thoughts also promote sadness. People in Western countries practice Yoga as a form of self-improvement. When people practice Yoga, they can gain alertness, greater awareness, and concentrate more on what needs to be done.

In Japan, a comparative study was conducted to assess the effect of Yoga on the mental health of subjects of different age groups. Participants were subjected to one and a half-hour Yoga session twice a week for one month. State-Trait Anxiety Inventory (STAI) was given before the start of Yoga and after one month of practice to record the variation. The results displayed a statistically substantial decrease in the scores, which signifies that Yoga helps to improve anxiety and overall mental health in both groups, i.e., immediately and in the long term also (Gururaja, Harano, Toyotake, & Kobayashi, 2011).

Another study investigated 90 individuals with stress and assessed the role of 8 and 16-week gym Yoga. The subjects were arbitrarily assigned to two groups. The first group had 16 weeks of Yoga, and the second crossover group did not practice Yoga for the initial 8 weeks and then practiced Yoga for the following 8 weeks. The variables were evaluated at the starting point, 8 and 16 weeks. Results exhibited significant reductions in stress, anxiety, depression, insomnia, and general mental health in the first group. The second group showed significant decreases in all the parameters after they crossed over and practiced Yoga for the last 8 weeks (Maddux, Daukantaité, & Tellhed, 2018). In a study, Musicians in a fellowship program were allotted to two groups. One group practiced Yoga and meditation while the others were assigned to the control group. The members were assessed for the effect of Yoga and meditation on dispositional flow, mindfulness, confusion, and anxiety during music performances. The Yoga and meditation group reported substantial reductions in confusion and increases in dispositional flow during the performance. The study thus confirmed the relation between positive psychology, human performance, and Yoga with meditation. The results also suggested that Yoga and meditation may increase the states of flow and mindfulness and lessen confusion (Butzer, Ahmed, & Khalsa, 2016).

2.4.4 YOGA AS A WAY OF LIFE

Yoga, as a "mode of life," comprises the practice of *Jnana* Yoga (knowledge of oneself), *Karma* Yoga (path of detached action), *Bhakti* Yoga (trust in the supreme), and *Raja* Yoga (asana, Pranayama, etc.). If a person follows all the 8 steps or branches of Yoga described by Sage Patanjali, he can achieve complete social and spiritual reforms and lead a happy and peaceful life. Continuous and regular practice of different types of Yoga may transform one's persona on physical, mental, emotional, and mystical levels, strengthening one's ability to cope with physical and mental pressure at all levels, which is important for the integral development of a person as a whole.

2.5 CONCLUSION

As described in this chapter, it can be understood that in today's fast and stressful life, people, especially the youth, face many problems affecting their social behavior and personal growth. We also know that a person's overall growth depends on physical strength and mental well-being. Although a commoner cannot attain a height at the yogic level but can surely train his mind to such an extent that it does not easily fall prey to his passions and desires and begins to thirst for inner peace by conquering his desires. Yoga may improve attention span, reduce impulsivity, decrease confusion, and increase patience and mindfulness. Or we can say that to lead a happy life, one has to overcome all these hurdles, and Yoga is proven to be a treatment that is safe, economic, free of side effects, and above all, supports the immune system. Yoga can be considered a complete super-specialty to deal with health-related problems, mental illnesses, and social reforms.

KEYWORDS

- mental illnesses
- muscular strength
- quality of life
- rehabilitation
- social life
- social reforms
- state-trait anxiety inventory
- Yoga

REFERENCES

Basavaraddi, I. V. (2015). Yoga: Its origin, history and development. *Public Diplomacy.* Available from: www.mea.gov.in/in-focus-article.htm?25096/Yoga+Its+Origin+History +and+Development (accessed on 5 July 2024).

Butzer, B., Ahmed, K., & Khalsa, S. B. (2016). Yoga enhances positive psychological states in young adult musicians. *Applied Psychophysiology and Biofeedback, 41*(2), 191–202. https://doi.org/10.1007/s10484-015-9321-x.

Gururaja, D., Harano, K., Toyotake, I., & Kobayashi, H. (2011). Effect of yoga on mental health: Comparative study between young and senior subjects in Japan. *International Journal of Yoga, 4*(1), 7–12. https://doi.org/10.4103/0973-6131.78173.

Hossain, A., & Ali, M. D. (2014). Relation between individual and society. *Open Journal of Social Sciences, 2*(8), 130–137.

Maddux, R. E., Daukantaité, D., & Tellhed, U. (2018). The effects of yoga on stress and psychological health among employees: An 8- and 16-week intervention study. *Anxiety, Stress & Coping, 31*(2), 121–134. https://doi.org/10.1080/10615806.2017.1405261.

Nagaratti, S. (2020). The study of yoga effects on health. *International Journal of Innovative Medicine and Health Science, 12,* 98–110.

Park, K. (2021). *Park's Textbook of Preventive and Social Medicine.* Banarsidas Bhanot Publisher, Jabalpur, India.

Psychology Today. (2022). Social life [Internet]. The United States. Available from: https://www.psychologytoday.com/us/basics/social-life#:~:text=A%20person's%20social%20 life%20consists,both%20in%20person%20and%20online (accessed on 5 July 2024).

Rao, M. V. (2011). *The Essence of Yoga* (1st ed.). Chaukhambha Orientalia, Varanasi, India.

Shroff, S., & Asgharpour, M. (2017). Yoga and mental health: A review. *Journal of Physiotherapy & Physical Rehabilitation, 2*(1), 1000132.

Telles, S., Kozasa, E., Bernardi, L., & Cohen, M. (2013). Yoga and rehabilitation: Physical, psychological, and social. *Evidence-Based Complementary and Alternative Medicine, 2013,* 624758. https://doi.org/10.1155/2013/624758.

Vivekananda, S. (2021). *Patanjali Yogasutra.* Srishti Publishers and Distributors, New Delhi, India.

Woodyard, C. (2011). Exploring the therapeutic effects of yoga and its ability to increase quality of life. *International Journal of Yoga, 4*(2), 49–54.

World Health Organization (WHO). (2022). *Constitution of the World Health Organization* [Internet]. Geneva: WHO. Available from: https://www.who.int/about/governance/constitution (accessed on 5 July 2024).

CHAPTER 3

Well-Being and Quality of Life Through Yoga: Rethinking Our Notions of Happiness

RICHA CHOPRA,[1] SHASHANK SHEKHAR TRIPATHI,[2] RAHUL SANAL,[3] and KASHINATH G. METRI[4]

[1]*Center of Excellence for Indian Knowledge Systems, Indian Institute of Technology (IIT), Kharagpur, West Bengal, India*

[2]*Pragyan Ritam Yog Aranya Nyas (PRYAN) Ashram, Udaipur, Rajasthan, India*

[3]*Freelancer, Sanal Kumar Foundation, Thiruvananthapuram, India*

[4]*Department of Yoga, Central University of Rajasthan, Ajmer, Rajasthan, India*

> "…[o]ut of bewildering Yogism must come the most scientific practical psychology–and all this must be put in a form so that a child may grasp it"
> —Vivekananda, 1896

ABSTRACT

Every individual aspires to a healthy, happy, and a satisfied life. Financial status, luxury, physical health, and overall well-being are generally considered to be the hallmarks of 'Quality of Life (QoL) and happiness.' However, it is an individual's perception that plays an even more momentous

Yoga and Meditation: Past and Present Evidence. Sachi Nandan Mohanty, Rabindra Kumar Pradhan, & Sugyanta Priyadarshini (Eds.)

role in determining gratification with one's life, QoL, and happiness. *Yoga* is a science of holistic health, well-being, and the 'Self[1]'– that can awaken the brilliance within by disintegrating the mind and making it ablaze with the light of Consciousness. According to the philosophy of *yoga, ānanda* or absolute happiness is inherent to or the very nature of the 'Self.' It is the deep rooted *samskāras*[2], *kleśas*[3] and *vṛttis*[4] in the mind that give rise to unlimited desires, restlessness, and negative emotions – diverting the mind from its 'Original Nature' towards the external world in search of happiness. Unfortunately, no worldly objects or events can lead to *ānanda*. Yoga teaches techniques such as *yama, niyama, āsana, prāṇāyāma, dhāyna,* etc., to overcome the *samskāras, kleśas,* and *vṛttis* – which then enables the individual to come back to its 'Source,' '*ānanda*.' An individual in such a state no longer craves external comforts or pleasures, thus experiencing the highest quality of life. This chapter aims to scheme out an understanding of well-being and happiness from *yogic* paradigms – excavating the profound philosophy and psychology embedded within various traditional Yoga and allied classical treatises (such as *Patañjali's Yogasūtras, Bhagavadgītā, Hatha Yoga, Yoga Vāsiṣṭha*) with an aim to re-approach and promote QoL, in light of modern-day challenges. Concepts such as the 'mind' as an 'instrument of human perception and experience,' as an 'object of one's Awareness' and 'happiness independent of all externalities' have been discussed. Extending these concepts to corroborate certain underlying yogic ideas centered around QoL (such as *sattvam, ārōgyam, nirmalam, samatvam, kauśalam, santōśam, sukham,* etc.) considering some of the predominant definitions and theories, the exploration has been furthered, and a universal schema on the indices of measurement of QoL has been suggested. Delineating holistic and practical methodology towards 'life quality-enrichment,' the thoughts presented can serve as theoretical foundations for future research on the subject.

---

[1]*Puruṣa.' 'ātman,' 'brahman,'* 'Consciousness,' 'Awareness,' 'Source,' 'Original Nature,' 'Seer;' that which verily enlivens the mind, but which cannot be tracked by the ordinary scattered mind – that is *brahman, ātman,* Self, or Pure Awareness – referred to as *saccidānanda. sat* is existence itself, not that is existing. *cit* is Consciousness itself not that it becomes conscious and *ānanda* is bliss and happiness itself not that it becomes happy. This source of all happiness is functioning through the body – mind complex.
[2]Psychological residues.
[3]Mental afflictions.
[4]Mental modifications.

3.1 QUALITY OF LIFE: A PONDERANCE

World War II and its consequences have shaped the current world order. Economic growth has been the most predominant goal for the world at large – encouraged due to its potential to 'upraise living standards' and enrich the 'QoL,' especially among the global south.

Advocates of hedonism[5] argue that pleasure is a natural signal (Veenhoven, 2003). It is therefore presupposed that economic advancement and linear development have fostered the need for the pursuit of pleasure, goading mankind to behave in advantageous ways. For many societies, higher economic resources have meant opportunities to seek and attain more pleasurable experiences in life by virtue of societal status, life expectancy, comfortable environs, physical health, etc. And thus, worldwide, these have conventionally served as some of the major determinants in the understanding of QoL, happiness, and the subsequent construct of various indices. Yet ironically, despite people having close to what the QoL benchmarks assume, there has been a burgeoning growth of mental illnesses and misery all around. While the global economy is soaring to new heights via technological, scientific, and industrial expansion cum advancement, modernity is also fast witnessing the rise of new crises in forms of lifestyle diseases encompassing anxiety, stress, depression, etc.

There has been a gradual shift from the Anthropocene to the humanitarian in recent times – a contemplation for a global insistence for attentiveness to happiness and well-being in shaping government policies (World Happiness Report, 2012). However, there is clearly a lack of awareness and the much-needed direction towards a life anchored on jubilance, harmony, and wholesomeness.

3.2 UNDERSTANDING QUALITY OF LIFE

The quality of life encompassing varied dimensions and attributes has been an area of prolonged investigation by scholars and organizations. For instance, QoL as studied under a few academic disciplines is depicted below:

---

[5]Represents the outlook w.r.t a 'good life' as being anchored on pleasures.

QoL as Understood across Disciplines

- Sociology - 'being happy'
- Economics - 'being rich'
- Medicine - 'staying normal on the disease'

(Lindstrom, 1992)

Social support, healthy life expectancy during birth, positive emotions, etc., have been included as some of the independent determinants of happiness[6] by the Sustainable Development Solutions Network in the World Happiness Report (2022) (Table 3.1).

TABLE 3.1 Regressions to Explain Average Happiness Across Countries (Pooled OLS)

	Dependent Variable			
Independent Variable	**Cantril Ladder (0–10)**	**Positive Affect (0–1)**	**Negative Affect (0–1)**	**Cantril Ladder (0–10)**
Log GDP per capita	0.36	−.013	0.0001	0.388
	(0.066)***	(0.009)	(0.007)	(0.065)***
Social support	2.420	0.316	−.328	1.778
	(0.368)***	(0.055)***	(0.049)***	(0.361)***
Healthy life expectancy at birth	0.029	−.0007	0.003	0.03
	(0.01)***	(0.001)	(0.001)***	(0.01)***
Freedom to make life choices	1.305	0.368	−.090	0.509
	(0.298)***	(0.041)***	(0.04)**	(0.284)*
Generosity	0.583	0.09	0.024	0.378
	(0.265)**	(0.032)***	(0.027)	(0.254)
Perceptions of corruption	−.704	−.006	0.094	−.704
	(0.271)***	(0.027)	(0.022)***	(0.259)***
Positive affect				2.222
				(0.333)***
Negative affect				0.173
				(0.395)
Year fixed effects	Included	Included	Included	Included
Number of countries	156	156	156	156
Number of obs.	1853	1848	1852	1847
Adjusted R–squared	0.753	0.439	0.322	0.777

Note: Reprinted from the World Happiness Report (p. 20) by J. F. Helliwell et al. (2022), Sustainable Development Solutions Network.

---

[6]Interconnected to and a measure of QoL.

3.2.1   SOME QoL DEFINITIONS AND THE VISIBLE CHASM

"Quality of life is the total existence of an individual, a group or a society"
(Lindstrom, 1992).

World Health Organization (WHO) defines quality of life as:

"An individual's perception of their position in life in the context of the culture and value systems in which they live and in relation to their goals, expectations, values, and concerns incorporating physical health, psychological state, level of independence, social relations, personal beliefs, and their relationship to salient features of the environment (WHOQOL Group, 1995, p. 11)."

WHO's definition, though seemingly balanced, has a dimension that creates challenges in enhancing the QoL, namely 'perception.' It is not sufficient that there is a mere upliftment in a being's measurable or material QoL alone, but that the persons themselves must also perceive an improvement in the same. And this perception will depend on the kind of personal and individual aspirations each one has in specific domains of life – ranging from marriage, interpersonal relations, work, leisure, health, and so on. This, therefore, leads one to ponder about the instrument of 'perception and experience,' i.e., the human 'mind,' and its role in the betterment of QoL.

3.2.2   THEORIES CONNECTED WITH QOL

A few theories dominating the discussions on QoL are listed in subsections.

3.2.2.1   HEDONISM, IDEALIST, AND PREFERENCE SATISFACTION THEORIES

In the context of hedonists, Shukla (2022) reiterates their belief that the "ultimate good for people is to undergo particular kinds of conscious experiences that can be characterized as pleasure, happiness, or enjoyment that typically accompanies the successful pursuit of one's desires." While the idealist theories focus on the "realization of specific, explicit normative ideals," the preference satisfaction theories center around the "satisfaction of people's desires or preferences" (p. 37).

3.2.2.2   SELF-DISCREPANCY THEORY

Higgins (1987) suggests through his theory that the mind simply cannot stop thinking about the gap between what exists and what more is needed to attain an enhanced quality of life. The self-discrepancy theory proposes that a poor QoL is the consequence of the discrepancy between an individual's actual and ideal self.

3.2.2.3   A DERIVATIVE FROM MASLOW'S THEORY

Maslow (1943) proposed a theory of development based on the hierarchical arrangement and fulfillment of human needs, namely "physiological, safety, love, and belonging, esteem, and self-actualization" (p. 370). Building on this, Sirgy (1986) defines QoL "as the hierarchical need satisfaction level of most of the members of a given society. The higher the need satisfaction of the majority in each society, the greater the quality of life of that society" (p. 329).

3.2.3   QoL: LEVELS AND INDICATORS

Before delving deeper into the subject, it is also important to understand the various levels and indicators of QoL, especially in current scenarios. The interconnectedness of QoL and development, though in a small way, is gradually catching the attention of policymakers and the implementing agencies as well – making ways to factor some of the QoL indicators so as to gauge the effectiveness of various programs. And thus, inching towards the desired outcomes – in the larger interest of the individual, state, and nation (Table 3.2).

3.2.3.1   DIRECT INDICATORS (USED EXTENSIVELY FOR THE PURPOSE OF FRAMING POLICIES AND THEIR EVALUATION)

1. **Physical Quality of Life Index (PQLI):** A computation that integrates three basic measures of well-being, namely "literacy rate, life expectancy, and infant mortality rate" (Morris, 1979), into one comprehensive index.

2. **Human Development Index (HDI):** A statistically compounded index by the United Nations Development Program encompassing "life expectancy, education, and per capita income indicators" (UNDP, 1990) for grading countries.
3. **Digital Quality of Life Index (DQLI):** Undertakes investigation into the "quality of digital well-being" by calibrating 117 countries on the indicators of "internet affordability, internet quality, electronic infrastructure, e-security, and e-government" (Surfshark, 2022).

TABLE 3.2   Levels of Quality of Life

	Objective (measured in numbers)	Subjective (expressed in words)
Individual level	Objective living conditions (e.g., income, place of living, mode of transportation)	Subjective well–being (e.g., satisfaction with income / home / transportation mode)
Societal level	Quality / livability of society (e.g., income disparities, housing density, air quality)	Perceived quality / livability of society (perceived importance of disparities / housing density)

Source: Reprinted from: Shukla (2022); Copyright 2022 by K. Shukla. Reprinted with permission.

3.2.3.2   *INDIRECT INDICATORS (VALUABLE INSIGHTS THAT CAN HELP IMPROVE THE QUALITY OF LIFE OF PEOPLE AT A GLOBAL LEVEL)*

1. **The Happy Planet Index (HPI):** It is a calculation of sustainable well-being using limited environmental resources across countries (Marks et al., 2006).
2. **The World Happiness Report:** This contemplates a global insistence for more recognition of "happiness and well-being as criteria for government policy" (Sustainable Development Solutions Network, 2012).

3.3   HAPPINESS AND QUALITY OF LIFE: THE LINKAGES

The modern conception of happiness and QoL is essentially centered on creating favorable external conditions that bring pleasure or a positive influence on mood. Despite experiencing levels of material comfort unknown to previous generations, the present generation seems to be caught in a paradox.

Neuroscientific Perspective of Happiness

"The thoughts that we think and the experiences we have determine the neural pathways or circuits in our brain. Neuroplasticity is the changes in the brain due to experiences. Experience is not external; it is always internal thought it may have an external stimulus. What we think is a subjective experience but the brian circuitry that we are creating as a result of it can be objectively tracked in a third person perspective. By doing this, researchers have concluded that positive thoughts of kindness-sharing, caring and love always keep one happy."

(Divyanandaprana, 2021)

Two interesting observations pointed out in the World Happiness Report (2012) lead us to think that there is more to happiness than previously conceived, intricately linked to the quality of life. Firstly, "individuals who put a high premium on higher incomes generally are less happy and more vulnerable to other psychological ills than individuals who do not crave higher incomes" (p. 5). Secondly, present-day advertising creates new material wants. The mind of the individual is constantly bombarded with powerful imagery to create a 'want' or desire in the mind that was not previously there. This perception of the 'want' creates the feeling in an individual's life of unfulfillment, that they do not have a good quality of life without these material objects.

The World Happiness Report (2012) goes to the extent of suggesting that we need a "very different model of humanity" (p. 5). Over the past two decades, development economists have started looking at including a new constituent in the quality of life – happiness.

Perhaps the QoL measure now seriously needs to take into consideration the inner harmony of an individual. Efforts at the individual level are of prime importance before policy changes can help societies grow. This might solve the paradox that we currently live in. Bhutan paved the way by formulating a new metric called the 'Gross National Happiness' index to measure the country's growth, prioritizing the happiness of its citizens rather than simply relying on numerical measures.

The foremost question then is – "what is happiness, and should the quality of life be re-approached and promoted through happiness?"

"Happiness is described as the experience of joy, contentment, or positive well-being, combined with a sense that one's life is good, meaningful, and worthwhile" (Lyubomirsky, 2008). Happiness is generally connected with the state of our mind–wherein the mind correlates itself with a sense of good mood and general well-being.

The definition of happiness thus can be a sense of well-being, along with a higher awareness, plus a positive affect[7]. This further implies that "each one of us understands and experiences happiness a little differently, according to the quality of our minds. Therefore, studying the mind is vital because one's happiness is the interpretation of one's mind. The kind of mind, the kind of samskaras we have, decides to a large extent, our experiences of happiness" (Divyanandaprana, 2021). And this in turn determines the QoL.

Though, there exist several models to understand happiness and quality of life, none of these provide a comprehensive solution. This is probably due to a lack of understanding of the nature, characteristics, and activities of the mind as well as the dimensions beyond the mind.

Plato[8] was perhaps one of the foremost philosophers who recognized that happiness could not be anchored on pleasure – for pleasure depended upon external objects, limited by time and space. He further emphasized that wisdom was the real source of happiness that could bring goodness across all dimensions of one's life. Perhaps, it is the lack of this wisdom today, which may be the root cause of anxiety, mental stress, and lifestyle illnesses among the current generation of people.

The perennial philosophy[9] of *yoga*, rooted in India is a treasure trove of knowledge that can help understand and culture the mind, go beyond its physical to the temporal and spiritual realms – towards eternal happiness, thus enriching the quality of life. The ancient *ṛṣis* had clearly understood the root cause of all miseries and unhappiness being in the disharmony that exists within a person.

3.4 YOGA

There is this remarkable thing about Indian philosophy – understanding the Subject (Self[10]), tapping into the powers of the Subject, by exploring deep within oneself. The famous *ekaśloki* by *Śaṅkarācārya* helps us to understand how to penetrate the Subject.

---

[7]Disposition to acquaint with positive emotions.
[8]A Greek philosopher.
[9]This article excavates the profound philosophy and psychology embedded within various traditional *yoga* and allied classical treaties (such as *Patañjali's Yogasūtras, Bhagavadgītā, Hatha Yoga, Yoga Vasishtha*) with an aim to re-approach and promote 'Quality of Life,' in light of modern-day challenges.
[10]The Experiencer. Also refer to footnote 1.

> *"kiṃ jyotistavabhānumānahani me rātrau pradīpādikaṃ*
> *syādevam ravidīpadarśanavidhau kiṃ jyotirākhyāhi me I*
> *cakṣustasya nimīlanādisamaye kiṃ dhīrdhiyo darśane*
> *kiṃ tatrāhamato bhavānparamakaṃ jyotistadasmi prabho"*

> By what light do we see the objects around us? The answer is 'by the light of the sun'. The next question then follows is 'by what light do we see the sun by the day and the moon by the night?' The answer is 'by the light of our eyes'. Then 'by what light do we see our eyes'? 'We see our eyes through our mind and we see our mind through the eyes of our Pure Awareness.

Yoga is a science that directly points towards our 'True Nature,' that can be discovered through the process of Self-inquiry. This is how *yoga* has penetrated the science of happiness. The philosophy of *yoga* says happiness is built right within us, right now. It is our very nature.

Chapter IV of the *Hatha Yoga Pradīpika*, verse 78 says:

> *"rasasya manasaśchaiva chanchalatvaṃ svabhāvataḥ |*
> *raso baddho mano baddhaṃ kiṃ na siddhyati bhutale"* || 4.26, Haṭha Yoga Pradīpikā ||

> "Mercury and mind are unstable by nature. By stabilizing (seizing or fixing) mercury and mind what cannot be perfected?" (Muktibodhananda, 2012).

Yoga abhyāsa is about enabling our body-mind complex to express our inner happy nature, to attains perfection, bliss, and highest wisdom (*pratibhā*).

3.4.1   THE PURPOSE AND ESSENCE OF YOGA

> *"yogaścittavṛttinirodhaḥ"* || 1.2, Patañjali's Yogasūtras ||
> *"tadā draṣṭuḥ svarūpe'vasthānam"* || 1.3, Patañjali's Yogasūtras ||

> yoga is a process of restraining the mental modifications and attaining tranquility. By doing so the 'Seer' establishes himself onto his Real Nature i.e *ānanda*[11] (unconditional happiness; bliss)

In *Yōga Vasiṣṭha* (one of the foremost expositions on *yoga* from *Rāmāyaṇa*), the essence of *yoga* is encapsulated as below:

> *"manaḥ praśamanopāyaḥ yoga ityabhidhīyate"* || 3. 9. 32, Yoga Vasiṣṭha ||

> yoga is called a contrivance trick to relax[12] the mind. It is an *upāyah*, a skilful subtle process and not brutal mechanical gross effort to stop the thoughts in the mind.

Sri Aurobindo enunciates *yoga* as a systematic and conscious endeavor towards self-growth and development of all the possibilities dormant in an

---

[11] *Ānanda* can be achieved only by overcoming the *samskāras, kleśas* and *vṛtti*. *yoga* philosophy encourages *vairāgya* (dispassion to overcome desire to such and move towards *ānanda*.
[12] A calm state of mind is devoid of desires, craving, anxieties, depression anger, hate etc. and it is only in such a state that there is contentment in the mind.

individual. He emphasizes holistic personality development encompassing the physical, mental, intellectual, emotional, and spiritual dimensions (Figure 3.1).

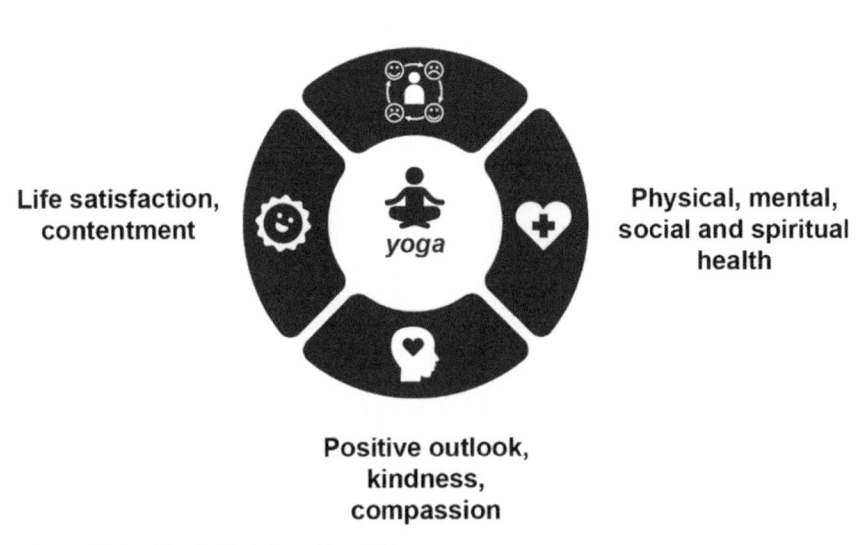

Emotional regulation

Life satisfaction, contentment

yoga

Physical, mental, social and spiritual health

Positive outlook, kindness, compassion

FIGURE 3.1   The holistic benefits of *Yoga*.

Thus, *yoga* is a methodical, step-by-step undertaking through which the growth and development of an individual is accelerated to higher dimensions of consciousness. Ceasing the mind to be the mind and culturing it towards vastness and tranquility is pivotal to this inward journey.

3.4.2   THE CONTEMPORARY REDUCTIONIST VIEW OF YOGA

The idea of *yoga* has shifted considerably, with its immortal essence being diluted. It is reduced simply to some form of physical exercise, breathing workouts, and perhaps a little meditation–undermining completely its spiritual and religious dimensions. Yogic postures (*āsanas*) have been elevated so much so as to encapsulate *yoga* in its entirety – misleading the world regarding the true, classical nature of *yoga*. Furthermore, the facet of *prāṇāyāma,* in current times, is forsaken and applied only for conquering a few ailments. The current state of affairs can thus be summarized as: *"yama niyama nirapekśa."*

The classical text, *Hatha*[13] *Yoga Pradīpikā*, clearly states *Râja Yoga*[14] as the culmination of *Hatha Yoga.*

"Śrī ādi nāthāya namostu tasmai yenopadishtā hathayogavidyā vibhrājate pronnatarājayogam ārodhumichchoraḍhirohinīva" **||1.1, Hatha Yoga Pradīpikā ||**

Obeisance to *Âdinâtha (Śiva)* having propounded the knowledge of *Hatha Yoga*, which as a stairwell ushers the seeker to the peak of *Râja Yoga*

Further, the interconnectedness of the two *Yoga* can be seen below:

"haṭhaṃ vinā rājayogho rāja-yoghaṃ vinā haṭhaḥ | na sidhyati tato yughmamānishpatteḥ samabhyaset" **|| 2.76, Hatha Yoga Pradīpikā ||**

No success in *Râja Yoga* without *Hatha Yoga*, and no success in *Hatha Yoga* without *Râja Yoga*. One should, therefore, practice both of these well, till complete success is gained

3.4.3   THE MIND ACCORDING TO YOGA

'Collective mind' according to *Patañjali's Yogasūtras* is called *citta*. Also known as *antaḥkaraṇa, citta* is composed of the *Manas, Buddhi*, and *ahaṅkāra. Manas* perceives the world through the senses while *buddhi* serves as the discriminating ability – formulating reactions and responses to the sense stimuli. *Ahaṅkāra* is the ego sense, which internalizes and stores all the incoming information as personal knowledge.

Analogy of the Mind with a Lake

The surface of a lake is lashed into waves or if the water is muddy, the bottom cannot be see. The lake represents the mind and the bottom of the lake the puruṣa, the Self. Whenever mind is made tranquil, knowledge of the Self is revealed.

3.4.4   NATURE OF THE MIND

According to Haṭha Yoga Pradīpikā,

---

[13]*ha* represents *prāna* and *tha* represents the mind.
[14]*Patañjali's Yogasūtras.*

"rasasya manasaśchaiva chanchalatvaṃ svabhāvataḥ |
raso baddho mano baddhaṃ kiṃ na siddhyati bhutale" || *4.26, Haṭha Yoga Pradīpikā* ||

"Mercury and mind are unstable by nature. By stabilizing (seizing or fixing) mercury and mind what cannot be perfected?" (Muktibodhananda, 2012).

The very nature of the mind is outgoing. It connects with the sense objects through the sense organs and creates *samskāras*. The experience of pain and pleasure is a consequence of the mind attached with the sensory organs. This leads to dependency on sensual pleasures, leading to the vicious cycle of desires and craving – which ultimately ends in misery. The *Bhagavadgītā* says:

"dhyāyato viṣayānpumsaḥ sangasteṣūpajāyate |
sangāt samjāyate kāmaḥ kāmātkrodho'bhijāyate" ||*2.62, Bhagavadgītā* ||
"krodhādbhavati sammohaḥ saṃmohātsmṛtivibhramaḥ |
smrtibhramśād buddhinaso buddhināśātpraṇaśyati" ||*2.63, Bhagavadgītā* ||

"When a man thinks of the objects, attachment for them arises; from attachment desire is born; from desire anger arises. From anger comes delusion; from delusion loss of memory; from loss of memory the destruction of discrimination; from the destruction of discrimination, he perishes (Sivananda, 1996)".

The *Haṭha Yoga Pradīpikā* categorically delineates the causes that give rise to the activities of the mind.

"hetu-dvayaṃ tu cittasya vāsanā ca samiraṇaḥ |
tayorvinaṣhṭa ekasmintau dvavapi vinaśyataḥ" || *4.22, Haṭha Yoga Pradīpikā* ||

There are two causes of the activities of the mind: (1) *vāsanā* (desires) and (2) the respiration (the *prāṇa*). Of these, the mastering of one is the mastering of both

According to *Patañjali's* Yoga*sūtras*, any perception modifies the mind. The modification is called *vṛtti* or whorl. That due to which the modification takes place is the thought, created by incoming data from the senses. This thought is called *pratyaya*[15]. When a stimulus from the outer world encroaches the senses, a *vṛtti* is formed in the mind. The *ahaṅkār* in turn recognizes itself with this thought. If the thought is agreeable, the ego feels happy, and if disagreeable, it feels perturbed. This is the root cause of transient feelings of joy, sadness, anxiety, etc.

The objects of insight and thoughts are numerous, and consequently, so are the *vṛttis*.

---

[15]Thought forms.

"vṛttayaḥ pañcatayyaḥ kliṣṭākliṣṭāḥ" **|| 1.5, Patañjali's Yogasūtras ||**

The modifications of the mind are of five types which may either be painful (*kliṣṭa*[16])
or non-painful (*akliṣṭa*[17]).

"pramāṇa-viparyaya-vikalpa-nidrā-smṛtayaḥ" **|| 1.6. Patañjali's Yogasūtras ||**

The *vrittis* are - correct understanding, incorrect understanding, imagination, sleep and memory.

As per the Yoga*sūtras*, the sufferance of the mind is due to the *kleśas* – a category of five afflictions which affect the human personality deeply and produce unhappiness in life.

kleśāḥ **|| 2.3, Patanjali's Yogasūtras ||**

* *avidyā*   ignorance of the True Self
* *asmitā*   identification of the Self with external objects
* *rāga*   strong likes, attachment to pleasures, desires
* *dveṣa*   strong dislikes, aversion to pain, hatred
* *abhiniveśa*   fear of death

If we look at the *kleśas* as a tree, then *avidyā* is like the root of the tree. Ignorance of the *puruśa*, i.e., the Self, is responsible for the entire tree of *kleśas*. Rooted in ignorance, this tree yields the four-fold afflictions of *asmitā, rāga, dveṣa,* and *abhiniveśa. Avidyā* leads to *asmitā,* a false sense of identity. The sense of *asmitā,* not as the pure being but as the ego with all its attachments and aversions (*rāga* and *dveṣa*), is responsible for much of the mental suffering (Figure 3.2).

As per *Vyāsa's Bhāṣya* on *Patañjali's* Yoga*sūtras*, the states of the mind can be:

i.   **Muḍha:** One with dullness and indolence. Generated from states of *tamas.*
ii. **Kṣipta:** Distracted or restless states of mind.
iii. **Vikṣipta:** A less scattered or preoccupied mind.
iv. **Ekāgra:** A concentrated mind generating flow.
v.   **Niruddha:** A mastered and restrained mind.

Yoga considers the veritable states of the mind along with the quiescent dispositions '*saṃskāras.* ' When one mental state transforms into the other, the earlier state is not altogether mitigated – the *saṃskāra* remains, which in turn births other similar states. The subconscious mind takes in every form of impression of the conscious mind. Thus, the actual states (conscious

---

[16]Marked by ignorance and bondage.
[17]That fosters the mind towards knowledge and liberation.

mind) activate the saṃskāras. As per *Vyāsa Bhāṣya,* the *saṃskāras* are a combination of both – conditioning and habits.

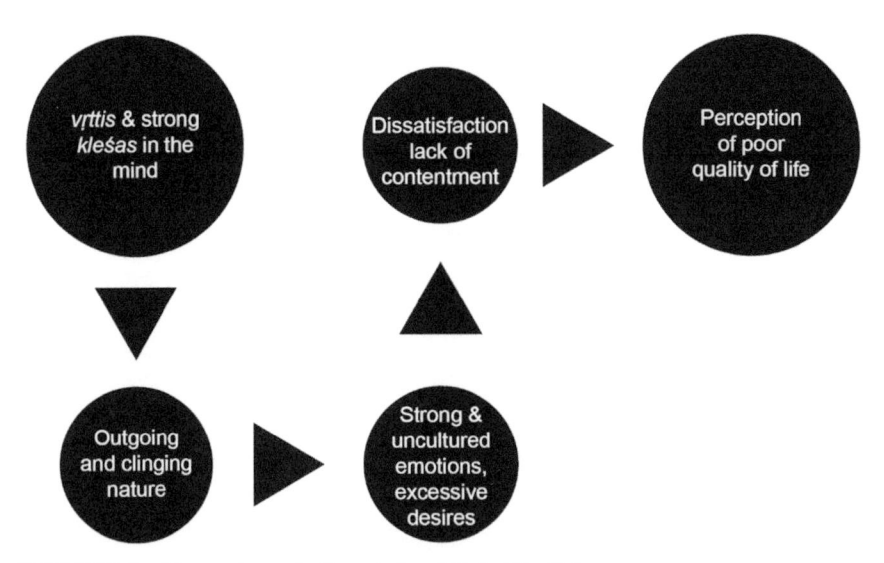

FIGURE 3.2 Despondency in the mind and QoL: The linkages.

Yoga therefore declares that our experience of life depends on the states of our mind – which in turn determines our quality of life.

3.4.5 MIND AND WELLBEING[18]: INTERLINKAGES

The mind – body connection is not unfamiliar. The thoughts, feelings, and the overall psychological construct can in direct proportions affect the physiological functions and vice versa.

According to *Patañjali's Yogasūtras,*

"vyādhistyānasamsayapramādālasyāviratibhrāntidarśanālabdha bhūmikatvānavasthitatvāni cittavikṣepāste'ntarāyāḥ" || 1.30, Patañjali's Yogasūtras ||

Disease, debility, doubt, inadvertence, sloth, sensuality, wrong understanding, non-attainment of the plane and instability are the mental obstacles

---

[18]Mental, physical, and psychosomatic.

And these mental distractions can manifest (*pariṇām*) in following ways:

"duḥkhadaurmanasyāṅgamejayatvaśvāsapraśvāsā vikṣepasahabhuvaḥ"
|| 1.31, Patañjali's Yogasūtras ||

Pain (physical), bitterness, tottering of limbs, irregular inhalation and exhalation.

Maharṣi çaraka[19] says:

"prajñaparādhāt sambhūte vyadhau karmaja ātmanah" || 7.21,nidāna sthāna, Caraka Samhita ||

Mistakes due to the carelessness of human intelligence are the root cause of diseases - the cause of mental diseases is definitely *prajñāparādha.*

"īrṣyāśokabhayakrodhamānadveṣādaśca ye|
manovikārāste'pyuktāḥ sarve prajñāparādhajāḥ"
|| 7.52, sūtra sthāna, Caraka Samhita ||

Jealousy, grief, fear, anger, hatred - All these disorders of the mind arise out of *prajñāparādha.*

The *Nirvāna Prakaraṇa* of the *Laghu Yōga Vasiṣṭha*, describes at length the dawning and ruination of both mental and body ailments.

"śrīvasiṣṭha uvāca |
"ādhayo vyādhayaścaiva dvayaṃ duḥkhasya kāraṇam |
tannivṛttiḥ sukhaṃ vidyāttatkṣayo mokṣa ucyate"
|| 12, Nirvāna Prakaraṇa, Laghu Yōga Vasiṣṭha ||

"dehaduḥkhaṃ vidurvyādhimādhyākhyaṃ vāsanāmayam |
maurkhyamūle hi te vidyāttattvajñāne parikṣayaḥ"
|| 14, Nirvāna Prakaraṇa, Laghu Yōga Vasiṣṭha ||

Sage *Vasiṣṭha* tells Lord *Rama* that there are two main categorizations of illnesses. *Ādhija vyādhi* (primary source by virtue of psychosomatic, stress disorders, etc.) are those caused by the mind while those which directly affect the body are *anadhija vyadhi* (secondary source based on infections, accidents, etc.). Both arise from inordinate desires – being ignorant of the Real Nature. Diseases are divided into *sāmānya* (physical) and *sāra* (the indispensable cycle of birth and rebirth which can be removed only by *ātma jñāna* or knowledge of brahman). *Sāmānya* diseases – those affecting the physical body may be cured through the balancing of mind-body disharmony.

---

[19]*Āyurveda* as a science of well-being is inseparable with *yoga*. Besides sharing a common philosophical ground, both systems share a similar approach w.r.t diet and nutrition, hygiene, lifestyle, cleansing as well as spiritual practices. Patañjali ' was also an *āyurvedāchārya*, all the *nāth yogis* had tremendous knowledge of herbs and life sciences.

3.5 YOGIC UNDERSTANDING OF HAPPINESS

Happiness is not merely a sensual pleasure that one experiences when the senses (with the mind) encounter with the objects. Rather, it is the *anubhūti*[20] of the joy within–when the mind dissociates itself from the senses (and the objects), and merges with the Self.

Yoga provides the necessary techniques to enable overcome the *kleśas* and *vṛttis* of the mind. The *abhyāsa* of yoga helps redirect the outward nature of the mind–turning it inward by restraining the *kāma* (desires) and the *vṛttis*. This deepens the journey–bringing oneself to abide in the unchanging 'Self,' in *ānanda*. Resting in one's True Nature brings a cessation to all desires–fountaining unconditional love, compassion, and happiness.

3.5.1 *ĀNANDA–UNCONDITIONAL HAPPINESS*

The *Taittirīya Upaniṣad* beautifully describes the attributes of brahman as *ānanda* in the following verse:

> **"āṇando brahmeti vyajānāt।**
> **ānandādhyeva khalvimāni bhūtāni jāyante।**
> **ānandena jātāni jīvanti। ānandaṃ prayantyabhisaṃviśantīti"**
> **|| 3-6, Bhrigu Valli, Taittirīya Upaniṣad ||**
>
> "brahman is ānanda, everything is born out of ānanda,
> everything lives in ānanda and at the time of dissociation,
> everything merges into ānanda. Hence, we are all the part of
> that ānanda" (Chinmayananda, 2014).

3.5.2 *SUKHA–CONDITIONAL HAPPINESS*

"How exactly we experience pleasure is interesting. Whenever we are seeking happiness, there is first a craving created for some particular object in our mind. And due to the mental hype, our expectations increase enormously. And when we actually experience the object, immediately our mind quiets down a little and then jumps to the next object of craving or passion. Thus, all the excitement was in the report which the mind gave us before we had the experience. This occurrence is known as the hedonic

---

[20]Experience.

treadmill. Hedonism is the theory of pleasure and treadmill signifies working hard and repeatedly on something while you remain in the same place. So, this is an exercise our mind engages in whenever we try to experience happiness. That is the reason why this category of experiences has been labeled transitory and ephemeral. These are not long-lasting, and they are addictive by nature" (Divyanandaprana, 2021).

3.6   YOGIC TECHNIQUES FOR HAPPINESS THROUGH MIND CULTURATION

In the preceding sections, we have recognized the nature of the mind, interlinkages of mind with wellbeing and the *yogic* paradigms of happiness. It is therefore pivotal to culture the mind to states of contentment and stability, awakening the brilliance within and making it ablaze with the light of Consciousness. This highest virtue is called *śanti*[21] and the being who embodies is *śanta puruṣa*[22].

Our conscious mind is the gateway to the *citta,* and our exposures thus become the content of our mind. We can therefore change the motifs of our mind by regulating and disciplining the conscious thought process. Mind control, for this reason, begins with the senses. Good intake ensures good content, '*āhāraśuddhau sattvaśuddhiḥ,*' it is said – which means that when food is *sāttvika*, calmness is generated in the system. Here *āhāra* includes all that we consume through all our five senses. In the succeeding sections, we will discuss a few *yogic* techniques on cultivating the mind.

3.6.1   *PRACTICE OF KRIYA YOGA*

The practice of *kriya yoga* consists of the following:

1. ***Tapas* (Austerity):** The regular practice of *āsana, prāṇāyāma* (breath regulation), *dhyāna* (meditation), following *yama* (moral disciplines) and *niyama* (observances).
2. ***Svādhāya:*** The study of the Real Nature, the 'Self' through scriptures, listening to knowledge and contemplation.

---

[21]Peace.
[22]As per *Yoga Vasiṣṭha.*

3. *Īśvarapraṇidhāna:* An attitude of surrender, a commitment to *īśvara* (God).

"samādhibhāvanārthaḥ kleśatanukaraṇārthaśca"
|| 2.2, Patañjali's Yogasūtras ||

The purpose of practicing *kriya yoga* is to minimize the *kleśas*. In doing so, the purified mind is habitually trained to enter into its natural state of *samādhi* (higher forms of concentration).

3.6.2 AṢṬĀṄGA YOGA AND ITS PRACTICE

3.6.2.1 YAMA AND NIYAMA

Restraining the *vṛttis* that possess the mind is neither a simple act nor can it be quickly achieved. *Patañjali* and the above-mentioned schools of *yoga* developed a method of self-reinvention where anchoring the mind on *yama* and *niyama* is critical for this endeavor. This state of *cittavṛttinirodaḥ* can be achieved through effective and unswerving *abhyāsa* (practice) and *vairagya* (dispassionate objectivity).

The *Haṭha Yoga Pradīpikā* elucidates *yama* and *niyama* as:

"atha yama-niyamāḥ
ahimsa satyamasteyam brahmacaryam kṣhamā dhṛtiḥ |
dayārjavam mitāhāraḥ śaucam caiva yamā daśa" ||16(ii), Hatha Yoga Pradīpika||

The ten rules of conduct are: *ahimsā* (non-injury), truth, non-stealing, continence, forgiveness, endurance, compassion, humility, moderate diet and cleanliness.

"tapaḥ santosha astikyam danamīśvara-pūjanam |
siddhanta-vākya-śravanam hrīmatī ca tapo hutam |
niyamā daśa samproktā yoga-śāstra-viśāradaiḥ" ||16(iii), Hatha Yoga Pradīpika||

The ten *niyamas* are penance, contentment, belief in the Supreme, worship of God, listening to recitations of sacred scriptures, modesty, a discerning intellect, *japa* (*mantra* recitation) and sacrifice.

3.6.2.2 ASANA

"sthirasukhamāsanam"
|| 2.46, Paṭañjali Yoga Sūtras ||

Āsana is 'to sit unwaveringly and agreeably.' This has come to be approved (by the commentators) as the attribute, and the know-how of '*āsana*' as a reverberation of this elucidation is seen in the next *sūtra*, *"prayatnaśaithi lyānantasamāpattibhyām"* || 2.47, *Patañjali Yoga Sūtras* ||, which implies that the unwinding of the effort and meditation on the infinite leads to the mastery of the *'āsana.'* The purpose of āsana is eventually to lift the mind from body consciousness through transcendence of the body by virtue of effort and relaxation.

The objective of *āsana* from *Haṭha Yoga Pradīpikā* is also described in the following śloka:

*"atha āsanam
haṭhasya prathamāṅgatvādāsanaṃ pūrvamucyate |
kuryāttadāsanaṃ sthairyamārogyaṃ cāṅga-lāghavam"* || 1.17, *Haṭha Yoga Pradīpikā* ||

Being the first appendage of *Haṭha Yoga*, *āsana* is delineated. It should be practiced for attaining balanced posture, health and lightness of body.

3.6.2.3   PRĀṆĀYĀMA

Prāṇa is the vital force in the body responsible for all physiological functions. Further, *prāṇa* and mind are deeply connected. Variation of one means alteration of the other. When either the mind or *prāṇa* becomes steady, the other is stabilized. *Hatha Yoga* enunciates on regulating the *prāṇa*, which spontaneously can control the mind.

*"cale vāte calaṃ cittaṃ niścale niścalaṃ bhavet||
yogī sthāṇutvamāpnoti tato vāyuṃ nirodhayet"* || 2.2, *Haṭha Yoga Pradīpikā* ||

Breath when disrupted, unsettles the mind. By channeling the breath, the *yogī* attains stability of mind.

Prāṇāyāma is the regulation of the *prāṇa* through the conscious regulation of the breath for mastering the mind. *Kumbhaka* is a state of natural cessation of breath by practice of *prāṇāyāma*.

*"kumbhaka-prāṇa-rodhānte kuryāccittaṃ nirāśrayam |
evamabhyāsa-yogena rāja-yoga-padaṃ vrajet"* || 2.77, *Haṭha Yoga Pradīpikā* ||

On the accomplishment of *kumbhaka*, the mind should be designated rest. By such *abhyāsa*, one succeeds in the attainment of *Rāja Yoga*.

Patañjali says that the root cause of the sufferance of the mind is *avidyā*, ignorance about our True Nature – ignorance about how the mind is functioning. Mitigation of *avidyā* (the root cause of sufferance) can lead to the mitigation of the other afflictions.

Thus, Patañjali emphasizes on stilling the fluctuations of *citta* by suspending the breath, following either inhalation or exhalation – breaking the rhythms of the breath. *"tasminsati śvāsapraśvāsayorgativicchedaḥ prāṇāyāmaḥ"* || 2.49, *Patañjali's Yogasūtras*||.

The *"śvāsa-praśvāsa"* which is one of the indicatives of *"cittavikṣepas"* ||1.31, *Patañjali's Yogasūtras*|| becomes disrupted – *"vicchedaḥ"* in a particular manner through *'prāṇāyāma'* – which helps in attenuating all awnings of the Consciousness || 2.52, *Patañjali's Yogasūtras*|| and the mind sets off the states of *dharaṇā*, i.e., concentration || 2.53, *Patañjali's Yogasūtras*||.

Haṭha Yoga Pradīpikā also emphasizes on the purification of the *nādis*[23] through various practices:

"āsanaṃ kumbhakaṃ citraṃ mudrākhyaṃ karaṇaṃ tathā |
atha nādānusandhānamabhyāsānukramo haṭhe" || 1.56, Haṭha Yoga Pradīpikā ||

The *nādis* should be cleansed of their impurities by performing the *mudrās*, etc., (which are the practices relating to the air) *āsanas, kumbhakas* and various *mudrās*.

Haṭha Yoga further state that when the *nādīs* are cleansed by well-ordered practices (such as *prāṇāyāma, bandhas,* and *mudrās,* etc.), the *prāṇa* can be directed upward through the *suṣmaṇa nādī* resulting in *manonmanī,* the most elevated realm of *yogic* Consciousness. || 2.41 & 2.42, *Haṭha Yoga Pradīpikā* ||

3.6.2.4 PRATYAHĀRA (WITHDRAWAL OF SENSES)

In *Kaṭhopaniṣad*, it is said that the sense organs are extrovert (*"parāñci khāni vyatṛṇat."*). Therefore, whenever these senses come in association with the world outside, the mind perceiving the stimuli, cogitates in varying forms. To steady the mind from varied distractions and turn it inward towards higher states of Consciousness, it needs a mental resolve to delink the senses from externalities.

3.6.2.5 DHĀRAṆĀ (CONCENTRATION) AND DHYĀNA (MEDITATION)

Through *dharaṇā*, the mind develops an ability to fix itself to a place, an object, or the idea of an object through volitional practice. And this

---

[23]Channels that carry *prāṇā.*

continued uninterrupted engrossment peaks into *dhyāna*. Further, there comes a stage wherein the mind takes on the attributes of the object of meditation '*samāpatti*' (engrossment). All traditional schools of *yoga* prepare the *sādhaka* (spiritual aspirant) to attain higher stages of meditation. However, the study and the fruition of *Rāja Yoga* or any *yoga* takes time that needs to be accompanied by diligent *abhyāsa*.

Food for Thought

The emphasis on the above stated preliminary disciplines makes self-directed neuroplasticity a possibility in our lives. These disciplines are targeted to condition our brain circuits in a particular way so as to reinforce positive pathways, yoga has become very easy to explain with the advancement of the neuroscience.

3.6.3   PRACTICE OF MODERATION

All schools of yoga also insist on the practice of moderation of the *jñānendriya* (organ of perception, i.e., the sense organs) and the *karmendriya* (motor organs) – to progress on the path of yoga.

"yuktāhāravihārasya yuktaceṣṭasya karmasu |
yuktasvapnāvabodhasya yogo bhavati duḥkhahā" || Bhagavadgītā.6.17 ||

One moderate in habits of eating, sleeping, working and recreation can
alleviate material pains through *yoga*

Moderation is the avoidance of overindulgences across all dimensions of life. Self-control is the key for making the body and the mind a perfect servant of the immutable 'self.'

3.7   SIGNS OF PROGRESS IN THE PRACTICE OF YOGA

Having deeply anchored on the philosophy and the praxis of *yoga*, what are the signs that one is progressing on the path?

The *Haṭha Yoga Pradīpikā beautifully elucidates:*

"vapuḥ kṛśatvaṃ vadane prasannatā
nāda-sphuṭatvaṃ nayane sunirmale |
arogatā bindu-jayo'gni-dīpanaṃ
nāḍī-viśuddhirhaṭha-siddhi-lakṣaṇam"

|| 2.78, Haṭha Yoga Pradīpikā ||

"Perfection of *Hatha Yoga* is accomplished when there is leanness of the body, reposeful expression, manifestation of the inner sound, clear eyes, free of illnesses, control of *bindu* (semen or ova), active digestive fire, and purification of *nādis*" (Muktibodhananda, 2012).

Further,

*"yadā saṃkṣhīyate prāṇo mānasaṃ ca pralīyate |
tadā samarasatvaṃ ca samādhirabhidhīyate"*

|| *4.6, Haṭha Yoga Pradīpikā* ||

When the *prāṇa* is enervated and the mind fully absorbed, that state is *samādhi*.

3.8 MEASUREMENT OF QOL FROM YOGIC PERSPECTIVES

In the following passages, we have taken a few parameters from *yoga* – reflective on the quality of life.

3.8.1 DHARMA

Dharma encompasses religious as well as the moral dutiful conduct of each individual, as well as behaviors that enable the maintenance of social order, and righteous conduct. This being the foremost goal of human life. In ancient India, *Dharmaśāstras* served as guidepost towards the path of *dharma*. *Viṣṇupurāṇa* says:

*"kṣamā satyaṃ damaḥ śaucaṃ dānamindriyasaṃyamaḥ |
ahiṃsā guruśuśrūṣā tīrthānusaraṇaṃ dayā ||
ārjavaṃ lobhaśūnyatvaṃ devabrāhmaṇapūjanam |
anabhyasūyā ca tathā dharmaḥ sāmānya ucyate iti"* || *2.16, Viṣṇupurāṇa* ||

dharma generally means *kṣamā* (forgiveness), *satya* (truth), *dama* (self-control), *śauca* (cleanliness in body and mind), *dāna* (charity), *indriyasaṃyama* (controlling all the senses), *ahiṃsā* (non-violence), *guruśuśrūṣā* (service to the master), *tīrthānusaraṇa* (pilgrimage), *dayā* (compassion/kindness), *ārjava* (honesty), *lobhaśūnyatva* (free from avarice), *devabrāhmaṇapūjana* (worship the God and respect the *brahmana*), *anabhyasūyā* (free from envy).

Manusmṛti says:

*"dhṛtiḥ kṣamā damo'steyaṃ śaucamindriyanigrahaḥ |
dhīrvidyā satyamakrodho daśakaṃ dharmalakṣaṇam"* || *6.92, Manusmṛti* ||

(1) Stability (2) pardoning (3) self-restraint, (4) abstaining from unlawful appropriation, (5) purity, (6) discipline of the sense-organs, (7) discrimination, (8) knowledge, (9) honesty, and (10) absence of anger —are the ten forms of duty.

"āhāra-nidrā-bhaya-maithunañca sāmānyametaṃ paśubhirnarāṇām|
dharmo hi teṣāmadhiko viśeṣo dharmeṇa hīnāḥ paśubhiḥ samānāḥ"
|| 25, Hitopadeśa/Mitralābhaḥ ||

Food, sleep, fear and mating, these acts of humans are similar to animals.
dharma is what is special to humans. Without *dharma*, human beings are as animals.

3.8.2   *CITTA PRASĀDANAM*

The following *sūtra* and *ślokas* elucidates the different virtues for a gracious
and a calm inner disposition:

"maitrīkaruṇāmuditopekṣāṇāṃ sukhaduḥkhapuṇyāpuṇyaviṣayāṇāṃ
bhāvanātaścittaprasādanam" || 1.33, Patañjali's Yogasūtras ||

By cultivating attitudes of friendliness toward the happy, compassion for the unhappy,
joyousness for the virtuous, and indifference toward the wicked, the mind assumes purity.

The *Bhagavad Gītā*, expounds on the spiritual nature of beings and
their concomitant qualities:

"abhayaṃ sattvasaṃśuddhirjñānayogavyavasthitiḥ|
dānaṃ damaśca yajñaśca svādhyāyastapa ārjavam"|| 16.1, Bhagavad Gītā ||
"ahiṃsā satyamakrodhastyāgaḥ śāntirapaiśunam|
dayā bhūteṣvaloluptvaṃ mārdavaṃ hrīracāpalam"|| 16.2, Bhagavad Gītā ||
"tejaḥ kṣamā dhṛtiḥ śaucamadroho nātimānitā|
bhavanti sampadaṃ daivīmabhijātasya bhārata" || 16.3, Bhagavad Gītā ||

The Blessed Lord said fearlessness, purity of heart, steadiness in knowledge and *yoga*,
charity, restraint of senses, sacrifice, study of scriptures, austerity and
straightforwardness. Harmlessness, truth, absence of anger, renunciation, peacefulness,
absence of crookedness, compassion towards beings, non-covetousness, gentleness,
modesty, absence of fickleness. Vigour, forgiveness, fortitude, purity, absence of hatred,
absence of pride – all these belong to the one born for a divine state, O Arjuna.

In *Yogavāśiṣṭha, Vaśiṣṭha* has enumerated a list of 26 virtues *'sadguṇa'*
– an aid to deal with emotions within and outside oneself.

sadguṇa

abhayam	fearlessness
sattvasaṃśuddhi	purity of heart
jñānayogavyavasthiti	steadfastness in knowledge and Yoga
dāna	charity
dama	control of the senses
yajña	Sacrifice
svādhyāya	the study of scriptures
tapa	austerity

ārjava	straight forwardness
ahiṃsā	nonviolence
satyam	truth
akrodha	absence of anger
tyāga	renunciation
śānti	serenity of mind
apaiśuna	absenity of crookedness
bhūtadayā	compassion towards beings
aloluptva	freedom from covetousness
mārdava	gentleness
hrī	modesty
acāpala	absence of fickleness
teja	vigour
kṣamā	forgiveness
dhṛtiḥ	fortitude
śauca	purity
adroha	absence of hatred
nātimānitā	absence of over weening/pride

Kaivalyam (True Knowledge and actualization of the Self) is a state of emancipation from all bondages (and hence sufferings) – the penultimate outcome and the aspired goal for a qualitative life.

SUMMARY

It is a natural human tendency to seek happiness, health, and comfort, the three most important determinants of the quality of one's life. However, individual attitudes, moods, and perceptions play a pivotal role in determining satisfaction towards life and the quality of life. Yoga is an ancient *Hindu* science of mind-body practice. It helps promote physical, mental, social, and spiritual well-being. Yoga recognizes *kleśas* and *vṛttis* that contribute to the restlessness in the mind and the constant creation of unlimited desires and dissatisfaction towards life and its aspects. According to the philosophy of Yoga, *ānanda* (everlasting happiness) is the nature of Self. The mind with *vṛttis* and *kleśas* diverts us from this everlasting nature of *ānanda* towards external momentary pleasures. Yoga provides tools (mind-body practices) that help to overcome these afflictions and modifications by which one can experience real happiness and a better quality of life (Figure 3.3).

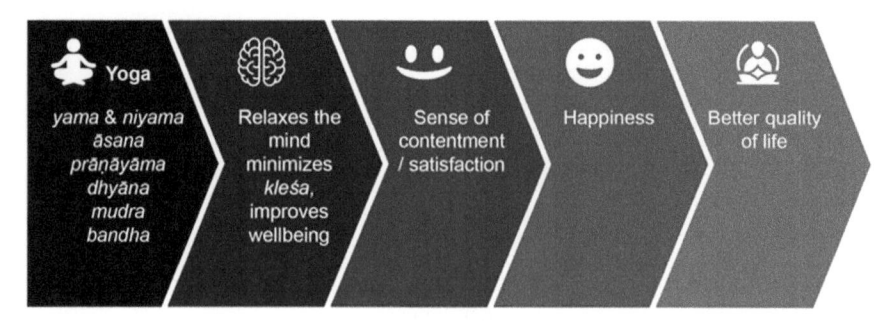

FIGURE 3.3 Well-being and quality of life through *yoga*: Rethinking our notions of happiness.

The current indices by which 'happiness' and QoL are measured seem myopic and confined to the material plane if considered according to the Indic worldview. The purely economic approach that gives weight to GDP, per capita income, and other financial benchmarks discounts the more spiritual and holistic markers that lend human life a dimension of happiness, contentment, and quality that perhaps cannot be adequately measured. This chapter has explored the various *yogic* paradigms that are possibly useful measures to gauge the true quality of life – aspiring to present an alternative lens, a credible and scientifically rooted framework through which these paradigms might be re-evaluated – complementing the happiness indices currently employed by studies worldwide.

Some of the metrics proposed as a result of this undertaking are delineated in Table 3.3.

In conclusion, there is much work to be done in this area of research. The exploration of *yogic* paradigms as markers of "quality of life" is presented as a method for the potential upliftment of mankind in general, without the dependence on the exploitation of nature and natural resources solely in pursuit of material goods as indicators of quality of life. Indian philosophy lays unique emphasis on spiritual knowledge being the remover of all blindness and enabling emancipation. This, along with existing psychological paradigms of well-being, can offer ground-breaking results in terms of true and holistic well-being. The sooner the world wakes up to the wisdom of Yoga and Indian traditions for their prescriptions regarding leading a spiritually and materially fulfilling, balanced life, the sooner we can make the world a happier place to live in.

TABLE 3.3 *Yogic* Indices of Measurement on QoL

01	*ārogyam*	Being free from disease
02	*samatvam*	Equanimity of mind,
03	*kauśalam*	Ability to learn and perform actions without anxiety and fear of result
04	*santoṣam*	Feeling of satisfaction, "happiness" in its truest sense
05	*cittaprsādanam*	A gracious mind
06	*abhayam*	Freedom from fear of death, uncertainty
07	*nirmalam*	Intellect free from judgement and prejudice
08	*ānandam*	Unconditional happiness
09	*samagram*	A holistic approach to life
10	*sampoṣaṇam*	The ability to understand and fulfill needs at one's individual, familial, societal and environmental level
11	*pūrṇam*	Feeling of completeness
12	*kaivalyam*	The freedom from ignorance, bondage and suffering; the complete revolution and transformation of human existence

"Happiness is within me, and Yoga leads the path within"

—Richa Chopra

ACKNOWLEDGMENT

Special acknowledgements to Grishma Raj Aryal, Sai Priya Chodavarapu, and Vineeta L. Dudgundi, Malvica Chopra.

KEYWORDS

- *aṣṭāṅga yoga*
- **conditional happiness**
- **dharma**
- **interlinkages**
- **mind culturation**
- **quality of life**
- **unconditional happiness**
- *yoga*
- **yogic techniques**

REFERENCES

Aranya, S. H. (2000). *Yoga Philosophy of Patanjali with Bhasvati*. University of Calcutta.

Bullinger, M. (1997). International validation and testing of quality-of-life scales in relation to Germany. *Quality of Life Research, 6*(3), 210.

Carr-Hill, R. (1991). Allocating resources to health care: Is the QALY (Quality Adjusted Life Year) a technical solution to a political problem? *International Journal of Health Services, 21*(3), 351–363.

Chaturvedi, B. K. (2017). *Vishnu Puran*. Diamond Pocket Books Pvt Ltd.

Chinmayananda, S. (2014). *Taittiriya Upanishad*. Central Chinmaya Mission Trust.

Divyanandaprana, P. (2021). *Science of Happiness: According to Yoga-Vedanta*. Sri Sarada Math.

Field, T. (2011). Yoga clinical research review. *Complementary Therapies in Clinical Practice, 17*(1), 1–8. [PubMed] [Google Scholar].

Field, T. (2016). Yoga research review. *Complementary Therapies in Clinical Practice, 24*(1), 145–161. [PubMed] [Google Scholar]

Gill, T. M., & Feinstein, A. R. (1994). A critical appraisal of the quality of quality-of-life measures. *JAMA, 272*(8), 619–626.

Group, T. W. (1998). The World Health Organization quality of life assessment (WHOQOL): development and general psychometric properties. *Social science & medicine, 46*(12), 1569–1585.

Helliwell, J. F., Layard, R., Sachs, J. D., De Neve, J.-E., Aknin, L. B., & Wang, S. (2022). *World Happiness Report 2022*. New York: Sustainable Development Solutions Network.

Helliwell, J., Layard, R., & Sachs, J. (2012). *World Happiness Report 2012*. New York: Sustainable Development Solutions Network.

Higgins, E. T. (1987). Self-discrepancy: A theory relating self and affect. *Psychological Review, 94*(3), 319.

Hunt, S. M. (1997). Quality of life claims in trials of anti-hypertensive therapy. *Quality of Life Research, 6*, 185–191.

Hunt, S. M. (1997). The problem of quality of life. *Quality of Life Research, 6*(3), 205–212. Retrieved from: https://www.jstor.org/stable/4035081 (accessed on 5 July 2024).

IIT Kanpur. (2020). *Srimad Bhagavad Gita*. Retrieved from: https://www.gitasupersite.iitk.ac.in/srimad?language=dv&field_chapter_value=4&field_nsutra_value=5&etsiva=1&choose=1 (accessed on 5 July 2024).

Jha, G. (2019). *Manusmriti with the Commentary of Medhatithi: Wisdom Library*. Retrieved from: https://www.wisdomlib.org/hinduism/book/manusmriti-with-the-commentary-of-medhatithi (accessed on 5 July 2024).

Lindström, B. (1992). Quality of life: A model for evaluating health for all. Conceptual considerations and policy implications. *Sozial-und Präventivmedizin, 37*, 301–306.

Lyubomirsky, S. (2008). *The How of Happiness: A Scientific Approach to Getting the Life You Want*. Penguin.

Marks, N., Abdallah, S., Simms, A., & Thompson, S. (2006). *The (un)Happy Planet Index: An Index of Human Well-Being and Ecological Impact*. London: NEF.

Maslow, A. H. (1943). A theory of human motivation. *Psychological Review, 50*(4), 370–396. doi:10.1037/h0054346.

Mishra, V. (1962). *Vācaspatyam* (Vol. 5, p. 3852). Varanasi: The Chowkhamba Sanskrit Series Office. Retrieved from: https://archive.org/details/vacaspatyam05tarkuoft/mode/2up (accessed on 5 July 2024).

Morris, M. D. (1979). *Measuring the Condition of the World's Poor: The Physical Quality-of-Life Index*. New York: Pergamon Press for the Overseas Development Council.

Muktibodhananda, S. (2012). *Hatha Yoga Pradipika*. Yoga Publications Trust, Munger, Bihar.

Muller, M. (1864). *The First Book of the Hitopadeśa*. London: Spottiswoode and Co.

Panshikar, V. L. S. (1985). *Laghuyogavāsistha: Text with the Sanskrit commentary Vāsistha-Candrikā*. Motilal Banarsisdass Publisher.

Ram, B. (2010). *The 8 Limbs of Yoga: Pathway to Liberation*. Delhi: Lotus Press. [Google Scholar].

Samhita, C. (1949). *Charaka Samhita*. Vols I-VI, Jamnagar, India: Shree Gulab Kunverba Ayurvedic Society.

Sarkar, S. (2020). Mannusmriti: A Critical Analysis. *International Journal of Humanities & Social Science Studies (IJHSSS)*, *8*, 255–260.

Sarvananda, S. (2022). *Katha Upanishad*. Sri Ramakrishna Math.

Shukla, K. (2022). *The Conceptual Frameworks on Quality of Life: A Go-to-Handbook for Quality-of-Life Research*. N.p.: Notion Press.

Sirgy, M. J. (1986). A quality-of-life theory derived from Maslow's developmental perspective: 'Quality' is related to progressive satisfaction of a hierarchy of needs, lower order and higher. *American Journal of Economics and Sociology, 45*(3), 329–342.

Sivananda, S. S. (1996). *Bhagavad Gita for Busy People*. Rishikesh, India: Divine Life Society.

Surfshark. (2022). *Digital Quality of Life Index*. Retrieved from: https://surfshark.com/dql2022 (accessed on 5 July 2024).

Susniene, D., & Jurkauskas, A. (2009). The concepts of quality of life and happiness–Correlation and differences. *Engineering Economics, 63*(3), 58–66. Retrieved from: https://www.researchgate.net/publication/228696715_The_concepts_of_quality_of_life_and_happiness_-_Correlation_and_differences (accessed on 5 July 2024).

Sustainable Development Solutions Network. (2012). *The World Happiness Report*. Retrieved from: https://worldhappiness.report/ (accessed on 5 July 2024).

Svatmarama, Y. (2002). *Hatha Yoga Pradipika*. Yogavidya.com.

United Nations Development Programme (UNDP). (2022). *Human Development Index* [Internet]. Available from: https://hdr.undp.org/data-center/human-development-index#/indicies/HDI (accessed on 5 July 2024).

Veenhoven, R. (2003). Hedonism and happiness. *Journal of Happiness Studies, 4*(4), 437–457.

Vivekananda, S. (1896). [Letter from Swami Vivekananda to Alasinga Perumal, 1896]. Retrieved from: http://www.ramakrishnavivekananda.info/vivekananda/volume_5/epistles_first_series/058_alasinga.htm (accessed on 5 July 2024).

Warburton, D. M. (1996). The functions of pleasure. In D. M. Warburton & N. Sherwood (Eds.), *Pleasure and Quality of Life* (pp. 1–15). Chichester: Wiley.

Wisdom Library. (2008). *For Translation: Wisdom Library*. Retrieved from: https://www.wisdomlib.org/hinduism/book/manusmriti-with-the-commentary-of-medhatithi/d/doc200653.html (accessed on 5 July 2024).

CHAPTER 4

Effect of Yoga and Meditation on "Quality of Life": Comparison among People Who Practice and Those Who Don't

MOUSUMI SETHY,[1] PALLABI MISHRA,[2]
PUSPITA BHARATI SAMANTARAY,[3] and RITUPARNA MITRA[3]

[1]*Assistant Professor, Department of Psychology, Utkal University, Bhubaneswar, Odisha, India*

[2]*Assistant Professor, Department of Business Administration, Utkal University, Bhubaneswar, Odisha, India*

[3]*Post-Graduate in Psychology, Department of Psychology, Utkal University, India*

ABSTRACT

The present study aimed to investigate the impact of yoga and meditation on the "quality of life" and "psychological well-being" among adults. A sample size of 180 adults within the age group of 23 to 46 years was selected for the study. The results were calculated using the WHO "Quality of Life" Scale-Brief (WHOQOL) and Ryff's psychological well-being. According to the results of the t-test, there is no significant difference between people who practice yoga and those who don't in terms of physical, psychological, social, and environmental "quality of life;" however, there is a significant difference in psychological well-being.

Yoga and Meditation: Past and Present Evidence. Sachi Nandan Mohanty, Rabindra Kumar Pradhan, & Sugyanta Priyadarshini (Eds.)

4.1 INTRODUCTION

4.1.1 YOGA

Yoga belongs to one of the six recognized schools of Indian philosophy. The yoga tradition does not originate with *Patanjali*, the creator of the yoga system. According to *Patanjali*, what he has provided is the explication of a previously established tradition. The first comprehensive explanation of Yoga that is still in existence is *Patanjali*'s Yogasutra, which dates back to around 300 AD. The *Bhagwad Gita, Upanishads*, and other works of literature that are considerably older than Yogasutra contain references to the Yoga tradition. The United Nations (UNO) has declared June 21 of each year as International Yoga Day in order to prioritize the importance of Yoga worldwide.

4.1.2 THE YOGA SYSTEM OF PATANJALI

Yoga is the prevention of mental modifications. This definition of Yoga, which *Patanjali* provided, uses four different terms. The first term is the one being defined; *citta, vrtti,* and *nirodha* are the other three words, respectively. As it was previously established, the Sanskrit root "*yuj*" which means "to join" or "union" is where Yoga first emerged. Yoga therefore requires a departure or detachment, called *viyoga*, which is accommodated in achieving Yoga.

4.2 TYPES OF YOGA

As was previously said, the goal of Yoga is to transcend individuality, and the condition of samadhi allows this to happen. For the practice of Yoga, ethical preparations are a vital requirement. This opens up the possibility of practicing Yoga in a variety of ways, and there are several Yoga lineages, including *Hatha* Yoga, *Raja* Yoga, *Jnana* Yoga, *Bhakti* Yoga, *Karma* Yoga, and *Laya* Yoga.

4.2.1 HATHA YOGA

Through the practice of asanas, *Hatha* Yoga is also known as the "forceful Yoga" that focuses on the development of the body's abilities to undergo the impacts of transcendental realization. *Hatha*-Yoga is distinct from other forms of Yoga in that it places a greater focus on the physical side of yogic practice. It is a technique for forcing focus through strenuous physical activity, certain postures, and similar things. According to *Hatha* Yoga, it must be interpreted as "psychospiritual technology in service of transcendental realization." *Hatha* Yoga is suitable for those with a healthy physical disposition. It frequently relates to *Patanjali* Yoga or *Raja*-Yoga.

4.2.2 JNANA YOGA

Realization is the goal of *Jnana* Yoga through knowledge. All schools of Indian philosophy view that ignorance is the fundamental reason for slavery, and *Jnana* Yoga is the technique for dispelling this ignorance by obtaining enlightenment. *Jnana* Yoga distinguishes between transcendental knowledge and empirical knowledge, believing the latter to be the true kind of knowing. One becomes identified with the supreme self through achieving *Jnana*. In other words, the goal of *Jnana* Yoga is to identify the empirical self (*jivatma*) and the transcendental self (*paramatma/Brahman*).

4.2.3 BHAKTI YOGA

The devoted devotion to God is known as bhakti. It makes it possible to think about things from a heavenly perspective, outside one's own personal boundaries. People with an emotional nature benefit from *bhakti* Yoga. The person purifies and directs their emotional energy toward the divine. *Bhakti* Yoga encourages selfless action in accordance with divine intent. It often thinks of God as being personal rather than being impersonal. There is therefore no total identification with God, even when the devotee entirely merges with Him. The individual's will be associated with his or her activity in the mystical fusion of *Bhakti* Yoga, enabling him or her to transcend the egoistic motivations of action.

4.2.4 MANTRA YOGA

Sound is a means of transcendence in mantra Yoga. *Mantras*, which are repeated repeatedly, can cause altered states of consciousness. A *mantra* might be made up of a single syllable or several syllables. The syllable AUM is the most significant of these mantras. Through continuous *mantra* chanting, the Vedic seers came to understand the concept of the "universal sound," with which the practitioner identifies.

4.2.5   LAYA YOGA

Through meditation, *Laya* Yoga allows the individual self to dissolve into the transcendental self. Laya is the process through which the cosmic principles are gradually absorbed into the transcendental spiritual principle. The way to do this is to focus intensely. By integrating his or her microcosmic existence into the transcendental Being, one aims to transcend their memories and sensory experiences through this focus.

4.3   IMPORTANT PRINCIPLES OF YOGA

1. **Yama**: It is interested in techniques for self-control. They allude to the behaviors that are forbidden. It is composed of the body, speech, and thinking. *Yama* is a part of the development of the social values in the previous developmental account. The five main pledges of *Yama* are to refrain from using violence, lying, stealing, acting impolitely, and possessing anything. These promises apply to all phases and are not contingent on class, location, time, or occasion. *Ahimsa* (non-violence), *Satya* (truthfulness), *Asteya* (non-stealing), *Brahmacharya* (celibacy), and *Aparigraha* are the *yamas* (non-progressiveness).

2. **Niyama**: It consists of the 'DOs.' They are observances that one must adhere to in order to develop individual values. Niyama includes *Sauca* (cleanliness), *Tapas* (penance), *Svadhyaya* (self-study), and *Isvarapranidhana* (surrendering oneself to God).

3. **Asana**: Known as the third limb of Yoga, *Asana* is a steady and comfortable posture. According to Yogasutra, *Asana* is said to be a steady and comfortable posture. In other words, it can be said as the preparation of the body by adopting prescribed postures of the body that aid in concentration and control of the mind. There are numerous different postures and practicing them will aid in achieving balance between the body and the mind. It also plays an

important role in developing mental equilibrium and preventing distractions of the mind. In a certain way, asanas help in the manipulation of the mind through the manipulation of the body.

4. ***Pranayama***: The fourth stage in *Astanga* Yoga is *Pranayama*, or the control over breath. It is aimed at attaining calmness of mind. *Pranayama* includes three stages which are as follows: *puraka* or inhaling; *kumbhaka* or retaining; and recaka or exhaling of breath. By practicing *Prana*yama, it increases concentration of the mind. Other than increased concentration, *Prana*yama also helps in maintaining good health and is often used for curing diseases.

5. ***Dharana, Dhyana,*** **and** ***Samadhi***: These are the final stages or phases in the practice of Yoga. Mostly, these are characterized by their concentration towards the object of meditation.

4.4 "QUALITY OF LIFE (QOL)"

Aristotle's writings on "the good life" and "living well" (as mentioned in Smith, 2000) are where the idea of "quality of life" (QoL) first emerged. In his work, he explores both the notion of individual and societal QoL. The term "quality of life" (QoL) was originally used in a scientific study by James Seth (as referenced in Smith, 2000) in 1889, which stated that "We must not consider the mere number, but also the quality of the life which forms the moral aim."

The concept of "quality of life" is very important in every area of global development, not just health psychology. The theoretical and practical implications of "quality of life" have been extensively studied in the context of health, and it is considered a significant and reliable outcome in a range of health situations. With a significant departure from the disease model of health, the inclusion of "quality of life" as a beneficial resource in an individual, society, or community has been emerging as a phenomenon.

According to the World Health Organization, "quality of life" refers to a broad concept that is intricately influenced by a person's degree of independence, physical and mental health, social connections, and interactions with significant environmental factors (WHO "quality of life" Group, 1993). The WHO states that a person's goals, expectations, standards, and concerns, as well as the value systems they live by, determine their perspective on their place in life. As a result, linking "quality of life" to health or happiness is insufficient.

The University of Toronto's "quality of life" research unit has defined "quality of life" as "the extent to which a person enjoys the significant possibilities of his/her life." Possibilities are the outcomes of the opportunities and constraints that each individual encounters in life and are a reflection of the interaction of environmental and personal factors. As demonstrated by the expression: "Enjoyment has two components: the experience of satisfaction and the possession or achievement of some characteristic." She is in excellent health. Being, belonging, and becoming are three of the basic life domains. From the ideas of numerous writers, the conceptualization of Being, Belonging, and Becoming as the areas of "quality of life" was established.

Three sub-domains make up the Being domain, which encompasses the fundamental components of "who one is." Personal hygiene, nutrition, exercise, grooming, clothing, and physical appearance are all parts of one's physical well-being. The phrase "psychological being" describes a person's emotional stability, psychological health, self-awareness, and self-control. Individual morality, ethics, and spiritual convictions that may or may not be linked to organized religions are expressed by Spiritual Being.

Along with having three sub-domains, belonging also refers to how well a person fits into their surroundings. Physical belonging refers to a person's connections to their immediate surroundings, including their home, place of employment, neighborhood, school, and community. Being accepted by intimate friends, family, co-workers, neighbors, and other community members are all aspects of social belonging. Community belonging is defined as having access to resources that are normally available to members of the community, such as sufficient income, health and social services, employment, educational, and recreational opportunities, and communal activities.

The term "becoming" refers to the intentional actions taken to fulfill one's own objectives, aspirations, and desires. Practical becoming can take many forms, including domestic duties, paid work, extracurricular or volunteer activities, and attending to social or health requirements. Leisure becoming includes activities that promote relaxation and stress reduction. These could be longer-term pursuits like card games, neighborhood strolls, family visits, or shorter-term ones like vacations or trips. Activities that promote improvement or maintenance of knowledge and skills.

There are typically three ways to evaluate life quality. The first strategy concentrates on traits of a decent existence in terms of particular normative values of society or culture. The second strategy is based on a person's preferences and level of pleasure. The third strategy places an emphasis on the experiences of the people.

Social science study was inspired by the biomedical model approach limitations that were initially suppressed by the medical establishment. Priority was placed on including subjective elements, which Maslow's Hierarchy of Needs Theory (Maslow, 1954) recommended. Currently, it is recognized that, in addition to strictly medical discourse, QoL incorporates fields including sociology, psychology, environmental studies, social work, and social policy.

In quality-of-life research, the subjective and objective "quality of life" are usually distinguished. Feeling pleased and optimistic about life in general is crucial for subjective "quality of life." What it means to live a life of objective quality is to fulfill societal and cultural ambitions for monetary prosperity, social status, and physical well-being.

The transition from objective to subjective experiences has broadened assessments of people's "quality of life" well beyond their physical and mental health. Quality evaluation has evolved from focusing solely on an individual's functional level to now take into account their sense of need fulfillment and contentment.

"Quality of life" is a metric that may be used to measure a wide range of characteristics and was validated based on consensus from numerous demographic groups. One's viewpoint on their "quality of life," their perception of their health, their physical and mental well-being, their social connections, and their environmental well-being are some of the elements that have been noted as key determinants of their "quality of life" (WHOQOL User Manual, 1998).

As a tangible aspect of health, physical health has been defined as being assessed by levels of exercise, dietary control, drug use or dependency, frequency of medical care, rest, and sleep. Some of the characteristics listed as indicators of psychological health, a crucial predictor of "quality of life," include the absence of any mental illnesses, negative orientation in thoughts and behavior, increased emotions of pleasant affect, high self-esteem, keen memory, and focus. The macro-domains that surround an individual are made up of social interactions and the environment, both of which are crucial components of "quality of life." Their constitution is made up of things like the caliber of their interpersonal relationships, the help they receive from friends and family, sexual activity, the accessibility of financial resources, knowledge, and skills, the opportunities for recreation, the availability of health and social care services, transportation, and the condition of their physical environment and home.

Since illness and its treatment have an impact on people's physical integrity as well as their emotional, social, and financial well-being, any definition should be broadly inclusive while allowing for the identification of specific parts. This enables evaluation of the overall impact of various illness states or therapeutic interventions on a number of "quality of life" parameters.

In clinical research, health psychology, primary care, and health promotion, it is vital to understand "quality of life" as a goal that is dynamically growing. This was highlighted in the discussion above. This promotes research into strategies that strive for longer lasting and more effective systems while also presenting the opportunity for a higher "quality of life" than merely longevity.

4.5   YOGA AND "QUALITY OF LIFE"

Yoga is both a science and an art. Yoga is a peaceful, methodical effort to achieve complete inner and outer perfection. The finest and quickest method to advance is through Yoga, which is also an end in and of itself. Thus, through the practicing of Yoga, "quality of life" experiences a quantum leap to the highest level of contentment as well as complete personality development on all levels: physical, mental, emotional, intellectual, and spiritual. As "quality of life" continues to rise to an impossibly high level, one can only wonder at the change that has occurred both within and externally (Nagendra HR, 2004). Research suggests that Yoga positively influences the common determinants of "quality of life" which are as follows: personal transformation, interpersonal relationships, spiritual realization, and a sense of purpose (Ross, Bevans, Friedmann, Williams, & Thomas, 2013).

Research provides a thorough evaluation of the benefits of traditional Yoga poses. The beneficial effects of Yoga are being investigated in various populations interacting with a wide range of special conditions and settings. Yoga that is used in therapy is defined as using Yoga postures and practices to treat health issues. It also involves receiving instruction in Yoga poses and poses to halt, lessen, or soothe physical, structural, mental, and emotional suffering, severe pain, or limits. The outcome of this investigation shows that Yoga exercises increase physical stamina and body elasticity, enhance, and improve breathing and cardiovascular functioning, promote addiction recovery and treatment, lessen stress, depression, anxiety, and chronic pain, establish sleep patterns, and generally improve prosperity and personal satisfaction (Woodyard, 2011).

4.6 REVIEW OF LITERATURE ON YOGA, MEDITATION, AND "QUALITY OF LIFE"

Many studies have been conducted to find out how Yoga and meditation impact both general "quality of life" and "quality of life" for those who are ill. These studies show that those who frequently practice Yoga or meditation tend to have improved their "quality of life" as well as their physical and mental health. While engaging in Yoga and meditation, the equilibrium between the sympathetic nervous system, which triggers the fight-or-flight response, and the parasympathetic nervous system, which triggers the relaxation response, is changed. Cortisol and vasopressin levels are decreased, respiration, and heart rate are slowed, blood supply to the body's organs is improved, and the person becomes calmer as a result (Desikachar et al., 2005; Woodyard, 2011; Bankar et al., 2013; Birdee et al., 2017; Oken et al., 2006). Yoga inhibits the posterior, or sympathetic, part of the hypothalamus. This inhibition improves the body's sympathetic reactions to stressful stimuli and recovers the stress-related autonomic regulating reflex systems. By suppressing the brain regions in charge of fear, aggression, and rage, Yoga practices increase the rewarding centers of pleasure in the middle forebrain and other locations, resulting in a happy and pleasurable experience. Yoga and meditation practitioners report lower levels of anxiety, as well as lower heart rates, respiration rates, blood pressure, and cardiac output. This inhibition also helps people from developing cancer, and their "quality of life" is improved (Bharshankar et al., 2003; Bhattacharjee, 2008; Wolff et al., 2013; Lin et al., 2011; Kizhak-keveettil et al., 2019).

The first and most obvious benefit of Yoga is improved flexibility. Because of the gradual relaxation of the muscular and skeletal systems that happens with regular practice, Yoga is thought to be associated with fewer aches and pains. Yoga encourages muscle development and/or strength maintenance, preventing conditions like osteoporosis, arthritis, and back pain. Numerous studies looking at how Yoga affects muscular pain have found that Yoga, meditation, or the two together, significantly reduce chronic pain in people with multiple sclerosis, arthritis, osteoporosis, chronic lower back pain, chronic pancreatitis, chronic pelvic pain in women, HIV, and even Carpal Tunnel Syndrome. They also improve the "quality of life" of these patients (Garfinkle et al., 1998; Gatantino et al., 2004; Williams et al., 2005; Sareen et al., 2006; Tekur et al., 2008; Haaz & Bartlett, 2011; Tul et al., 2011; Woodyard, 2011; Cramer et al., 2013, Dehkordi & Jivad, 2014; Moonaz et al., 2015; Rusell et al., 2019). Numerous research looking into how Yoga and meditation affect people with diabetes have discovered that it lowers the waist-hip ratio in diabetics. Additionally, it was discovered that consistently performing Yoga, meditation, or a combination of the two reduced insulin levels to normal ranges, indicating improved insulin sensitivity and lower insulin resistance. The asanas of Yoga also assisted in the release of the pancreatic insulin that had been stored, aiding in glycemic management. As a result, the people's "quality of life" is improved (Malhotra et al., 2005; Innes & Vincent, 2007; Sahay, 2007; Kosuri & Sridhar, 2009; Aljasir et al., 2010; Thangasami et al., 2015; Pal et al., 2017; Cui et al., 2017; Ravindran et al., 2018).

4.7 THE PRESENT STUDY

- ➢ **Aim:** To study the "quality of life" of people who practice Yoga and those who do not practice Yoga.
- ➢ **Objectives:** To find out the distinction between "quality of life" of people who practice Yoga and those who do not practice Yoga.
- ➢ **Hypothesis:** From the above literature it is assumed that people who practice Yoga will have better "quality of life" than the people who do not practice Yoga.

4.8 METHOD OF INVESTIGATION

- ➢ **Research Design:** To investigate if the subjects were currently doing Yoga and how it had influenced their "quality of life" at the time, a cross-sectional research methodology was chosen.
- ➢ **Selection Criteria of Sample:** Inclusion criteria: Individuals above the age of 23 and below the age of 46 were selected. Exclusion criteria: Individuals below the age of 23 and above the age of 46 were excluded from the study.

- ➤ **Sampling Technique:** After establishing the selection criteria, a sample of 180 was selected through non-probability purposive sampling.
- ➤ **Sample Description:** The sample consisted of 180 individuals from Bhubaneswar, who were between the ages of 23 and 46.
- ➤ **Variables Used for the Study:** Yoga, "quality of life."
- ➤ **Operational Definition of Variables:**
  - **Yoga:** It is a spiritual practice based on an incredibly delicate science that aims to harmonize the body and mind.
  - **"Quality of Life":** The viewpoint of a person's position in life in light of their goals, ideals, and concerns, as well as the culture and value systems in which they are raised.
- ➤ **Tools Used for the Study:**
  - **WHO "Quality of Life" Scale-Brief:** The WHOQOL Group worked concurrently with 15 international field centers to establish the WHOQOL in an effort to construct a "quality of life" evaluation that would be culturally universal. It evaluates a person's "quality of life" in relation to four different areas: their physical health, psychological health, social health, and environmental health. Additionally, it rates the person's general QoL. The 26-item self-administered questionnaire evaluates a person's impression of their health and well-being over a period of two weeks. Each statement requires a response from the subject on a 5-point Likert scale. The WHO has conducted extensive study and validated the psychometric qualities. According to Skevington et al. (2004), the WHOQOL-BREF is a reliable tool in the cross-cultural area. It has demonstrated strong test-retest reliability, internal consistency, concurrent validity, and discriminant validity.
  - **Procedure of Data Collection:** 180 people between the ages of 23 and 45 who were personally contacted and informed of the study's goal make up the sample. The secrecy of their answers was then confirmed to them, and participants were informed that they could withdraw from the study whenever they wanted to. Then permission was sought from them. After obtaining their agreement, the WHOQOL-BREF was handed to them along with instructions on how to complete the form. The completed questionnaires were then gathered.

- **Statistical Analysis Used in the Study:** In order to compare the "quality of life" of individuals who practice Yoga to those who did not, the data was computed using an independent t-test.

4.9 ANALYSIS OF RESULTS

In this chapter, a detailed analysis of the collected data has been presented as per the objectives stated earlier, and the results are presented.

Table 4.1 shows that from the data obtained by the "quality of life" questionnaire, the mean score along with SD of individuals who practice Yoga in terms of overall "quality of life" are 6.36 and 1.23, respectively, and the mean score along with SD of individuals who do not practice Yoga in terms of overall "quality of life" are 5.96 and 1.58, respectively. In order to find out the mean difference, an independent t-test was computed. At a 99% confidence interval, it was discovered that there is no discernible difference in overall "quality of life" between those who do Yoga and those who do not, i.e., $t = 1.887$ ($p > 0.01$).

TABLE 4.1 t-Test Result Comparing the Individuals Who Practice Yoga and Those Who Do Not Practice Yoga in Terms of Overall "Quality of Life"

"Quality of Life"	N	Mean	SD	df	t-Score	p
Practice yoga	90	6.36	1.23	178	1.89	$p > 0.01$
Do not practice yoga	90	5.96	1.58			

Table 4.2 shows that from the data obtained by the "quality of life" questionnaire, the mean score along with SD of individuals who practice Yoga in terms of physical "quality of life" are 24.60 and 3.69, respectively, and the mean score along with SD of individuals who do not practice Yoga in terms of physical "quality of life" are 22.40 and 4.9, respectively. In order to find out the mean difference, an independent t-test was computed. At a 99% confidence level, it was discovered that there is a considerable difference in terms of physical "quality of life" between those who do Yoga and those who do not, i.e., $t = 3.4$ ($p < 0.001$).

Table 4.3 shows that from the data obtained by the "quality of life" questionnaire, the mean score along with SD of individuals who practice Yoga in terms of psychological "quality of life" are 20.07 and 2.95, respectively, and the mean score along with SD of individuals who do not practice Yoga in terms of psychological "quality of life" are 17.83 and 4.33, respectively. In order to find out the mean difference, an independent t-test was computed. However, it was found that there is a significant difference between the individuals who practice Yoga and individuals who do not practice Yoga in terms of psychological "quality of life" at a 99% confidence interval, i.e., t = 4.04 (p < 0.001).

TABLE 4.2 t-Test Result Comparing the Individuals Who Practice Yoga and Who Do Not Practice Yoga in Terms of Physical "Quality of Life"

Physical "Quality of Life"	N	Mean	SD	Df	t-Score	P
Practice yoga	90	24.60	3.69	178	3.4	p < 0.001
Do not practice yoga	90	22.40	4.9			

TABLE 4.3 t-Test Result Comparing the Individuals Who Practice Yoga and Who Do Not Practice Yoga in Terms of Psychological "Quality of Life"

Psychological "Quality of Life"	N	Mean	SD	Df	t-Score	P
Practice yoga	90	20.07	2.95	178	4.04	p <0.01
Do not practice yoga	90	17.83	4.33			

Table 4.4 shows that from the data obtained by the "quality of life" questionnaire, the mean score along with SD of individuals who practice Yoga in terms of social "quality of life" are 12.03 and 1.23, respectively, and the mean score along with SD of individuals who do not practice Yoga in terms of social "quality of life" are 9.93 and 2.58, respectively. In order to find out the mean difference, an independent t-test was computed. However, it was found that there is a significant difference between the individuals who practice Yoga and individuals who do not practice Yoga in terms of social "quality of life" at a 99% confidence interval, i.e., t = 6.96 (p < 0.01).

TABLE 4.4 t-Test Result Comparing the Individuals Who Practice Yoga and Who Do Not Practice Yoga in Terms of Social "Quality of Life"

Social "Quality of Life"	N	Mean	SD	df	t-Score	P
Practice yoga	90	12.03	1.23	178	6.96	p < 0.01
Do not practice yoga	90	9.93	2.58			

Table 4.5 shows that from the data obtained by the "quality of life" questionnaire, the mean score along with SD of individuals who practice Yoga in terms of environmental "quality of life" are 29.60 and 3.39, respectively, and the mean score along with SD of individuals who do not practice Yoga in terms of environmental "quality of life" are 24.17 and 4.98, respectively. In order to find out the mean difference, an independent t-test was computed. However, at a 99% confidence interval, it was discovered that there is a substantial difference between those who practice Yoga and those who do not in terms of environmental "quality of life," i.e., $t = 8.55$ ($p < 0.01$).

TABLE 4.5 t-Test Result Comparing the Individuals Who Practice Yoga and Who Do Not Practice Yoga in Terms of Environmental "Quality of Life"

Environmental "Quality of Life"	N	Mean	SD	df	t-Score	P
Practice yoga	90	29.60	3.39	178	8.55	$p < 0.01$
Do not practice yoga	90	24.17	4.98			

4.10 DISCUSSION AND CONCLUSION

This research was done in an effort to learn more about how Yoga and meditation affect "Quality of life." The primary goal of the study was to compare the characteristics of Yoga practitioners and non-practitioners using responses to the WHO's "Quality of life" Questionnaire. Around 180 participants in the study, ranging in age from 23 to 45, participated. The approach of non-probability purposeful sampling was employed to choose possible respondents. With the aid of Google Forms, data collection was carried out by distributing the questionnaire over social media platforms.

First, the WHO's "Quality of life" survey was given to all 180 people. To determine the outcomes, the independent samples t-test was used.

4.10.1 MAJOR FINDINGS OF THE STUDY

1. Within a 99% confidence interval, there is no discernible difference in overall "Quality of life" between Yoga practitioners and non-practitioners.

2. At a 99% confidence level, there is a significant difference in physical "quality of life" between people who practice Yoga and others who do not.
3. At a 99% confidence level, there is a significant difference between Yoga practitioners and non-practitioners in terms of psychological "quality of life."
4. At a 99% confidence level, there is a considerable difference in social "quality of life" between people who practice Yoga and others who do not.

At a 99% confidence level, there is a significant difference in environmental "quality of life" between people who practice Yoga and others who do not.

4.10.2   LIMITATIONS OF THE PRESENT STUDY

No study is free of limitations, and this study is also not an exception. The following are some of the limitations of the study:

1. In the present study, the sampling method was purposive sampling, which is a non-probability sampling and not as valid as probability sampling or random sampling.
2. The sample was collected from people within a limited age group.
3. The administration of questionnaires through the online mode may question the validity of the study and may involve self-selection bias.
4. Extraneous variables were not controlled.
5. The sample size was limited.

4.10.3   SUGGESTIONS FOR FUTURE RESPONSE

Future research should attempt to steer clear of all the restrictions outlined above. Additionally, more research should be done in an Indian environment in order to reduce cultural differences and facilitate easy generalization. Future studies on the effects of Yoga and meditation on "Quality of life" should be undertaken more frequently.

KEYWORDS

- **environmental health**
- *jnana yoga*
- **meditation**
- **Patanjali**
- **psychological well-being**
- **quality of life**
- **social health**
- **t-test**
- **yoga**

REFERENCES

Aljasir, B., Bryson, M., & Al-Shehri, B. (2010). Yoga practice for the management of type II diabetes mellitus in adults: A systematic review. *Evidence-Based Complementary and Alternative Medicine: ECAM, 7*(4), 399–408. https://doi.org/10.1093/ecam/nen027.

Arora, S., & Bhattacharjee, J. (2008). Modulation of immune responses in stress by yoga. *International Journal of Yoga, 1*(2), 45–55. https://doi.org/10.4103/0973-6131.43541.

Bankar, M. A., Chaudhari, S. K., & Chaudhari, K. D. (2013). Impact of long-term yoga practice on sleep quality and quality of life in the elderly. *Journal of Ayurveda and Integrative Medicine, 4*(1), 28–32. https://doi.org/10.4103/0975-9476.109548.

Bharshankar, J. R., Bharshankar, R. N., Deshpande, V. N., Kaore, S. B., & Gosavi, G. B. (2003). Effect of yoga on cardiovascular system in subjects above 40 years. *Indian Journal of Physiology and Pharmacology, 47*(2), 202–206.

Birdee, G. S., Ayala, S. G., & Wallston, K. A. (2017). Cross-sectional analysis of health-related quality of life and elements of yoga practice. *BMC Complementary and Alternative Medicine, 17*(1), 83. https://doi.org/10.1186/s12906-017-1599-1.

Cramer, H., Lauche, R., Langhorst, J., & Dobos, G. (2013). Yoga for rheumatic diseases: A systematic review. *Rheumatology (Oxford, England), 52*(11), 2025–2030. https://doi.org/10.1093/rheumatology/ket264.

Cui, J., Yan, J.-H., Yan, L.-M., Pan, L., Le, J.-J., & Guo, Y.-Z. (2017). Effects of yoga in adults with type 2 diabetes mellitus: A meta-analysis. *Journal of Diabetes Investigation, 8*(2), 201–209. https://doi.org/10.1111/jdi.12548.

Desikachar, K., Bragdon, L., & Bossart, C. (2005). The yoga of healing: Exploring yoga's holistic model for health and well-being. *International Journal of Yoga Therapy, 15*(1), 17–39. https://doi.org/10.17761/ijyt.15.1.p501l33535230737.

Galantino, M. L., Bzdewka, T. M., Eissler-Russo, J. L., Holbrook, M. L., Mogck, E. P., Geigle, P., & Farrar, J. T. (2004). The impact of modified Hatha yoga on chronic low back pain: A pilot study. *Alternative Therapies in Health & Medicine, 10*(2), 56–59.

Garfinkel, M. S., Singhal, A., Katz, W. A., Allan, D. A., Reshetar, R., & Schumacher, H. R., Jr. (1998). Yoga-based intervention for carpal tunnel syndrome: A randomized trial. *JAMA, 280*(18), 1601–1603.

Haaz, S., & Bartlett, S. J. (2011). Yoga for arthritis: A scoping review. *Rheumatic Diseases Clinics of North America, 37*(1), 33–46. https://doi.org/10.1016/j.rdc.2010.11.001.

Hassanpour-Dehkordi, A., & Jivad, N. (2014). Comparison of regular aerobic and yoga on the quality of life in patients with multiple sclerosis. *Medical Journal of the Islamic Republic of Iran, 28*, 141.

Innes, K. E., & Vincent, H. K. (2007). The influence of yoga-based programs on risk profiles in adults with type 2 diabetes mellitus: A systematic review. *Evidence-Based Complementary and Alternative Medicine: ECAM, 4*(4), 469–486. https://doi.org/10.1093/ecam/nel103.

Kizhakkeveettil, A., Whedon, J., Schmalzl, L., & Hurwitz, E. L. (2019). Yoga for quality of life in individuals with chronic disease: A systematic review. *Alternative Therapies in Health and Medicine, 25*(1), 36–43.

Kosuri, M., & Sridhar, G. R. (2009). Yoga practice in diabetes improves physical and psychological outcomes. *Metabolic Syndrome and Related Disorders, 7*(6), 515–517. https://doi.org/10.1089/met.2009.0011.

Lin, K.-Y., Hu, Y.-T., Chang, K.-J., Lin, H.-F., & Tsauo, J.-Y. (2011). Effects of yoga on psychological health, quality of life, and physical health of patients with cancer: A meta-analysis. *Evidence-Based Complementary and Alternative Medicine: ECAM, 2011*, 659876. https://doi.org/10.1155/2011/659876.

Malhotra, V., Singh, S., Tandon, O. P., & Sharma, S. B. (2005). The beneficial effect of yoga in diabetes. *Nepal Medical College Journal: NMCJ, 7*(2), 145–147.

Moonaz, S. H., Bingham, C. O., 3rd, Wissow, L., & Bartlett, S. J. (2015). Yoga in sedentary adults with arthritis: Effects of a randomized controlled pragmatic trial. *The Journal of Rheumatology, 42*(7), 1194–1202. https://doi.org/10.3899/jrheum.141129.

Oken, B. S., Zajdel, D., Kishiyama, S., Flegal, K., Dehen, C., Haas, M., Kraemer, D. F., Lawrence, J., & Leyva, J. (2006). Randomized, controlled, six-month trial of yoga in healthy seniors: Effects on cognition and quality of life. *Alternative Therapies in Health and Medicine, 12*(1), 40–47.

Pal, D. K., Bhalla, A., Bammidi, S., Telles, S., Kohli, A., Kumar, S., Devi, P., Kaur, N., Sharma, K., Kumar, R., Malik, N., Thakur, V., Bhargava, G. G., Goyal, A. K., Devi, G., Chauhan, S., Singh, G., Ahmad, S., Joshi, M., & Anand, A. (2017). Can yoga-based diabetes management studies facilitate integrative medicine in India: Current status and future directions. *Integrative Medicine International, 4*(3–4), 125–141. https://doi.org/10.1159/000479816.

Raveendran, A. V., Deshpandae, A., & Joshi, S. R. (2018). Therapeutic role of yoga in type 2 diabetes. *Endocrinology and Metabolism (Seoul, Korea), 33*(3), 307–317. https://doi.org/10.3803/EnM.2018.33.3.307.

Russell, N., Daniels, B., Smoot, B., & Allen, D. D. (2019). Effects of yoga on quality of life and pain in women with chronic pelvic pain: Systematic review and meta-analysis.

Journal of Women's Health Physical Therapy, 43(3), 144–154. https://doi.org/10.1097/jwh.0000000000000135.

Sahay, B. K. (2007). Role of yoga in diabetes. *The Journal of the Association of Physicians of India, 55,* 121–126.

Skevington, S. M., Lotfy, M., O'Connell, K. A., & WHOQOL Group. (2004). The world health organization's WHOQOL-BREF quality of life assessment: Psychometric properties and results of the international field trial. A report from the WHOQOL group. *Quality of Life Research: An International Journal of Quality-of-Life Aspects of Treatment, Care and Rehabilitation, 13*(2), 299–310. https://doi.org/10.1023/B:QURE.0000018486.91360.00.

Tekur, P., Singphow, C., Nagendra, H. R., & Raghuram, N. (2008). Effect of short-term intensive yoga program on pain, functional disability and spinal flexibility in chronic low back pain: A randomized control study. *Journal of Alternative and Complementary Medicine (New York, N.Y.), 14*(6), 637–644. https://doi.org/10.1089/acm.2007.0815.

Thangasami, S. R., & Chandani, A. L. (2015). Emphasis of yoga in the management of diabetes. *Journal of Diabetes & Metabolism, 6*(10), 1–11. https://doi.org/10.4172/2155-6156.1000613

Tul, Y., Unruh, A., & Dick, B. D. (2011). Yoga for chronic pain management: A qualitative exploration. *Scandinavian Journal of Caring Sciences, 25*(3), 435–443. https://doi.org/10.1111/j.1471-6712.2010.00842.x.

Williams, K. A., Petronis, J., Smith, D., Goodrich, D., Wu, J., & Ravi, N. (2005). Effect of Iyengar yoga therapy for chronic low back pain. *Pain, 115*(1–2), 107–117.

Wolff, M., Sundquist, K., Larsson Lönn, S., & Midlöv, P. (2013). Impact of yoga on blood pressure and quality of life in patients with hypertension: A controlled trial in primary care, matched for systolic blood pressure. *BMC Cardiovascular Disorders, 13*(1), 1–9.

Woodyard, C. (2011). Exploring the therapeutic effects of yoga and its ability to increase quality of life. *International Journal of Yoga, 4*(2), 49–54. https://doi.org/10.4103/0973-6131.85485.

CHAPTER 5

Mental Component Study to Ensure Sustainable Health Through Quality of Life of Participants in Challenging Situations of the 21st Century

ROHIT RASTOGI, TRIBHUVAN MISHRA, VAISHNAVI MISHRA, SARANSH CHAUHAN, ROHAN TYAGI, and UTKARSH PRATAP SHAHI

Department of CSE, ABES Engineering College, Ghaziabad, Uttar Pradesh, India

ABSTRACT

From the ages, the human race is evolving and trying to find the different means to improve the Quality of Life. This was a subjective and vague term earlier but with statistical tools and advancement in process and methodologies of analysis, this is made measurable and quantified. It has been found in research that physical and mental fitness both play an important role to ensure the good human health. Earlier IQ and EQ are leading towards SQ too. The present manuscript is an effort to validate the need of mental component and with standardized study, the encouraging results have been obtained. It has been established with the study over 500 people and using modern NumPy, Matplotlib libraries and SF-36 Questionnaire, the various dimensions have been covered. In 21st century, the health is a global concern and human wellness is being studied with various models. To develop smart cities with smart residents, this study presents a scientific approach for sustainable living.

Yoga and Meditation: Past and Present Evidence. Sachi Nandan Mohanty, Rabindra Kumar Pradhan, & Sugyanta Priyadarshini (Eds.)

> **Motivation:** Lifestyle of people living in the 21st century has totally oriented towards the materialistic world. People are working relentlessly in order to achieve success, but in this phase of working day and night what mostly people forgot is the consequences of this work on their health. Working for 8–10 hours permanently in front of laptop or mobile phone screens by just sitting at one place can lead to many diseases, some of them being weakening of eyesight, headache, diabetes, spinal pain, etc.

To tackle these problems, instead of taking pills and drugs, an ancient Indian practice can be followed which is called Yoga and Meditation. Yoga and Meditation not only maintain our physical health but also prove to be a helpful practice to maintain mental peace and hence improve the factors affecting the quality of life. Depression and mental illness can be very well treated with medications. The increase in various issues regarding physical and mental health motivated the author team to study the scientific effects of Yoga and Meditation on the human body. Thus, the author team contributed towards their fundamental responsibility for society and hence provided the results which have shown the quality of life of the people living in the 21st century.

> **Scope of the Study:** In this study, we will explore how physical and mental exercises, along with Yoga techniques, help improve the quality of life. We will also statistically analyze the quality of life to validate the 21st Century Smart City and urban infrastructure development and lifestyle with a blend of Indian Vedic sciences. Additionally, we aim to understand how physical and mental fitness are negatively impacted and threatened by today's medical treatments and processes. To achieve this, a proper SF-36 Questionnaire was prepared and distributed among 250–300 people to analyze the overall health status of the community. The gathered information was then analyzed using advanced algorithms, focusing on various aspects such as physical functioning, emotional well-being, social functioning, pain, and general health. Our study also references other research conducted by authors in this field. In addition to providing an analysis and study on activities that improve quality of life, our study also encourages readers to explore more dimensions of QoL that may vary.

- ➢ **Topic: Organizations:** The methodology described by the author team involves the use of ML and data sciences. The author team collected the data themselves through the SF-36 questionnaire. The data was then analyzed using Python and machine learning. Further details on the methodology and experimental requirements are discussed.

  In the results and discussion, the important highlights of the analysis are given, and inferences made are discussed. Furthermore, in the most important section of any research paper, the recommendation section, suggestions have been made for specific applications to handle the issues and problems identified in the research. The novelty section gives details about the unique elements in the research. In the conclusion section, the final assessment and concluding remarks have been given.

- ➢ **Ethical Committee and Funding:** The experiment does include human-related experiments, but it is ensured that no ethical constraints are violated. Since the research work is related to the health of humans, the data has been collected by the authors' team, but it is ensured that the study doesn't violate any ethical laws. The research work only works with the data collected through the survey; there were no experiments directly performed on human beings. The study is not financially governed by any external body.

- ➢ **Role of Authors:** Dr. Rohit Rastogi conceptualized the content and structured it. Mr. Tribhuvan analyzed the data and plotted various graphs. Mr. Utkarsh prepared the SF 36 Questionnaire used for the survey and provided input in the analysis. Ms. Vaishnavi researched various types of scales and questionnaires that can aid the analysis, prepare the flow chart, and outline the methodology steps. Mr. Rohan critically analyzed the writings, made necessary changes, and did the editing. Mr. Saransh worked on the referencing, and Mr. Utkarsh did the image editing, both contributing to the data collection by distributing the form among people and recording their responses.

5.1 INTRODUCTION

Modern lifestyle has led to a poor standard of living and has badly affected the essence of human life. The lifestyle of the 21st century is the cause of many diseases, both physical and mental, and it is high time that we started thinking about ways to improve our way of living. There are many ways to do so, and Yoga is one of them. We can also use technologies like AI and ML to analyze and improve lifestyle; for example, various sensors can be used to analyze Yoga poses and correct the wrong posture. Besides Yoga, meditation can also increase the quality of life and is especially effective in mental well-being.

5.2   WORLD HEALTH INDEX AND THE SITUATION IN INDIA

In 2021, the USA ranked first in the Global Health Index with a health index score of 75.9, followed by Australia and Finland. India's rank is 66 with a health index score of 42.8. If we compare India's index score in 2021 with that of 2019, it has reduced by 0.8. Therefore, India needs to invest more in health services to meet the future health demands (Evolution and Importance of the GHS index, article on ghsindex.org); (Health index of countries worldwide by health index score, article on statista.com).

The structure of Global Health Index. The 6 categories present the indicators, sub-indicators, questions in GHS index for overall scores.

5.3   YOGA AND MEDITATION: A BOON FROM INDIAN RISHI-MUNI TO WORLD

Yoga is the gift of Indian Rishi-Muni to the world. Yoga mainly originated from the Northern part of India around 3000 BC. Yoga keeps everyone healthy and physically fit. Meditation refers to the process of recognizing the inner soul and silently watching one's own mind. Meditation keeps us stress-free and helps in controlling one's emotions and activities. Life without meditation is just like a body without a soul.

Also, Yoga and Meditation help in reducing depression, anxiety, and stress. Various health clubs and organizations have started including Yoga and meditation in their therapies for curing various diseases, and many people only go there for Yoga and Meditation (Naragatti et al., 2020; Rastogi et al., 2022; Sagar et al., 2021).

The *Chakras* which refer to the energy centers in the body. There are mainly seven chakras in the body named as *Muladhara, Svadishthana, Manipura, Anahata, Vishuddhi, Ajna,* and *Sahasrara.*

5.4   MEDITATIVE TECHNIQUES AND THEIR BENEFITS

Meditation helps in keeping the mind calm and cool. Various methods of meditation such as transcendental meditation, mantra meditation, etc. Some of the meditation techniques are described as follows: Transcendental meditation introduced by Maharishi Mahesh focuses on reaching a state from where the thoughts are originating. It improves creative intelligence and consciousness of mind. *Vipassana* Meditation technique was given by Gautama Buddha. *Vipassana* means to observe things in their true states or special states. This technique helps in improving awareness of mind. Mindfulness meditation technique focuses on the movement of breath while we inhale and exhale. It helps in relaxing from the state of depression. *Mantra* Meditation is a meditation in which a person chants a mantra and tries to reach toward the inner soul. In this technique, generally, the word 'OM' is used for chanting. All these meditation techniques help in improving psychological, physical, and spiritual levels of human beings (Pathath, 2017; Rastogi et al., 2021).

Different emotional benefits of meditation such as increased happiness and optimism, reduced stress and anxiety, and increased resilience in hard times.

5.5   NEED OF SCIENTIFIC STUDIES IN BENEFICIAL EFFECTS OF YOGA AND MEDITATION

Yoga and Meditation are not newly invented scientific processes. They are practices of ancient India, and the word Yoga originates from the Sanskrit word "YOG," which means union of physical, mental, and spiritual domains in order to maintain the balance of all three in the body, to have control over the human mind, and to live a healthy life. Nowadays, people often treat Yoga as a set of physical exercises only, necessary for maintaining physical health. This highlights the need for scientific studies on Yoga and Meditation, so that the actual benefits can be examined and proven through relevant research results (Rastogi et al., 2022).

Studying the scientific aspects of Yoga and Meditation is important because it directly impacts the body of the most complex creature in the universe, the human being. Various research results have shown that Yoga and Meditation are not only important for physical health but also play a crucial role in maintaining mental peace. Therefore, having knowledge of the scientific aspects and beneficial effects of all the *Asanas* and *Mudras* of Yoga and Meditation is important, so that people follow the process correctly and do not view it as a mere ancient practice (Scientific research on Yoga, article from Yogaalliance.org; Rastogi et al., 2019).

Figure 5.4 describes the scientific relation of Yoga on physical health and mental health of the human body. It also shows that Yoga unites understanding and coordination of functions of the mind and also works upon inner wisdom of the person. The impact of Yoga can be seen as a form of outer actions of the person. The two pillars of yoga are self-discipline and self-realization.

5.6 CALM, COOL, AND HEALTHY PEOPLE WILL BE REQUIRED IN 21ST CENTURY SMART CITIES 4.0 TO DEVELOP INDUSTRY 5.0

It is a need of time to have calm, cool, and healthy people to work for the development of smart cities and industries keeping the needs of the environment in mind. This is only the human who exploited earth so badly, so if we could not get people with a good and healthy mindset then this exploitation will continue. Yoga and meditation are a great way to connect with oneself and to connect with nature (as per Figure 5.5) (Rastogi et al., 2022).

Meditation helps in releasing stress and eases tension. People regularly doing Yoga and meditation are found to be more relaxed and efficient in workplaces. Calm and Cool people have the ability to make decisions which are beneficial for themselves as well as for others and surroundings (Grabowska et al., 2022; Rastogi et al., 2022).

Development and environment can move hand in hand. The plants present outside the houses keep the environment clean and healthy and normalize Air Quality Index (AQI).

5.7 LITERATURE REVIEW

Here, the author team read some research made in the related areas and provided a brief description of the data, methodology, results, and conclusion. The author team also compiled the insights gained in a tabular form in order to make it easy for readers to get the gist of reviews.

Cohen et al., explained depression as a simple yet most misunderstood disorder. Unlike an illness, depression doesn't affect any specific part of the body, but it stays in the person as a state which, if persists, becomes more of a habit through the circadian rhythm. We start shaping our behavior according to the disorder rather than what separates us from it. Our mind is very easy to get habituated to something, and the habituation is what separates normal depression from severe. Consider it like an addiction; you're suffering while taking the substance, but you'll also suffer when the substance is not present. So is our mind; if a habit is taken away from someone, we start seeking the activity again as the mind starts feeling empty. In most cases of depression, there's a trigger in the world that surrounds us that reminds us of a repressed memory or an action. There are also instances where depression can be self-inflicted to hide something bigger. Identifying the trigger plays a massive role in managing depression. The false hope of thinking we can treat something that doesn't have a physical attribute is what makes patients more agitated through the phase of treatment.

The best way of managing depression is therapy, which can only be conducted by a trained psychologist. Another way is through understanding projection and building your self-esteem. There are aspects of life that we want to be true, and then there's the absolute truth. We mostly get depressed because the aspects of the truth we seek, and the absolute truth don't align. We try so hard to shape it to our liking that we start deforming our self-worth, and we do it on a daily basis. If we start identifying when we're doing it, it stops automatically. We can start doing this by questioning the things that aren't going our way and questioning our wishes. Are our wishes the things we need, or are they something we want to fulfill our un-needing desire? An example would be trying to understand what a person is thinking at the moment. There's no actual way of knowing. When there's no way of knowing the truth, our brain starts creating lies that we state as truth. And then when things don't align, we get depressed. Start by questioning your decisions and then understand what might have made you make those decisions. Write them down and work on things that you actually want and need, rather than working on what you might need to fix about yourself. Trying to fix something that doesn't have a physical being only molds you into a fault. Shape yourself to your own will, not the will of your desires.

Another simple thing is thinking about how to drive it away constantly. It's a thought. The more you're trying to get rid of the thought, the more you're thinking of it, and the more persistent it gets. Mindfulness over Forcefulness, a way of understanding what makes depression (Shahidi J. Construct validity of the quality of life in life-threatening illness patient questionnaire (QOLLTI-P) in cancer patients (McGill University, 2010; Cohen et al., 2019).

Connell et al., performed research to find the parameters for the quality of life of people suffering from mental health problems. The researchers noticed that common preference-based quality of life measures are being used for each group of people. However, it was observed that the definition of quality of life for a person with a mental health problem cannot be similar to that of a person living a normal life. Therefore, the research team stated that there must be different quality of life measures for people suffering from mental health issues. To obtain quality of life measures, the team qualitatively interviewed 19 individuals who were recruited from UK mental health services and were experiencing various mental health issues with different levels of severity. In the research, the researchers identified seven measures that were found to be important for mental health problems. The identified seven measures include: self-perception, hope and hopelessness, relationships and a sense of belonging, well-being and ill-being, physical health, autonomy, and activity. The researchers' team claimed that these measures were consistent, and they showed differing emphasis on the quality of life of the person depending upon the severity of mental health issues. It is mentioned in the study that they interviewed only 19 people, due to which it may be possible that various other disorders were not included and also research did not include any woman having psychosis disorder, which may give some other domains for quality of life, so these were some of the limitations of the study. The author team claimed that the domains they found through their research are the fundamentals for the development of quality-of-life measures addressing the life of a person having mental health issues in the future (Connell et al., 2014).

Huang et al. in their paper "Development and Validation of Parameters of QoL Standards for Elementary School Students" discuss working on the quantitative and qualitative aspects of research that can validate the Quality of Life (QoL) Scale for children in Taiwan. They collected data from 711 students in the fifth and sixth grades. The data was collected from students aged 10–12 years from 14 different schools. According to the World Health Organization, students should be physically, mentally, and emotionally strong. The WHO also defines QoL as an individual's perception with respect to culture, values, relationships, goals, etc. The authors mention that the scale is based on six factors, including environmental life, learning ability, family function, school function, peer relationships, and vitality of life. Pearson's correlation coefficient, LISREL 8.8 software, EFA, item analysis, and descriptive analysis were used on the collected data. The results showed a 44% variation in the factors mentioned above. A satisfactory outcome was achieved using the Elementary School Quality of Life (ESQoL) instrument, which could help in understanding the factors responsible for the emotional well-being of students (Huang et al., 2017).

Haraldstad et al. described in their paper the importance of quality of life in the field of health and medicine, that is, Health-related quality of life (HRQOL). Quality of life can be used to identify the number of problems that can affect patients. QOL is important for improving health-related factors such as care, symptom relief, and making patients fit for habitation. The authors also stated that there is a lack of conceptual clarity about the meaning and evaluation of QoL parameters, which may further be a danger to the validity of QOL research.

The authors have dealt with depression for a while and there are a multitude of things they have learned, but the most important one is "trying to run away from something that's attached to you rather than something that's following you only tires you, and when you're tired, the power of depression increases. It's not a body part you can cut off; you're rather your own depression, and you have to be your own cure. Understanding it is what drives it away, not trying to force it away" (Haraldstad et al., 2019).

Davenport et al. in their studies discuss the use and applications of Artificial Intelligence in the field of health. The author team also discusses the impact of AI on the healthcare workforce and ethical issues related to Artificial Intelligence in this field. Artificial Intelligence (AI) has great potential in the automation of healthcare, but there are still some barriers that restrict its speedy implementation in all dimensions of healthcare. Artificial Intelligence consists of several technologies. The technologies useful in this field include Natural Language Processing (NLP), Rule-based expert systems, Physical robots, Machine learning-neural networks and deep learning, and Robotic process automation. These technologies are integrated together when designing a system related to healthcare. Artificial intelligence is used in Diagnosis and treatment applications. There are AI-based systems that help in the identification of diseases and also suggest their treatment. Patient engagement and adherence application is one of the issues where there is a need for an AI-based system that can alert and notify the patient to follow the health schedule prepared by the doctor for better health. AI has administrative applications through the use of chatbots that can interact with patients and can be used in dealing with payment, health insurance, etc. There is immense potential for AI in the field of health in the future (Davenport et al., 2019).

5.8 METHODOLOGY AND SETUP OF EXPERIMENT

This experiment was done by the author's team in order to examine the quality of life of the persons living around in the cities. A series of steps has been followed in order to obtain conclusive results. The following flow-chart shows the methodology used by the author team (as per Figure 5.1).

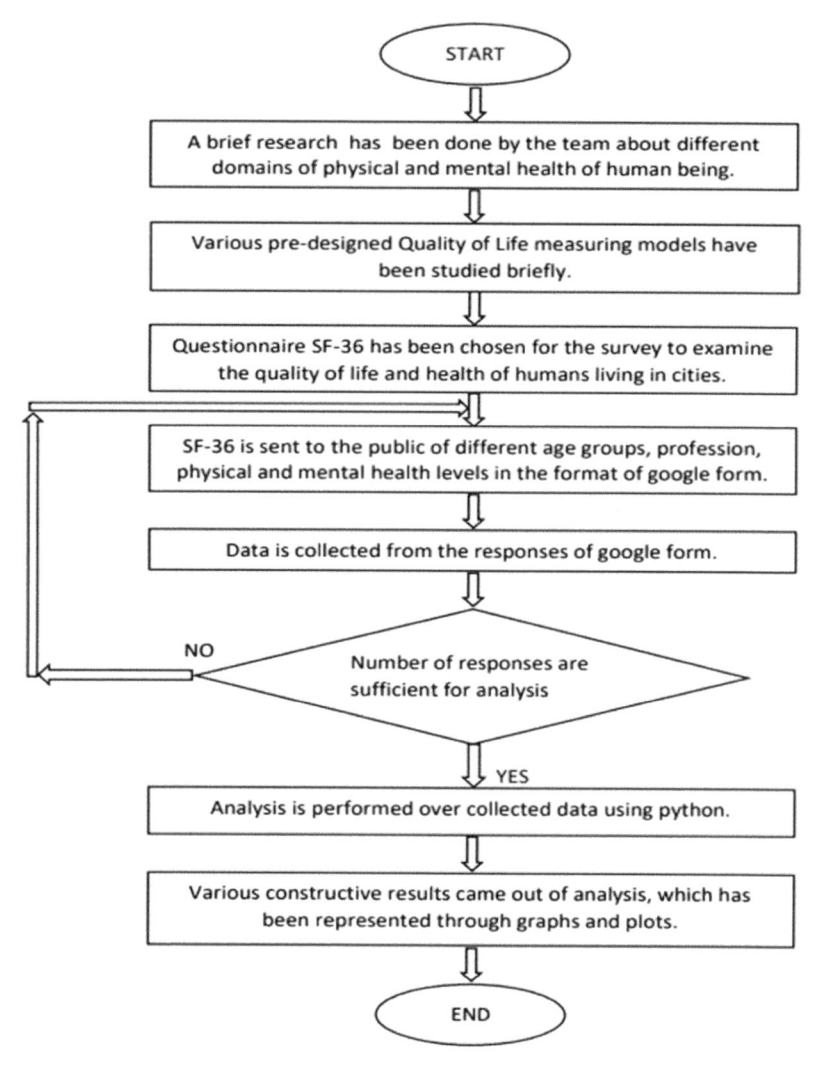

FIGURE 5.1   Flow chart of proposed experiment.

5.8.1   SF-36 QUESTIONNAIRE IN OR PROPOSED APPROACH

Short Form-36 (SF-36) was standardized in 1990. It is a health status profile designed to measure the health status of people. It contains 36 questions. This scale has been found reliable and valid for measuring the quality of life of individuals suffering from chronic health conditions. This scale has been used for several decades to measure quality of life. It can be applied to any age group regardless of age. The score in SF-36 ranges from 0 to 100, with 100 being the highest. The higher the score, the better the health status (SF-36 Questionnaire); (Rastogi et al., 2018).

5.8.2   SETUP AND FLOW CHART

The analysis is performed by the research team on the collected data by following some crucial steps represented in the flow chart below (as shown in Figure 5.2).

5.9   RESULTS AND DISCUSSIONS

The implementation work has been shown in subsequent steps.

5.9.1   RESULTS OF MCS CALCULATIONS

Figure 5.8 pie chart represents the male and female ratio of people who took the survey. From Figure 5.3, it is seen that number of females is more than males (as per Figure 5.3).

Figure 5.4 pie chart represents the age of people who took the survey. From Figure 5.4, it is seen that nearly half of the population is adults and rest is teenagers and seniors.

Figure 5.5 pie chart represents the occupation of people who took the survey. From Figure 5.5, it is seen that there is an equal number of students, people who have jobs, business owners, and those who are unemployed.

Figure 5.6 pie chart represents the occupation of people who took the survey. From Figure 5.6, it is seen that there is equal number of people who did graduation, post-graduation, intermediate, and research.

Figure 5.7 bar graph represents the number of males and females with different professions who have less vitality, i.e., a vitality score of less than 60. It is observed that the maximum number of people with less vitality are in the job category. People with other occupations are fewer in number. In

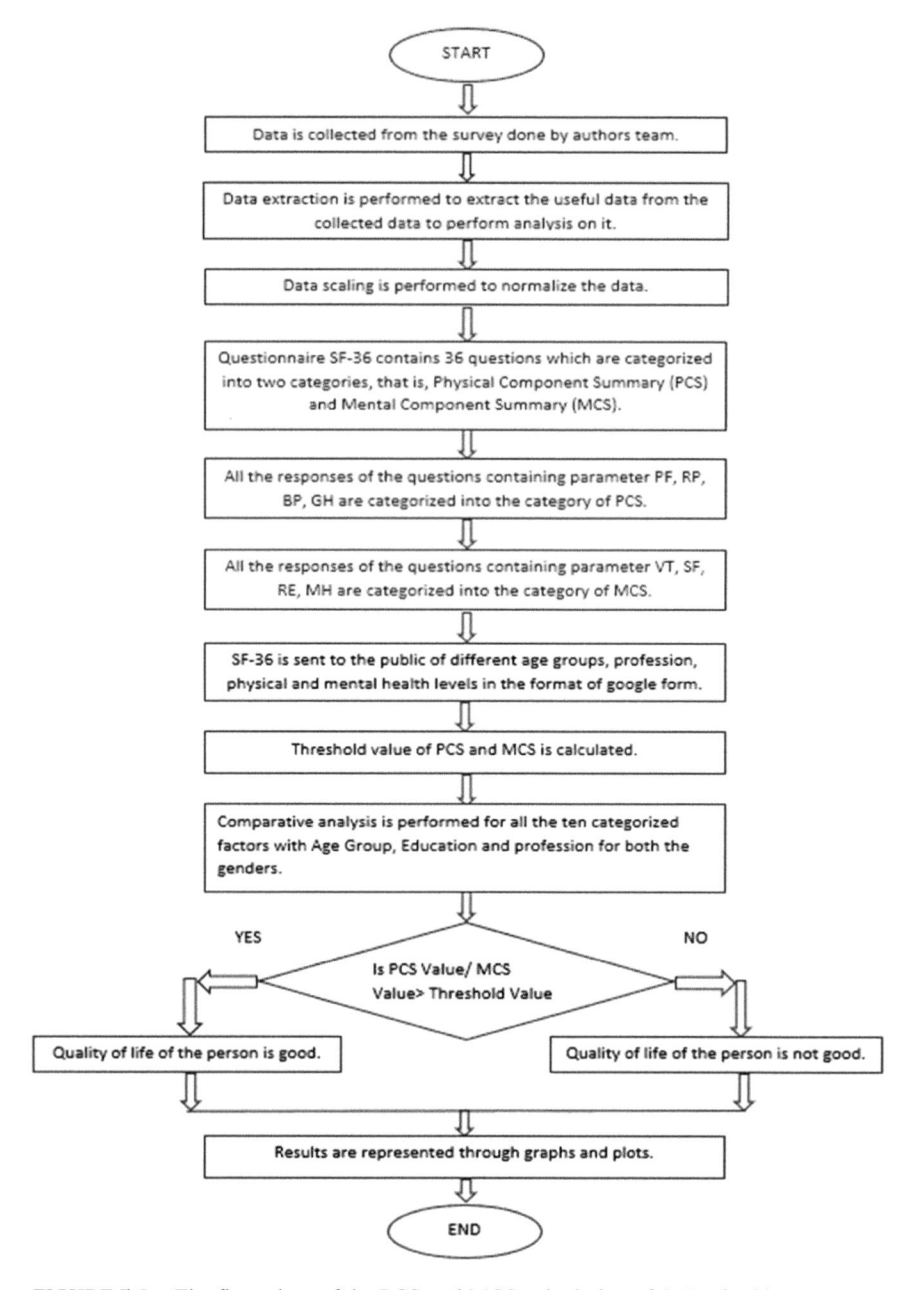

FIGURE 5.2 The flow-chart of the PCS and MCS calculation of QoL of subjects.

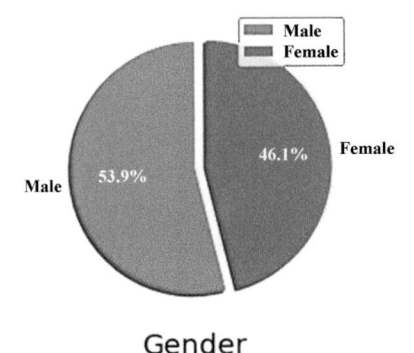

FIGURE 5.3 Visualization of gender.

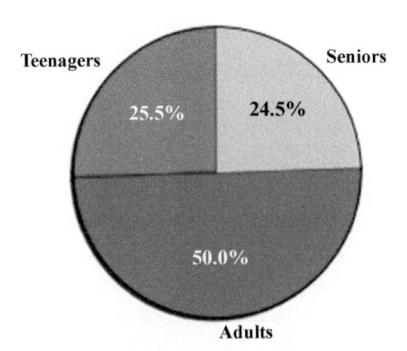

FIGURE 5.4 Visualization of age categories.

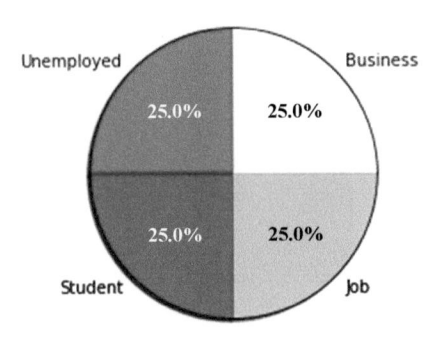

FIGURE 5.5 Visualization of occupation.

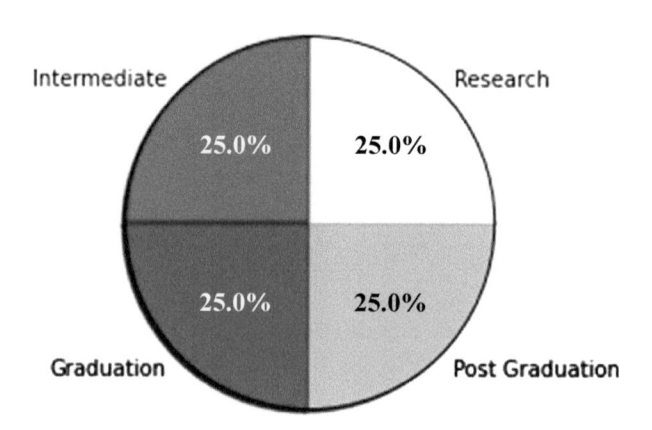

FIGURE 5.6   Visualization of education.

every profession, it can be seen that females are fewer in number except in the student category where they are more numerous (as per Figure 5.12).

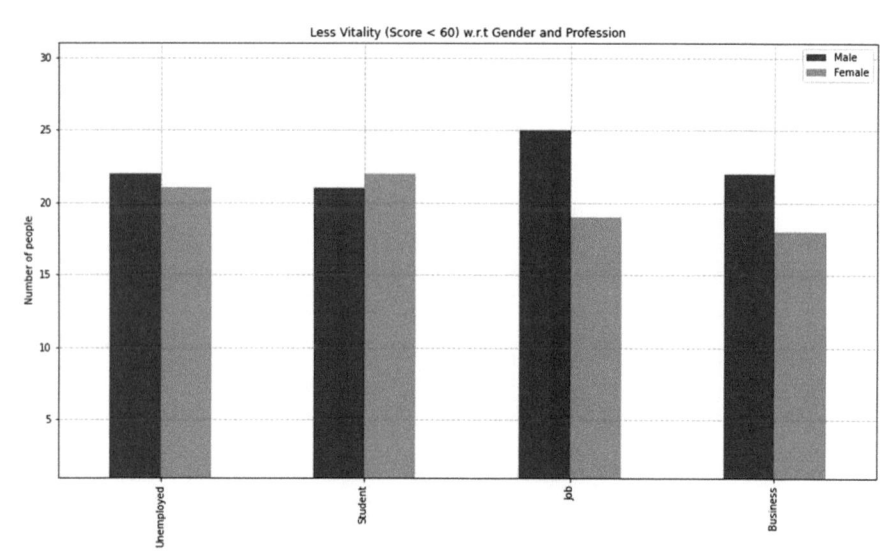

FIGURE 5.7   Visualization of number of people with less vitality w.r.t gender and profession.

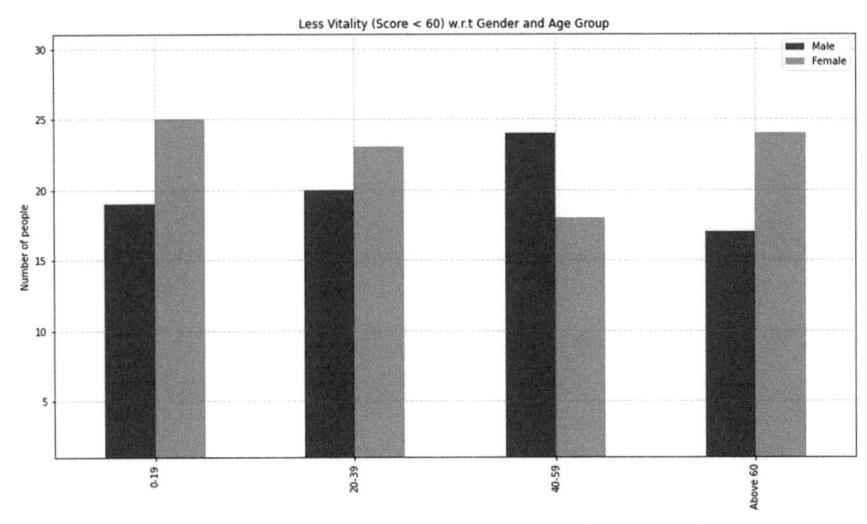

FIGURE 5.8 Visualization of number of people with less vitality w.r.t gender and age group.

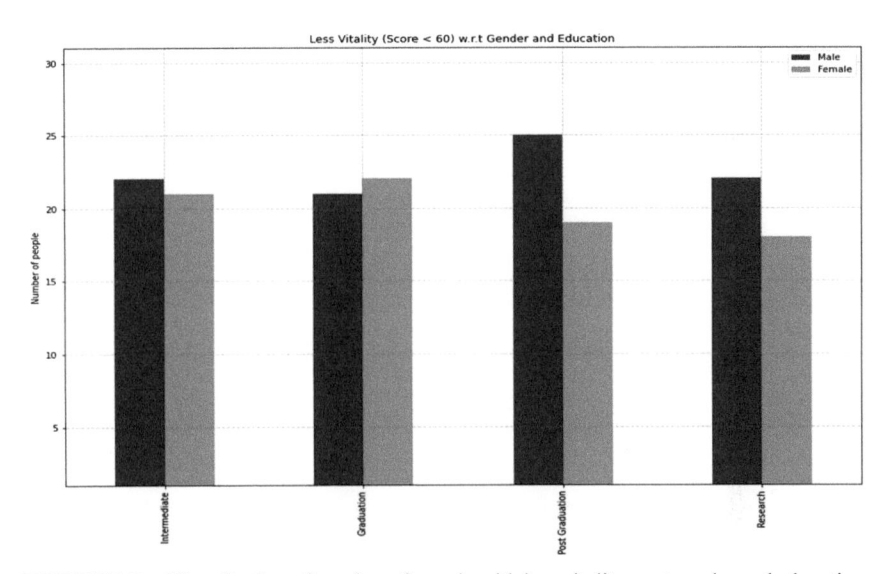

FIGURE 5.9 Visualization of number of people with less vitality w.r.t gender and education.

Figure 5.8 bar graph represents the number of males and females in different age groups who have low vitality, meaning a vitality score of less than 60. It can be observed that in every age group except for 40–59 years, the number of females with low vitality exceeds the number of males. In the age group 40–59 years, the number of males is greater than the number of females (as shown in Figure 5.8).

Figure 5.9 bar graph represents the number of males and females with different educational backgrounds who have less vitality, i.e., a vitality score of less than 60. It can be seen that the number of males is greater than the number of females in every educational background except for graduation. In graduation, the number of females is greater than males (as per Figure 5.9).

Figure 5.10 bar graph represents the number of males and females with different professions who have declined social functioning, i.e., a social functioning score of less than 60. It is observed that the maximum number of people with declined social functioning are in the student category. People with other occupations are fewer in number. In every profession, it can be seen that females are fewer in number except in the student category where they outnumber males (as per Figure 5.10).

Figure 5.11 bar graph represents the number of males and females in different age groups who have declined social functioning, i.e., a social functioning score of less than 60. It can be seen that in teenagers and people above 60, the number of females is greater than males. In the age group of 20–60 years, the number of males is greater than the number of females (as per Figure 5.11).

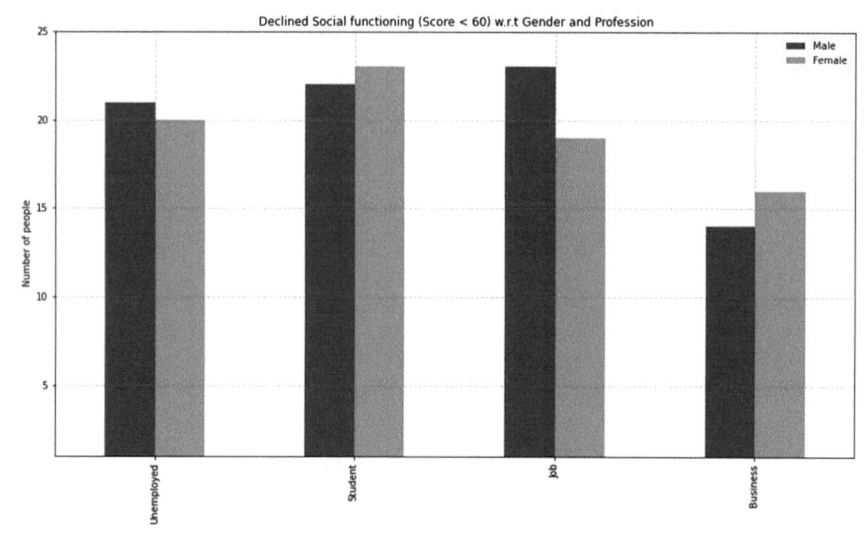

FIGURE 5.10　Visualization of number of people with declined social functioning w.r.t gender and profession.

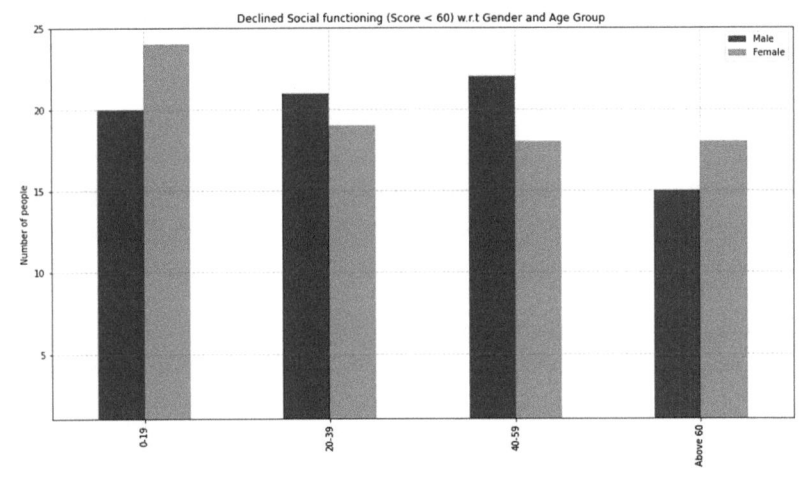

FIGURE 5.11   Visualization of number of people with declined social functioning w.r.t gender and age group.

Figure 5.12 bar graph represents the number of males and females with different educational backgrounds who have declined social functioning, i.e., a social functioning score of less than 60. It can be seen that the number of females is greater than the number of males in every educational background except post-graduation. In post-graduation, the number of males is greater than females (as per Figure 5.12).

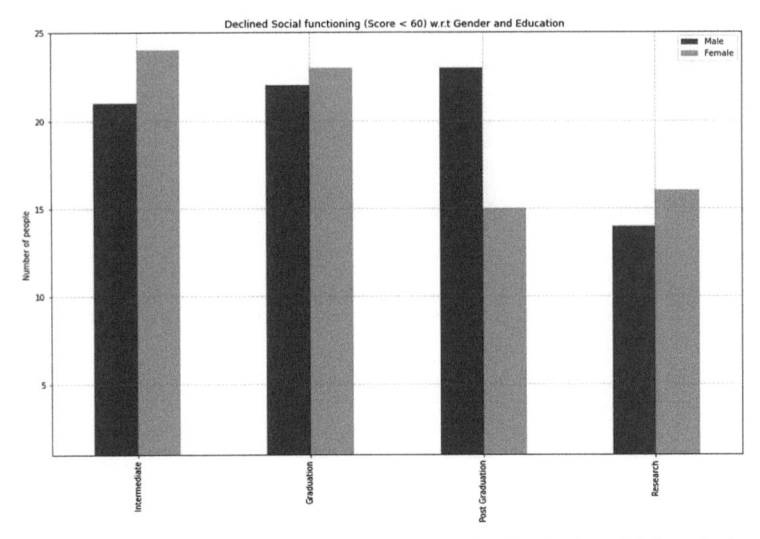

FIGURE 5.12   Visualization of number of people with declined social functioning w.r.t gender and education.

Figure 5.13 bar graph represents the number of males and females with different professions who are experiencing role limitations due to emotional health, i.e., role limitation due to emotional health score is less than 60. It is observed that the maximum number of people who have role limitations due to emotional health are employed. People with other occupations are fewer in number. In every profession, other than the unemployed category, it can be seen that females are fewer in number, except in the unemployed category where they are more numerous (as per Figure 5.13).

Figure 5.14 bar graph represents the number of males and females in different age groups who are experiencing role limitations due to emotional health, i.e., a role limitation due to emotional health score of less than 60. It can be observed that in teenagers and in people above 60 years, the number of females is greater than males. In the age group of 20–39 years, the number of females is equal to the number of males. In the age group of 40–59 years, the number of males is greater than the number of females (as per Figure 5.14).

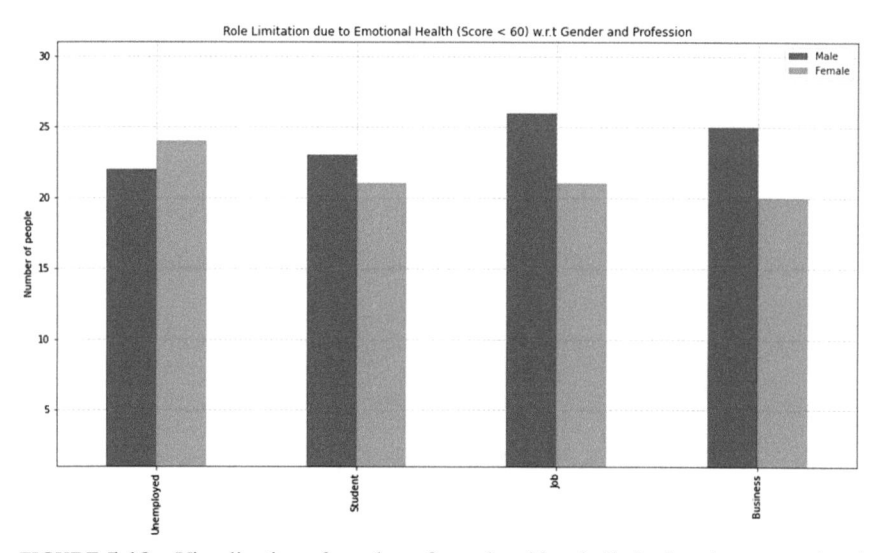

FIGURE 5.13   Visualization of number of people with role limitation due to emotional health w.r.t gender and profession.

Figure 5.15 bar graph represents the number of males and females with different educational backgrounds who are experiencing role limitations due to emotional health, i.e., role limitation due to emotional health score is less than 60. It can be seen that the number of males is greater than the

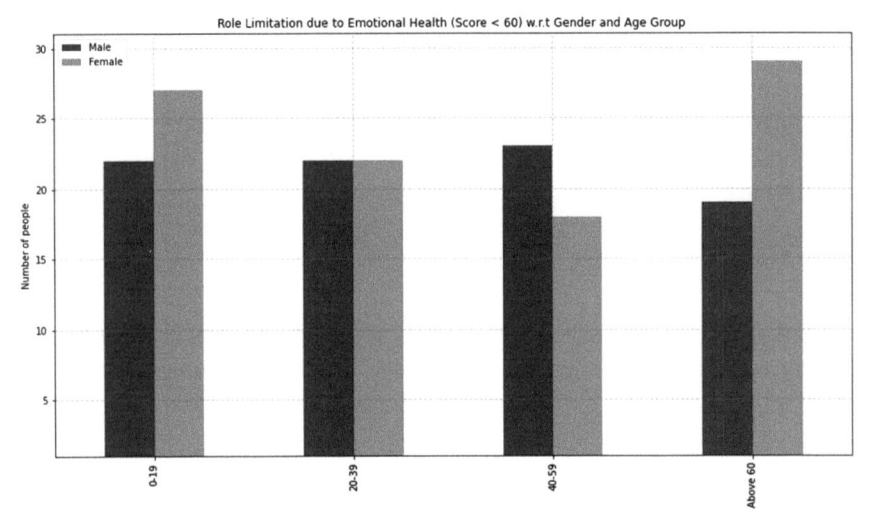

FIGURE 5.14 Visualization of number of people with role limitation due to emotional health w.r.t gender and age group.

number of females in every educational background except intermediate. In intermediate, the number of females is greater than the number of males (as per Figure 5.15).

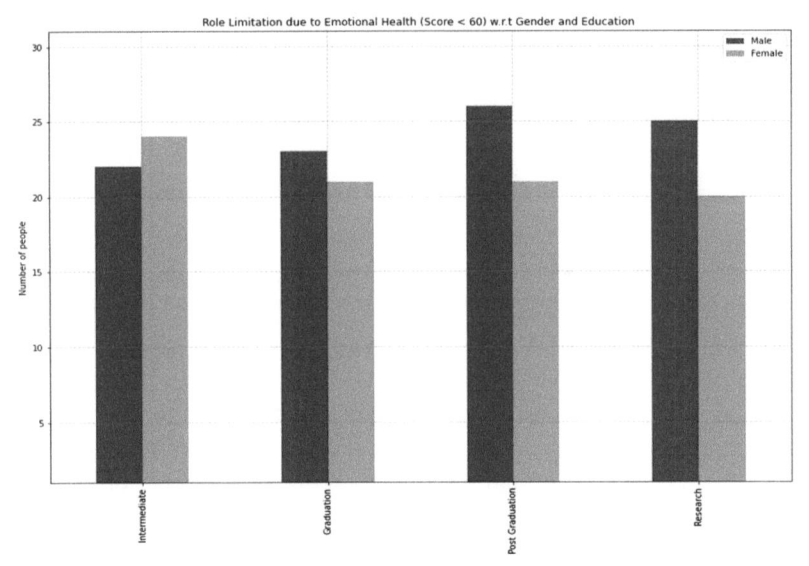

FIGURE 5.15 Visualization of number of people with role limitation due to emotional health w.r.t gender and education.

Figure 5.16 bar graph represents the number of males and females with different professions who have declined emotional well-being, i.e., an emotional well-being score of less than 60. It can be seen that in every profession, other than the unemployed category, the number of males with declined emotional well-being is higher compared to females. In the unemployed category, the number of males and females is higher (as per Figure 5.16).

Figure 5.17 bar graph represents the number of males and females in different age groups who have declined emotional well-being, i.e., an emotional well-being score of less than 60. It can be observed that in every age group, except for the 40–59 age group, the number of males is greater than the number of females. In the 40–59 age group, the number of females is greater than the number of males. The behavior of teenagers and senior citizens is almost similar (as per Figure 5.17).

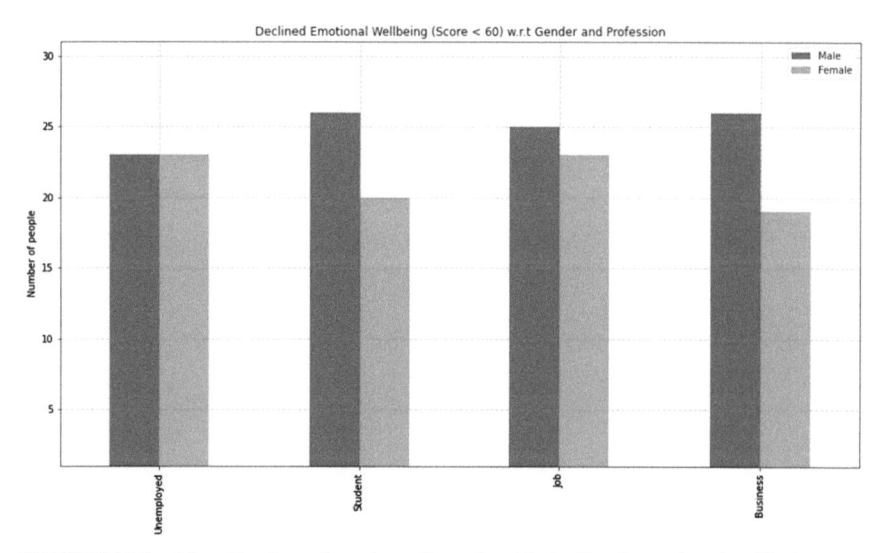

FIGURE 5.16   Visualization of number of people with declined emotional wellbeing w.r.t gender and profession.

Figure 5.18 bar graph represents the number of males and females with different educational backgrounds who have declined emotional well-being, i.e., an emotional well-being score of less than 60. It can be seen that the number of males is greater than the number of females in every educational background except for intermediate. In intermediate, the number of females is equal to males (as per Figure 5.18).

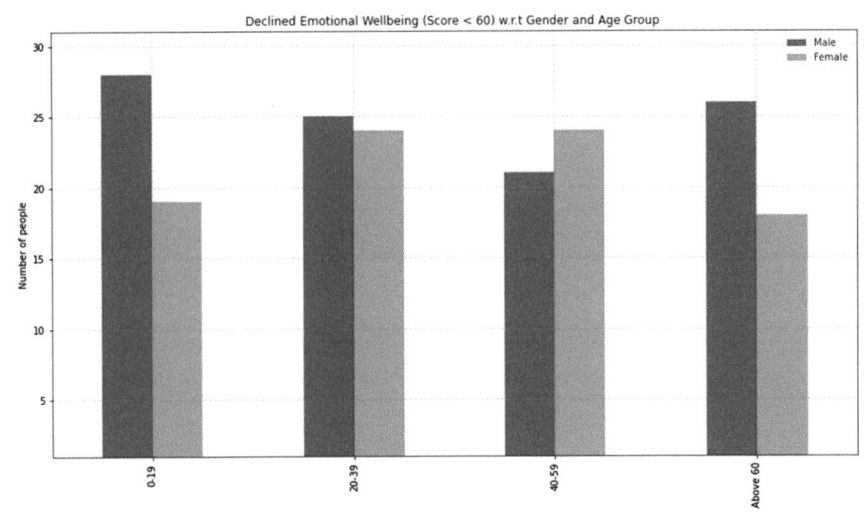

FIGURE 5.17 Visualization of number of people with declined emotional wellbeing w.r.t gender and age group.

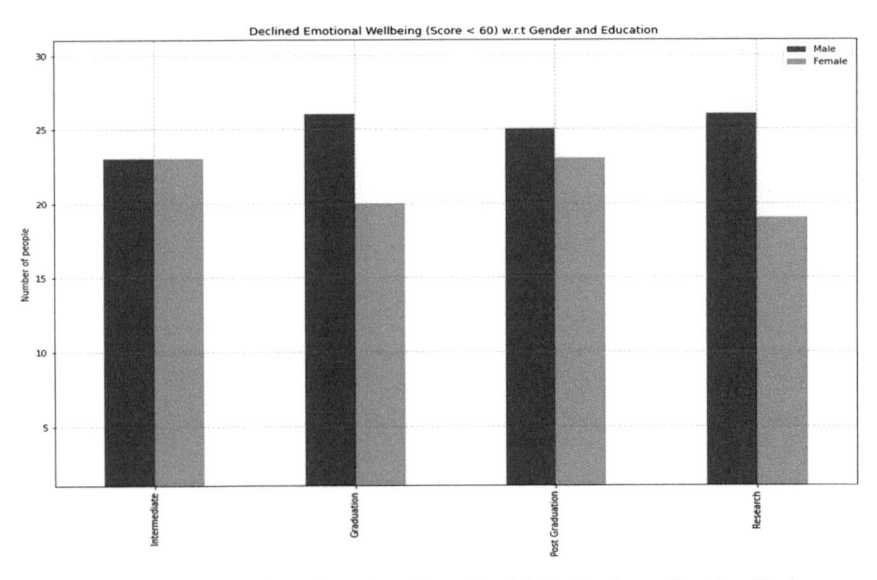

FIGURE 5.18 Visualization of number of people with declined emotional wellbeing w.r.t gender and education.

Figure 5.19 bar graph represents the number of males and females with different professions who have a low MCS value, i.e., MCS value score is less than 60. It is seen that in the job and business category, the number of females with a low MCS value is higher compared to males, whereas in the unemployed and student categories, the number of females and males are equal (as per Figure 5.19).

Figure 5.20 bar graph represents the number of males and females in different age groups who have declined general health, i.e., a general health score of less than 60. It can be seen that the number of females in the age groups above 60 and 0–19 years is much higher compared to the number of males in the same categories. In the age group 20–39 years, the number of males and females is equal. The number of males is higher in only one age group, i.e., 40–59 years (as per Figure 5.20).

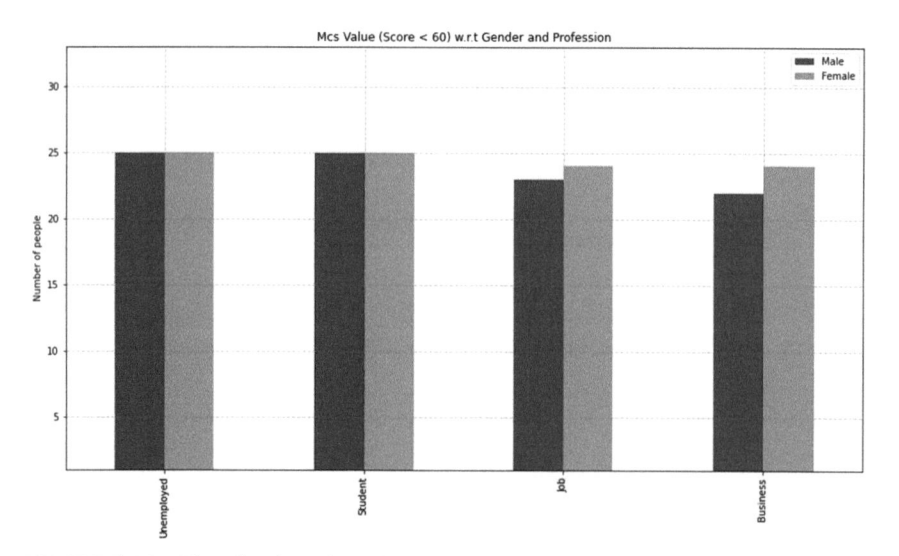

FIGURE 5.19 Visualization of number of people with less MCS value w.r.t gender and profession.

Figure 5.21 bar graph represents the number of males and females with different educational backgrounds who have a lower MCS value, i.e., MCS value score is less than 60. It can be seen that the number of females is greater than the number of males in every educational background except in intermediate. In intermediate, the number of males and females is equal (as per Figure 5.21).

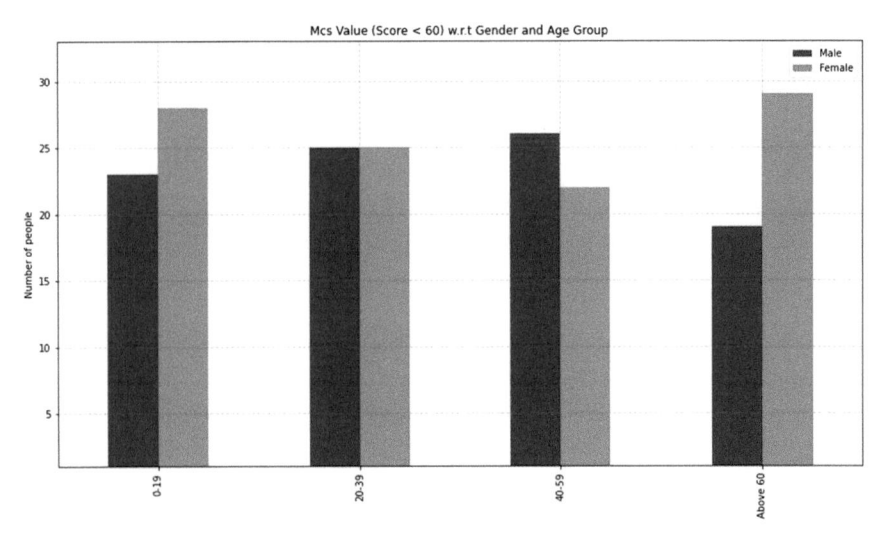

FIGURE 5.20   Visualization of number of people with less MCS value w.r.t gender and age group.

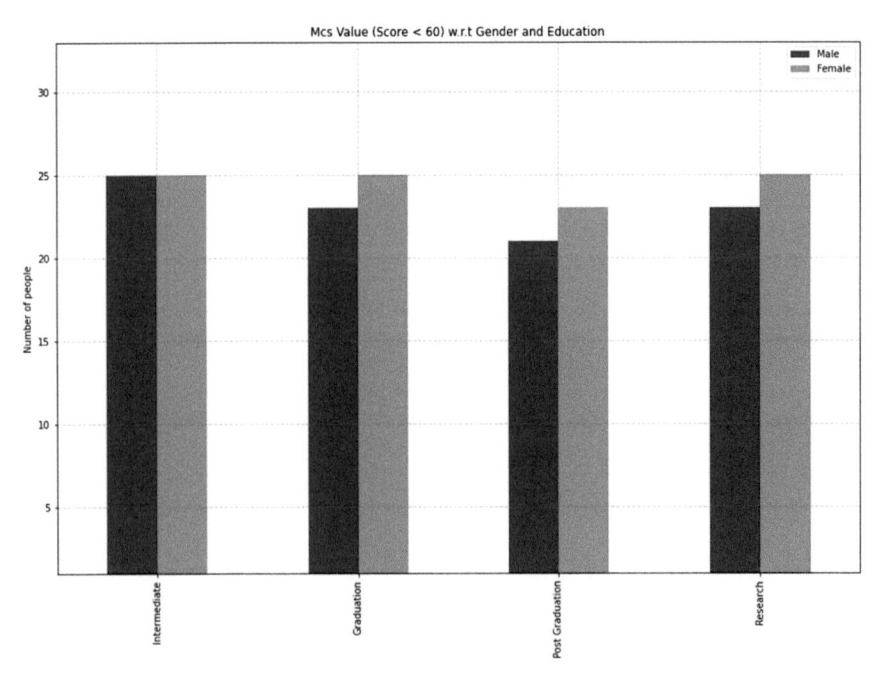

FIGURE 5.21   Visualization of number of people with less MCS value w.r.t gender and education.

Figure 5.22 chart shows the value of mean, median, and mode of various parameters which were taken into consideration for analyzing data and drawing conclusions. Cronbach's Alpha value is also calculated, and the negative score of Cronbach's Alpha is due to the recoding of scores in parameters. While recoding, the author team has taken high scores to denote positive results; for example, 5 is recoded to 100. Therefore, the negative value of Cronbach's Alpha actually denotes positive results. For the originality of results, the author team did not alter the negative scores (as per Figure 5.22).

	PhysicalFunctions	PhyHealthLim	EmoProbLim	Energy/fatigue	Emotionalwellbeing	Socialfunctioning	Pain	Generalhealth	pcsvalue	mcsvalue
count	204.000000	204.000000	204.000000	204.000000	204.000000	204.000000	204.000000	204.000000	204.000000	204.000000
mean	31.470588	35.600490	35.375817	50.214461	47.328431	48.161765	69.252451	52.941176	47.316176	45.270118
std	26.064417	20.757462	23.305645	10.275977	8.500651	14.722082	23.537754	10.489332	9.370674	8.168269
min	0.000000	0.000000	0.000000	12.500000	25.000000	0.000000	0.000000	20.000000	25.000000	22.500000
25%	5.000000	25.000000	22.916667	43.750000	40.000000	37.500000	55.000000	45.000000	40.000000	39.973958
50%	30.000000	37.500000	33.333333	50.000000	45.000000	50.000000	68.750000	50.000000	46.875000	44.583333
75%	50.000000	50.000000	50.000000	56.250000	55.000000	50.000000	90.000000	60.000000	52.578125	50.000000
max	100.000000	100.000000	100.000000	81.250000	90.000000	87.500000	100.000000	85.000000	78.750000	79.062500
alpha	0.910049	0.728900	0.793000	-0.570000	-0.940000	-1.225330	0.720000	-0.140000	-0.350000	0.160000

FIGURE 5.22   Chart showing reliability, central tendency, and variability of scales.

5.9.2 *DISCUSSIONS ON MCS*

From the results obtained from the data, we can clearly see that irrespective of their age group, educational background, and profession, approximately the same number of people have a lower MCS (Mental Component Summary) value. If we focus on profession, we can see that there are the same number of males and females in each category (i.e., Unemployed, Student, Job, and Business) who have a lower MCS score, and that the number of males and females is small when compared to the Education and age group category. In both the education and age groups categories, there are more males and fewer females.

The results clearly show that males are living a more dissatisfied life and do not have sound mental health. There may be various factors responsible for this, like in the case of age group males between the ages of 0–19 years and above 60 years being very large in number, and there is also a significant difference between the number of males and females in terms of a lower MCS score. This may be because of more stress at home and improper living conditions. In terms of profession, we can see that there are comparatively fewer males and females with respect to other divisions.

5.10 NOVELTIES

- This research document analyzes various techniques that can be used to improve the QoL.
- The author team has used MCS (Mental Component Summary) values and plotted various graphs taking these two values into consideration and found that people with higher values of these have better QOL.
- The author team has also studied the application of AI and ML in improving quality of life.

5.11 RECOMMENDATIONS

1. One should include Yoga in daily practice as it helps in improving mental health.
2. One should encourage family members, society members and every other known person for performing exercise and Yoga daily to ensure a healthy living.
3. One should find time in a day to follow one's passion for ensuring peace of mind (Rastogi et al., 2021).

5.12 FUTURE RESEARCH DIRECTIONS AND LIMITATIONS

5.12.1 *LIMITATIONS*

- Algorithm used for analysis may be less efficient.
- Time duration of study is less.

5.12.2 *FUTURE DIRECTIONS*

- The next research should be conducted for a longer duration with more data sets.
- The experiment should be made constant using a controlled environment method and other uncontrollable factors should be also taken into consideration during the experiment.

5.13   CONCLUSION

The above studies show that the quality of life is greatly influenced by physical activities. The results obtained show that people engaging in physical activities are happier, more active, and live a healthy life. Living in a healthy, fresh, and unpolluted environment makes a person physically, mentally, and socially well-being. Additionally, it has been observed that people with more involvement in physical activities (sports, Yoga, and meditation) are more satisfied with the quality of life they live. Some methods suggested by the author team for remaining physically and mentally active are Yoga and meditation. Yoga and meditation not only help us keep our bodies fit but also rejuvenate the heart and soul. Sports activities are also a good and engaging way to keep oneself healthy.

This chapter critically analyzes all 36 items of the SF-36 questionnaire and averages them to form 8 scales. From these 8 scales, two summaries, namely PCS (Physical Component Summary) and MCS (Mental Component Summary), are made by averaging 4 scales out of 8 for each of these two component summaries. It then analyzes all 8 scales and 2 component summaries with respect to gender, age group, occupation, and profession, and gives out meaningful results about the quality of life of people involved in various occupations, from different educational backgrounds, or from different age groups according to gender.

KEYWORDS

- **data sciences**
- **holistic health**
- **machine learning**
- **mental component summary**
- **quality of life**
- **questionnaire**
- **smart cities**
- **sustainable development**

REFERENCES

Burckhardt, C. S., Anderson, K. L., & Archenholtz, B. (2003). The Flanagan Quality of Life Scale: Evidence of construct validity. *Health and Quality of Life Outcomes, 1*(1), 59. https://doi.org/10.1186/1477-7525-1-59.

CDC HRQOL–14 "Healthy Days Measure" Article on HRQOL. (2022). https://www.cdc.gov/hrqol/hrqol14_measure.htm (accessed on 5 July 2024).

Cohen, S. R., Russell, L. B., Leis, A., Shahidi, J., Porterfield, P., Kuhl, D. R., Gadermann, A. M., & Sawatzky, R. (2019). More comprehensively measuring quality of life in life-threatening illness: The McGill Quality of Life Questionnaire–Expanded. *BMC Palliative Care, 18*(1), 92. https://doi.org/10.1186/s12904-019-0473-y.

Connell, J., O'Cathain, A., & Brazier, J. (2014). Measuring quality of life in mental health: Are we asking the right questions? *Social Science & Medicine, 120,* 12–20. https://doi.org/10.1016/j.socscimed.2014.08.026.

Davenport, T., & Kalakota, R. (2019). The potential for artificial intelligence in healthcare. *Future Healthcare Journal, 6*(2), 94–98. https://doi.org/10.7861/futurehosp.6-2-94.

Evolution and Importance of the GHS Index, Article in ghsindex.org. (2022). https://www.ghsindex.org/about/#Evolution-and-Importance-of-the-GHS-Index (accessed on 5 July 2024).

Grabowska, S., Saniuk, S., & Gajdzik, B. (2022). Industry 5.0: Improving humanization and sustainability of Industry 4.0. *Scientometrics, 127*(6), 3117–3144. https://doi.org/10.1007/s11192-022-04370-1.

Haraldstad, K., Wahl, A., Andenæs, R., Andersen, J. R., Andersen, M. H., Beisland, E., Borge, C. R., Engebretsen, E., Eisemann, M., Halvorsrud, L., Hanssen, T. A., Haugstvedt, A., Haugland, T., Johansen, V. A., Larsen, M. H., Løvereide, L., Løyland, B., Kvarme, L. G., Moons, P., & Norekvål, T. M., LIVSFORSK network. (2019). A systematic review of quality-of-life research in medicine and health sciences. *Quality of Life Research, 28*(10), 2641–2650. https://doi.org/10.1007/s11136-019-02214-9.

Health Index of Countries Worldwide by Health Index Score, Article in Statista.com. (2022). https://www.statista.com/statistics/1290168/health-index-of-countries-worldwide-by-health-index-score/ (accessed on 5 July 2024).

Huang, C. H., Wang, T. F., Tang, F. I., Chen, I. J., & Yu, S. (2017). Development and validation of a quality-of-life scale for elementary school students. *International Journal of Clinical and Health Psychology, 17*(2), 180–191. https://doi.org/10.1016/j.ijchp.2017.01.001.

Naragatti, S. (2020). The study of yoga effects on health. *International Journal of Innovative Medicine and Health Science, 12,* 98–110. https://www.whitesscience.com/product/the-study-of-yoga-effects-on-health/ (accessed on 5 July 2024).

Pathath, A. W. (2017). Meditation: Techniques and benefits. *International Journal of Current Research in Medical Science, 3*(6), 162–168. http://dx.doi.org/10.22192/ijcrms.2017.03.06.021.

Rastogi, R., Chaturvedi, D. K., Verma, H., Saini, H., Mehlyan, K. S., & Varshney, Y. (2018). Statistical analysis of EMG and GSR therapy on visual mode and SF-36 scores for chronic TTH. *IEEE Uttar Pradesh Section International Conference on Electrical, Electronics and Computer Engineering (UPCON),* 43684, 1–6. https://doi.org/10.1109/UPCON.2018.8596851.

Rastogi, R., Rastogi, A. R., Sharma, D., Rastogi, M., Garg, P., & Srivastava, P., (2022). Detection of air pollution and its adverse effects on human health: Analytical approach of different data particles in NCR, India. *International Journal of Social Ecology and Sustainable Development, 13*(1), 1–18. https://doi.org/10.4018/IJSESD.289645

Rastogi, R., Sagar, S., Tandon, N., Rajeshwari, T., & Dhamija, L., (2021). Vedic systems and their scientific aspects to sustain mental health: A solution for challenging issues for human race in epidemic time. *Journal of Natural & Ayurvedic Medicine, 5*(1), 1–8. https://doi.org/10.23880/jonam-16000299.

Rastogi, R., Sagar, S., Tandon, N., Rajeshwari, T., & Singh, B., (2021). Computational statistics on stress patients with happiness and radiation indices by Vedic Homa therapy: South Asian heritage with scientific aspects in global pandemic. *Journal of Natural & Ayurvedic Medicine, 5*(1), 1–10. https://doi.org/10.23880/jonam-16000295.

Rastogi, R., Saxena, M., Chaturvedi, D. K., Sagar, S., Rastogi, A. R., Sharma, D., Gupta, H., Gupta, N., Bhardwaj, M., & Sharma, M., (2022). Surveillance on emission of herbal woods and cow dung for refinement of atmosphere with Vedic mantra: A scientific regression to roots amidst pandemic threats. *International Journal of Social Ecology and Sustainable Development, 13*(1), 1–24. https://doi.org/10.4018/IJSESD.293242.

Rastogi, R., Saxena, M., Chaturvedi, D. K., Sagar, S., Tandon, N., Rajeshwari, T., & Singh, B., (2022). Verifying the effects of Homa therapy with herbal woods on air quality in the Indian festive season: Prediction and analytical approach amidst unlocking the society in pandemic challenges. *International Journal of Social Ecology and Sustainable Development, 13*(1), 1–16. https://doi.org/10.4018/IJSESD.292071.

Rastogi, R., Saxena, M., Chaturvedi, D. K., Sagar, S., Tandon, N., Rajeshwari, T., & Singh, B., (2022). Fundamental aspects of Vedic sciences by Yajna Vijnan and mantra therapy: An interdisciplinary study in light of the second wave of the pandemic. *International Journal of Social Ecology and Sustainable Development, 13*(1), 1–34. https://doi.org/10.4018/IJSESD.296689.

Rastogi, R., Saxena, M., Sharma, S. K., Muralidharan, S., Beriwal, V. K., Singhal, P., Rastogi, M., & Shrivastava, R. (2019). Evaluation of efficacy of Yagya therapy on T2-Diabetis Mellitus patients. *International Conference on Industry Interactive Innovations in Science, Engineering and Technology, 1*(1), 1–13. https://papers.ssrn.com/sol3/papers.cfm?abstract_id=3514326 (accessed on 5 July 2024).

Sagar, S., Vikas Garg, B., Gupta, B., & Rastogi, R. (2021). Impact of meditation quality of life of employees & business performance: An empirical study for innovative management with Industry 5.0. *IIM Bodh Gaya Management Conference 2021, 1*(1), 241–242.

Scientific Research on Yoga, Article from Yogaalliance.org. (2022). https://www.yogaalliance.org/About_Yoga/Scientific_Research_on_Yoga (accessed on 5 July 2024).

SF-36 Questionnaire. https://clinmedjournals.org/articles/jmdt/jmdt-2-023-figure-1.pdf (accessed on 5 July 2024).

ANNEXURES

➢ **Additional Readings:**
1. Benchmarking life quality support interventions in long-term care using the long-term care quality of life scale (https://pubmed.ncbi.nlm.nih.gov/30536944/).
2. Health-related quality of life and influencing factors in drug addicts based on the scale QLICD-DA: A cross-sectional study (https://hqlo.biomedcentral.com/articles/10.1186/s12955-022-02012-x).
3. Improving quality of life in hospitalized children (https://pubmed.ncbi.nlm.nih.gov/25084722/).
4. Quality of life (https://www.statpearls.com/ArticleLibrary/viewarticle/28144).
5. Reliability and validity of an HIV-specific health-related quality-of-life measure for use with injecting drug users (https://journals.lww.com/aidsonline/Abstract/1996/12000/Reliability_and_validity_of_an_HIV_specific.15.aspx).

➢ **Key Terms and Definitions:**
- **Yoga:** It is a group of physical, mental, and spiritual practices or disciplines which originated in ancient India and aim to control and still the mind, recognizing a detached witness-consciousness untouched by the mind and mundane suffering.
- **Meditation:** It is a practice in which an individual uses a technique – such as mindfulness, or focusing the mind on a particular object, thought, or activity – to train attention and awareness, and achieve a mentally clear and emotionally calm and stable state. Meditation is practiced in numerous religious traditions.
- **Fitness:** It is a state of health and well-being and, more specifically, the ability to perform aspects of sports, occupations, and daily activities. Physical fitness is generally achieved through proper nutrition, moderate-vigorous physical exercise, and sufficient rest along with a formal recovery plan.
- **Quality of Life (QoL):** It is defined by the World Health Organization as "an individual's perception of their position in life in the context of the culture and value systems in which they live and in relation to their goals, expectations, standards, and concerns."

- **Mental Peace:** It refers to the deliberate state of spiritual calm and the potential of stressors such as the burden arising from pretending to perform at an optional level with a positive mind (inner peace). Peace of mind is generally associated with joy, happiness, calmness, prayer, Yoga, meditation, etc., many spiritual practices refer to this peace as an experience of knowing oneself.
- **Indian Culture:** It is the heritage of social norms, ethical values, traditional customs, belief systems, political systems, artifacts, and technologies that originated in or are associated with the ethno-linguistically diverse Republic of India. The term also applies beyond India to countries and cultures whose histories are strongly connected to India by immigration, colonization, or influence, particularly in South Asia and Southeast Asia. India's languages, religions, dance, music, architecture, food, and customs differ from place to place within the country.
- **Human Health:** Health, according to the World Health Organization, is "a state of complete physical, mental, and social well-being and not merely the absence of disease and infirmity."

➢ **Data Sets:**

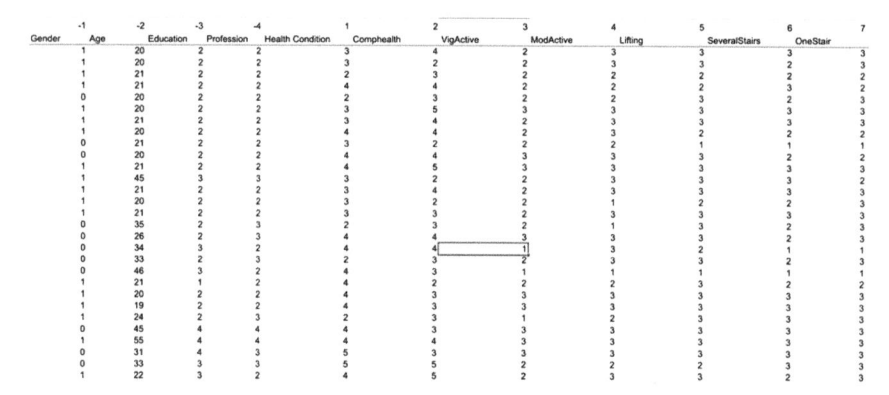

-1	-2	-3	-4	1	2	3	4	5	6	7
Gender	Age	Education	Profession	Health Condition	Comphealth	VigActive	ModActive	Lifting	SeveralStairs	OneStair
1	20	2	2	3	4	2	3	3	3	3
1	20	2	2	3	2	2	3	3	2	3
1	21	2	2	2	3	2	2	2	2	2
1	21	2	2	4	4	2	2	3	3	2
0	20	2	2	2	3	2	2	3	2	3
1	20	2	2	3	5	3	3	3	3	3
1	21	2	2	3	4	2	3	3	3	3
1	20	2	2	4	4	2	3	2	2	2
0	21	2	2	3	2	2	2	1	1	1
0	20	2	2	4	4	3	3	3	2	2
1	21	2	2	4	5	3	3	3	3	3
1	45	3	3	3	2	2	3	3	3	2
1	21	2	2	3	4	2	3	3	3	3
1	20	2	2	3	2	2	1	2	2	3
1	21	2	2	3	3	2	3	3	3	3
0	35	2	3	2	3	2	1	3	2	3
0	26	2	3	4	4	3	3	3	2	3
0	34	3	2	4	4	1	3	2	1	1
0	33	2	2	2	3	2	3	3	2	3
0	46	3	2	4	3	1	1	1	1	1
1	21	1	2	4	2	2	2	3	2	2
1	20	2	2	4	3	3	3	3	3	3
1	19	2	2	4	3	3	3	3	3	3
1	24	2	2	2	3	1	2	3	3	3
0	45	4	4	4	3	3	3	3	3	3
1	55	4	4	4	4	3	3	3	3	3
0	31	4	3	5	3	3	3	3	3	3
0	33	3	3	5	5	2	2	2	3	3
1	22	3	2	4	5	2	3	3	2	3

FIGURE A   Sample Dataset-1 with Column 1–7.

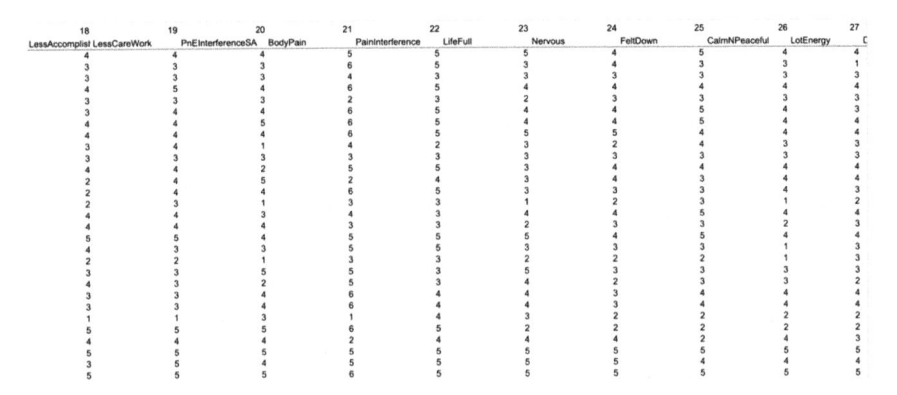

FIGURE B   Sample Dataset-2 with Column 8–17.

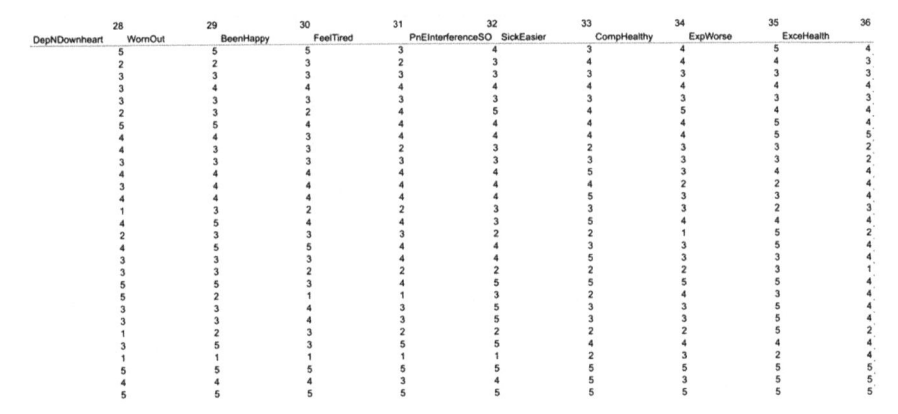

FIGURE C   Sample Dataset-3 with Column 18–27.

FIGURE D   Sample Dataset-4 with Column 28–36.

Physical Functions	PhyHealthLim	38	EmoProbLim	39	Energy/fatigue	40	Emotional wellbeing	41 Social functioning	Pain	42	43	44 General healt
10	18.75		25		56.25		40	50		90		50
10	62.5		41.66666667		50		50	50		100		45
50	50		50		50		50	50		55		45
35	18.75		16.66666667		50		50	50		100		55
30	31.25		50		43.75		50	50		35		45
0	56.25		33.33333333		50		40	37.5		100		55
10	31.25		16.66666667		43.75		35	62.5		100		45
45	25		25		56.25		35	50		100		55
85	43.75		33.33333333		56.25		45	25		42.5		50
55	100		50		50		50	50		45		50
0	12.5		16.66666667		43.75		45	25		90		45
25	37.5		50		43.75		55	62.5		47.5		50
5	37.5		50		37.5		55	50		100		45
65	43.75		66.66666667		37.5		50	25		45		55
5	25		25		43.75		40	50		55		45
45	31.25		25		43.75		50	75		45		25
15	12.5		8.333333333		50		45	50		90		50
65	50		33.33333333		43.75		40	37.5		90		50
15	56.25		75		50		45	37.5		45		35
100	50		50		43.75		40	50		65		50
55	100		58.33333333		68.75		35	37.5		65		70
0	25		41.66666667		62.5		55	37.5		87.5		50
0	25		41.66666667		62.5		55	37.5		87.5		50
25	37.5		100		56.25		65	62.5		37.5		30
0	37.5		0		12.5		55	50		100		55
0	31.25		25		81.25		55	87.5		47.5		70
0	0		0		50		40	50		90		60
20	18.75		25		62.5		40	50		90		50
10	0		8.333333333		50		40	50		100		55

FIGURE E   Sample Dataset-5 with 8 derived features.

➢ **Snapshots of Coding:**

```
labels = 'Unemployed', 'Student', 'Job', 'Business'
sizes = [u, s, j, b]
colors = ( "red", "green", "#cab8c4",
          "white")

fig1, ax1 = plt.subplots()
explode = (0, 0, 0, 0)
font = {'family': 'serif',
        'color': 'darkred',
        'weight': 'normal',
        'size': 20,
        }
plt.xlabel("Occupation",loc="center",fontsize=20)
ax1.pie(sizes, colors = colors, explode=explode, labels=labels,autopct='%1.1f%%', shadow=True, startangle=90,wedgeprop
                      'linewidth': 2,
                      'antialiased': True))
patches, texts, auto = ax1.pie(sizes, colors=colors, shadow=True, startangle=90,explode=explode, autopct='%1.1f%%' )

plt.show()
plt.savefig('Occupation_per.jpeg')
```

FIGURE F   Coding snippet for pie graph representing various occupational categories.

Bar graph showing Medium body pain accoring to gender and professions

```
plotdata = pd.DataFrame({

    "Male":[9,14,13,12],

    "Female":[7,13,5,5]},

    index=["Unemployed", "Student","Job","Business"])
y=[1,2,3,4,5,6,7,8,9,10,11,12]
#y=[1,2,3,4,5,6,7,8,9,10,11,12,13,14,15,16,17,18,19,20]
plotdata.plot(kind="bar",figsize=(15, 8))

plt.title("Medium Body Pain (Score < 60) w.r.t Gender and Profession")
plt.xlabel("Profession")
max_ylim = max(y) + 3
min_ylim = min(y) -1
plt.ylim(min_ylim, max_ylim)
plt.ylabel("Number of people")
plt.grid(b = True, color ='grey',
         linestyle ='-.', linewidth = 0.5,
         alpha = 1)

plt.savefig("Pain_Profession.jpg")
```

FIGURE G   Coding snippet for bar graph showing medium body according to gender and professions.

```
plotdata = pd.DataFrame({

    "Male":[25,25,28,26],

    "Female":[25,24,23,21]},

    index=["Unemployed", "Student","Job","Business"])
#y=[1,2,3,4,5,6,7,8,9,10,11,12]
y=[2,4,6,8,10,12,14,16,18,20,22,24,26,28,30]
plotdata.plot(kind="bar",figsize=(15, 8))

plt.title("Mcs Value (Score < 60) w.r.t Gender and Profession")
plt.xlabel("Profession")
max_ylim = max(y) + 3
min_ylim = min(y) -1
plt.ylim(min_ylim, max_ylim)
plt.ylabel("Number of people")
plt.grid(b = True, color ='grey',
        linestyle ='-.', linewidth = 0.5,
            alpha = 1)

plt.savefig("mcsvalue_Profession.jpg")
```

FIGURE H   Coding snippet for bar graph showing variation of PCS-value according to gender and profession.

```
plotdata = pd.DataFrame({

    "Male":[22,21,25,22],

    "Female":[21,22,19,18]},

    index=["Intermediate", "Graduation","Post Graduation","Research"])
#y=[1,2,3,4,5,6,7,8,9,10,11,12]
y=[2,4,6,8,10,12,14,16,18,20,22,24,26,28,20]
plotdata.plot(kind="bar",figsize=(15, 10))

plt.title("Less Vitality (Score < 60) w.r.t Gender and Education")
plt.xlabel("Education")
max_ylim = max(y) + 3
min_ylim = min(y) -1
plt.ylim(min_ylim, max_ylim)
plt.ylabel("Number of people")
plt.grid(b = True, color ='grey',
        linestyle ='-.', linewidth = 0.5,
            alpha = 1)

plt.savefig("Vitality_Education.jpg")
```

FIGURE I   Coding snippet for bar graph showing less vitality according to gender and educational background.

Bar graph showing variation of mcs value accoring to gender and educational backgrounds

```
plotdata = pd.DataFrame({

    "Male":[25,25,28,26],

    "Female":[25,25,23,21]},

    index=["Intermediate", "Graduation","Post Graduation","Research"])
#y=[1,2,3,4,5,6,7,8,9,10,11,12]
y=[2,4,6,8,10,12,14,16,18,20,22,24,26,28,30]
plotdata.plot(kind="bar",figsize=(15, 10))

plt.title("Mcs Value (Score < 60) w.r.t Gender and Education")
plt.xlabel("Education")
max_ylim = max(y) + 3
min_ylim = min(y) -1
plt.ylim(min_ylim, max_ylim)
plt.ylabel("Number of people")
plt.grid(b = True, color ='grey',
        linestyle ='-.', linewidth = 0.5,
            alpha = 1)

plt.savefig("mcsvalue_Education.jpg")
```

FIGURE J   Coding snippet for bar graph showing variation of MCS-value according to gender and educational.

CHAPTER 6

Female Adolescents are a Step Ahead of Male Adolescents in Decision-Making via Yoga-Cultivated Attentiveness: Pedagogy Interventions in Indian Settings

SUGYANTA PRIYADARSHINI,[1] SARTHAK DASH,[1] SUKANYA PRIYADARSHINI,[2] and NISRUTHA DULLA[1]

[1]*School of Humanities, KIIT Deemed to be University, Bhubaneswar, Odisha, India*

[2]*Berhampur University, Odisha, India*

ABSTRACT

In-depth literature survey examined the very limited research available on the differential impact of mindfulness Yoga training in both genders and hence needed detailed research and investigation. The current research work highlights the responsiveness of male and female adolescent students to college-based Yoga training, with a specialized focus on self-reported changes in positive and negative affect and the mechanisms underlying these changes. The sample comprises undergraduate engineering students (n = 42, 21 women, 22 men) enrolled at Kalinga Institute of Industrial Technology, deemed to be a university. Participants were requested to fill out the questionnaire before (pre-Yoga intervention) and after (post-Yoga intervention) the 15-week meditation course from November 2021 to March 2022. Every class was followed by a question-answer session to

Yoga and Meditation: Past and Present Evidence. Sachi Nandan Mohanty, Rabindra Kumar Pradhan, & Sugyanta Priyadarshini (Eds.)

open up about the feelings deep inside the heart and thoughts obstructing the mind's focus. This practice focused on attention allocation, mindful thinking, weakening negative emotions, and adding positive vibes to life. The mindfulness-based intervention for adolescents is analyzed with the help of two instruments named Positive Affect and Negative Affect Scale (PANAS) and Mindful Attention Awareness Scale (MAAS). However, their mindfulness intervention after practicing yoga is interpreted using the Decision Difficulty Scale (DDS). The research found that there are differential effects of mindfulness-based interventions (MBIs) for both male and female adolescent students, with female students showing a greater response to the training and improvement in positive and negative affect compared to their male counterparts. This difference in affect suggests that gender-specific coping methods must be applied. Furthermore, it can be predicted that different MBIs must be practiced for male and female students in order to achieve a higher efficacy of yoga training.

6.1 INTRODUCTION

The age-old practice of Yoga has currently become the most researched domain of existing psychotherapeutic methods (Walsh & Shapiro, 2006). The practice of Yoga can be defined as the manifestation of multiple mental upskilling practices that boost voluntary control over one's mental processes on one hand and the escalation of psychological potential comprising attentiveness and emotional self-modulation on the other (Tang et al., 2015). One of the multi-complex practices of Yoga with several positive outcomes and little evidence behind its practice is mindfulness Yoga (Pepping et al., 2016), which revolves around paying non-judgmental attention to the current moment by focusing on one's breath (Kabat-Zinn, 2005). The practice of mindfulness Yoga aids individuals to have robust control over their emotions by accepting their current status without any diversion towards unpleasant events (Teasdale et al., 2000). Moreover, the incorporation of clinical interventions in mindfulness training through mindfulness-based intervention (MBI) is identified as the potent treatment to prevent depression and its recurrence (Segal et al., 2002). Furthermore, MBI also prevents the occurrence of rumination that exaggerates dysphoric moods (Broderick, 2005). Multiple research works are being conducted on the application of MBI on stress and anxiety (Chang et al., 2004; Khusid & Vythilingam, 2016; Goldin & Gross, 2010), anger, and aggression accompanied by schizophrenia (Davis et al., 2015; Singh et al., 2014), heavy substance use and addictions (Brewer et al., 2013), and even learning disabilities and ADHD (Haydicky et al., 2012; Mitchell et al., 2015). However, in the academic scenario, schools have acted as the perfect setting for the implementation of mindfulness programs (Felver & Jennings, 2016). The mindfulness intervention programs have gained popularity because of the promising positive association of mindfulness practices and the reduction of stress and anxiety (van de Weijer-Bergsma et al., 2014), mood disorders (Bluth et al., 2015), and substance use/ addiction (Volanen et al., 2016). MBI is shown to be effective in helping children focus on the current moment non-judgmentally, in order to pay full attention (Sciutto et al., 2021) and create a mental breathing space to observe, respond, and react to the stimulus (Nelson et al., 2022). Mindfulness training has the potential to regulate emotions (Arch and Craske), reduce emotional reactivity (Mendelson et al., 2010), resolve behavioral issues and stress disorders (Klatt et al., 2013), increase attentiveness (Poehlmann et al., 2015), and improve mental well-being (Carsley et al., 2018). But this intense research and investigation are limited by poor methodological practices (Greenberg & Harris, 2012).

A substantial body of research over the past decades suggests that gendered social practices have created a divide in psychological distress between men and women (Matud et al., 2015; Rosenfield & Smith, 2010; Turner & Lloyd, 1995). Evidence suggests that there is a difference in the type of psychological symptoms displayed by men and women, but the overall degree of psychological distress is nearly the same in both genders (Viertiö et al., 2019; Osayomi & Adegboye, 2016; Rosenfield & Mouzon, 2013). The difference in psychological symptoms begins in childhood (Kessler et al., 2005), heightens in adolescence, and then continues into adulthood, with a higher incidence in women compared to men (Matud, 2004; Saluja et al., 2004). Research suggests the existence of two factors, i.e., internalizing and externalizing, reflecting the difference in psychopathological symptoms of both men and women (Carragher et al., 2015; Willner et al., 2016; Askari et al., 2022). Men have a higher level of the externalizing factor, while women have a higher level of the internalizing factor (Malhotra & Shah, 2015). The internalizing factors result in the internalization of multivariate problems of women and their conversion into depression, anxiety, stress, a sense of hopelessness, multiple phobias, and panic attacks. Whereas the externalizing factors cause men to externally reflect their myriad problems in the form of hyper-activity, aggression, substance abuse or addiction, antisocial, aberrant, and aggressive behavior, which are often problematic for others (Cotto et al., 2010; Rosenfield, 2012; Bask, 2014; Mendez & Bozzay, 2021). However, epidemiological data suggest the co-occurrence of both internalizing and externalizing factors in both genders (Caron & Rutter, 1991; Essau, 2002; Lilienfeld, 2003; Sallis et al., 2019).

The efficiency and efficacy of mindfulness training are reflected in the improvement of psychiatric and stress-related symptoms. Hence, mindfulness training is being integrated into psychotherapeutic interventions (Holzel et al., 2011). Studies suggest that mindfulness training has improved the overall psychological well-being in both genders by shaping the coping strategies adopted to deal with their myriad emotions (Weinstein et al., 2009; Donald & Atkins, 2016). However, the adoption of different coping strategies for the cultivation of mindfulness in both genders has resulted in contrasting results (Brown et al., 2021). Further, the divergent impact of mindfulness training on both genders is clearly evident by the pilot study conducted on the feasibility of qigong Yoga in the residential treatment for substance addiction. This study clearly supports the fact that after treatment, women reflect higher mitigation for anxiety, stress, and withdrawal symptoms as compared to men (Chen et al., 2010). Moreover, Katz & Toner (2013), had conducted a systematic review that confirmed that mindfulness treatment for substance abuse is more beneficial for women as compared to men. However, very limited research is available on the differential impact of mindfulness training in both genders and hence needs detailed research and investigation. The current study focuses on different ways in which male and female adolescent students respond to the college-based Yoga training, with a specialized focus on self-reported changes in (positive and negative) affect and the mechanisms underlying these changes. We hypothesized that there are differential effects of mindful-based interventions (MBIs) for both male and female adolescent students; with female students showing a greater response to the training and improvement in (positive and negative) affect as compared to their male counterparts. This difference in affect suggests gender-specific coping methods must be applied. Further, we can predict that different MBIs must be practiced for male and female students, so as to bring a higher efficacy of Yoga training. Therefore, it can be predicted that the improvement in affect in the case of women is associated with increased self-acceptance, whereas improvement in affect in the case of men is associated with diminishing distraction.

6.2 MATERIALS AND METHODOLOGY

6.2.1 SAMPLE SIZE

The participants (n = 42, 21 women, 22 men) enrolled in the study are undergraduate engineering students from Kalinga Institute of Industrial Technology, deemed to be a university. The participants were asked to register for a 15-week Yoga Training course which comprised weekly moralistic workshops and practice-based learning via "Yoga labs." Participants were requested to fill out the questionnaire before and after the 15-week meditation course from November 2021 to March 2022. Staff were recruited to describe the study and circulate sign-up sheets with a written consent form from each participant. In the initial stage, 68 students enrolled in the study, but 24 were excluded based on their passive participation, inadequate attendance, discontinuity in the course, critical psychological issues (suicidal tendency, extreme aggression, and panic), and irrelevant answers in the questionnaire, resulting in a 38% attrition rate.

6.2.2 INSTRUMENTS

6.2.2.1 AFFECT SCALE

PANAS, widely known as Positive and Negative Affect Scale devised by Watson et al. (1988), is used in the current study to analyze the impact of Yoga before and after the Yoga session. The 20-item scale is used to analyze the participants' current mental affective state with the help of 10 items (attentive, interested, alert, excited, enthusiastic, inspired, proud, determined, strong, and active) weighing positive affect, and the other 10 items (distressed, upset, hostile, irritable, scared, afraid, ashamed, guilty, nervous, jittery) weighing negative affect, ranging from very slightly or not at all (1) to very much (5). The 20-item PANAS scale has high reliability (Crawford & Henry, 2004) with appreciable internal consistency both at pre (0.88) and post (0.98) time points.

6.2.2.2   MINDFUL ATTENTION SCALE

MAAS, broadly known as the Mindful Attention Awareness Scale introduced by Brown & Ryan (2003), is used in the current study to analyze the extent of open and receptive mindfulness among the participants before and after the Yoga procedure with an overall satisfactory consistency (0.89). Participants rated the 15-item scale comprising certain queries (e.g., Difficulty in remaining focused in the present time, doing certain things without paying attention to it) from 1 (at all times) to 6 (not once).

6.2.2.3   DECISION MAKING SCALE

DDS, otherwise known as the decision difficulty scale, formulated by Shin et al. (2021), is a 29-item highly reliable and consistent compassion scale (α=0.90) used to analyze the degree of decision-making strength in an individual. The scale comprises 3 sub-scales named 5-item Maximization Goal (α= 0.93), 12-item Maximization Strategy (α= 0.93), and 12-item Decision Difficulty (α= 0.95). Participants were asked to rate the sub-scales such as Maximization Goal (e.g., am not okay with good enough), Maximization Strategy (e.g., take time to come to a decision after considering all alternatives), Decision Difficulty (e.g., keep wondering if decision-making could be easier) ranging from 1 (almost always) to 7 (almost never). However, the reverse scores of the 3 subscales under items such as Maximization Goal (e.g., do not believe in asking more than what I deserve), Maximization Strategy (e.g., comfortable making a decision before exploring other options), and Decision Difficulty (e.g., not worried about making any hasty decision) are computed as 1 = 7, 2 = 6, 3 = 5, 4 = 4, 5 = 3, 6 = 2, 7 = 1, and hence the mean of the responses is calculated at the end for interpretation.

6.2.3   YOGA WORKSHOP ASSESSMENT

Yoga labs were conducted twice a week for a period of 2 hours comprising of training on focusing on open monitoring practices such as breathing and analyzing the body sensations. Every class ended with a question-answer session to encourage sharing feelings and thoughts, helping to focus the mind. This practice aimed to improve attention, promote mindful thinking, reduce negative emotions, and bring positivity into life.

6.3 RESULTS

6.3.1 POSITIVE VS. NEGATIVE AFFECT IN MINDFUL INTERVENTION

The data obtained revealed that there is a significant gender divergence on the measures of Negative Affect but not Positive Affect. Such differentiation can be explained by the essence of Yoga training which involved practices quintessential to generate awareness, deep concentration and calmness in order to maintain an equilibrium in every situation. This exhibits a complete contrast to other clinical Yoga training practices (Hofmann et al., 2011; Zeng et al., 2015) that applied love-kindness and self-compassion to promote positive emotion. Hence, it can be considered that the training resulted in decline of negative emotions but maintained neutrality in positive emotions. It was also noted that no individual of particular gender showed any improvement in positive affect. And even if the entire group was taken into consideration, no improvement was observed in either positive or negative affect. This study strongly contradicts the results of the improved positive and negative affects through mindfulness training (Chambers et al., 2008; Menezes & Bizarro, 2015; Sedlmeier et al., 2018). There was no improvement in either positive or negative affect in the whole sample or all the individuals of a sample. Therefore, gender may be a determinant in the differential response to mindfulness training.

Table 6.1 represents the mean and standard deviation values of the age of female and male participants, along with the entry (Before Yoga) and exit (After Meditation) scores of PANAS, MAAS, and DDS. Table 6.1 also represents the before and after Yoga time effect and BAMTE × GS value with all the scales. A paired t-test was performed to trace the relationship between the entry and exit scores of all the scales. It is found that female participants showed a significant change in both the negative [$t(21) = 0.63$, $p = 0.03$] and positive affect [$t(21) = 1.46$, $p = 0.04$]. The test also reveals that female participants exhibited a significant change in the Mindful Attention Awareness Scale [$t(21) = 1.34$, $p = 0.004$] and in two sub-scales of the Decision Difficulty scale, i.e., in Maximization Strategy [$t(21) = 1.24$, $p = 0.02$] and Decision Difficulty [$t(21) = 1.68$, $p = 0.03$]. Whereas male participants showed significant change only in the decision difficulty [$t(21) = 1.87$, $p = 0.03$]. Further, ANOVA analysis was also performed, and the outcome showed a significant BAMTE × GS interaction effect for the negative affect that specifies that female participants have a greater reduction of negative affect [F $(1,42) = 8.24$, p $= 0.001$] in the post-Yoga period in comparison to the male participants. Similarly, there is a significant BAMTE × GS interaction effect with Mindful Attention Awareness [F $(1,42) = 7.43$, p $= 0.002$] that specifies the score of MAAS of female participants is more than that of male participants. Further, ANOVA analysis shows a significant BAMTE × GS interaction with the gender effect for the two subscales of the Decision Difficulty Scale, i.e., for Maximization Strategy [F $(1,42) = 1.12$, p $= 0.02$] and for decision difficulty [F $(1,42) = 5.28$, p $= 0.001$]. This indicates that women have a greater reach in maximization strategy and lesser difficulty in decision making.

6.3.2   CORRELATION BETWEEN PRE-POST CHANGES IN POSITIVE AFFECT AND OTHER MEASURES FRAGMENTED BY GENDER

In Table 6.2, the Pearson Product Moment correlation is calculated to trace the relationship between the positive affect and other measures among the female and male participants. The analysis found a negative correlation between positive affect and the Mindful Attention Awareness Scale in male participants, whereas female participants showed a positive correlation. Secondly, male participants showed a significant positive correlation only in the Maximization Strategy, whereas female participants showed a significant positive correlation only with Maximization Goal. In the decision difficulty measure associated with positive affect, male participants showed a positive correlation. In contrast, female participants showed a significant negative correlation indicating a better decision-making strategy in the post-Yoga period.

6.3.3   MINDFUL ATTENTION AWARENESS (MAAS) AND POSITIVE AFFECT AND NEGATIVE AFFECT (PANAS) ON THE DECISION DIFFICULTY

Table 6.3 analyzes the strength of influence of mindful attention awareness (MAAS) and positive affect and negative affect (PANAS) on the decision difficulty of the Female and Male Participants. Table 6.3 shows that the MAAS (2.240) and PANAS (0.000101) significantly influence the score of decision difficulty scale (DDS) for male participants. In contrast, there

TABLE 6.1 Descriptive Statistics (Mean and SD) of All the Scales Before and After Yoga Training in Female and Male Participants, with Analysis of Variance (ANOVA) Result

Measures	Female ($n = 21$)	Male ($n = 21$)	F (1, 42)		
Demographics			BAMTE	GS	BAMTE × GS
Age (years)	24.71 (4.63)	25.05 (4.24)	2.66	–	–
Affect (PANAS)					
Entry positive affect	16.24 (1.37)	15.48 (2.09)	2.17	2.69	0.166
Exit positive affect	41.67 (0.97)*	24.57 (3.16)	–	–	–
Entry negative affect	44.10 (1.26)	40.81 (3.25)	4.71	2.56	8.24**
Exit negative affect	17.14 (1.74)*	31.00 (3.00)	–	–	–
Mindful Attention Awareness Scale (MAAS)					
Entry MAAS	27.38 (5.11)	35.05 (2.27)	23.86***	1.33	7.43**
Exit MAAS	71.71 (4.01)**	66.71 (1.85)	–	–	–
Decision Difficulty Scale (DDS)					
Entry maximization goal	11.43 (2.04)	14.85 (1.88)	16.44***	0.89	5.62
Exit maximization goal	29.90 (1.55)	29.14 (1.90)	–	–	–
Entry maximization strategy	28.48 (2.62)	32.90 (2.21)	13.31**	0.65	1.12*
Exit maximization strategy	70.48 (3.17)**	69.29 (3.07)	–	–	–
Entry decision difficulty	68.52 (2.87)	69.19 (2.84)	37.16***	3.65	5.28**
Exit decision difficulty	30.38 (3.26)**	33.19 (2.80)**	–	–	–

*p < 0.05; **p < 0.01; ***p < 0.001; BAMTE: Before and after yoga time effect; and GS: Gender slot.

is no significant relationship between MAAS and PANAS with DDS in the case of female participants. The analysis also reveals that the R^2 value is 0.922 with a corresponding F-value of 257.225, which is significant at 0.000 for the male participants. Here, the value of R^2 explains that the independent variables together explained 92% of the variance in the Decision Difficulty Scale score.

TABLE 6.2 Pearson Product Moment Correlation between Pre-Post Changes in Positive Affect and Other Measures Fragmented by Gender

Measures	Positive Affect (PANAS Positive)	
	Female	Male
MAAS	0.014	−0.011
DDS (maximization goal)	0.113*	0.118
DDS (maximization strategy)	0.171	0.048*
DDS (decision difficulty)	−0.090*	0.174

*$p < 0.05$.

TABLE 6.3 Multiple Liner Regression Analysis of Female and Male Participants

Unstandardized Coefficients			Standardized Coefficient		
Model	B	Std. Error	Beta	t-Stat	Sig.
Male					
Constant	34.913	2.649	–	22.662	0.000
MAAS	2.240	0.307	0.268	2.249	0.002
PANAS	0.000101	0.003	0.275	1.225	0.001
Female					
Constant	1.102	3.497	–	32.223	0.000
MAAS	−1.410	−0.395	−0.237	−1.037	0.134
PANAS	1.153	0.413	0.385	6.372	0.156

N = 42 (21 female, 21 male); R^2 = 0.922 (F), 0.462 (M); F = 257.225 (F), 98.597 (M); MAAS: Mindfulness attention awareness scale; and PANAS: positive affect negative affect scale.

6.3.4 IMPROVING STATUS OF WOMEN AS COMPARED TO MEN IN MINDFULNESS TRAINING

Figure 6.1 depicts the change in the mean score of negative effects on female and male participants in the pre-mediation period and the post-Yoga period. It shows that female participants have a larger negative effect in the pre-mediation period whereas male participants have a lesser negative effect in the pre-Yoga period. In the post-mediation period, female participants showed a significant reduction in the negative effect in comparison to the male participants as shown in Figure 6.1.

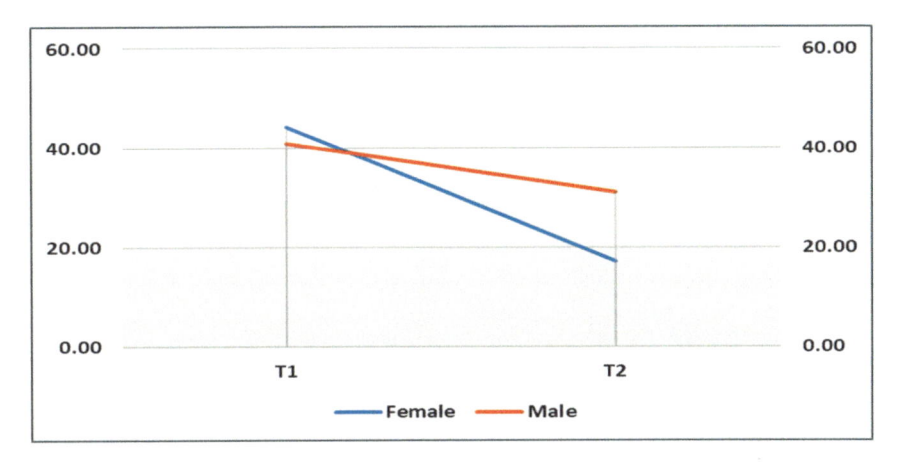

FIGURE 6.1 Negative effect in female and male participants before and after yoga.

Figure 6.2 depicts the change in the mean score of all the measures in female and male participants in the pre-Yoga (T1) and post-meditation (T2) periods. The blue bar in Figure 6.2 represents the mean score in the T1 time period for all the measures of female and male participants. In the T1 time period, the mean score for all the measures among female participants is lower in comparison to the male participants. Similarly, the orange bar represents the mean score in the T2 time period for all the measures among female and male participants. In the T2 time period, female participants have slightly higher mean scores for all the measures than the male participants which are shown in Figure 6.2. In addition, the gray line represents the difference between the mean score of the T1 and T2 time periods. The line indicates that the difference between the pre- and post-Yoga scores for all the measures of female participants is higher than the male participants. It specifies that meditation has a greater impact on the female than the male participants.

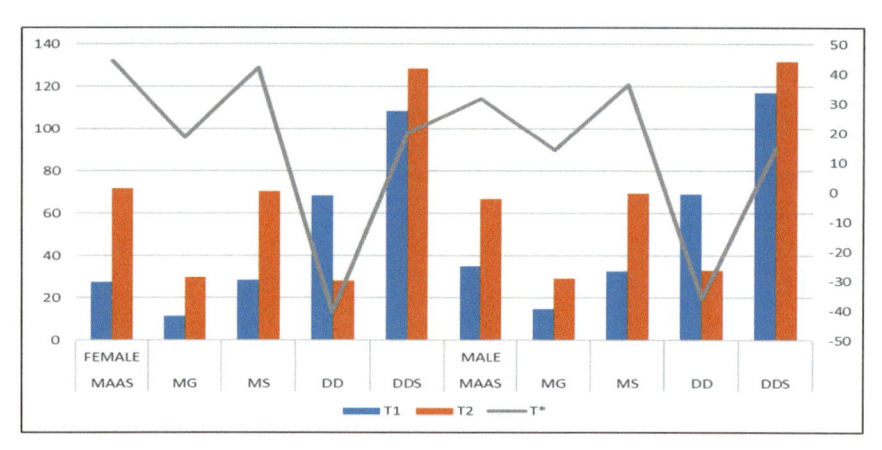

FIGURE 6.2   Change in the mean score of all the measures in female and male participants before and after yoga.

Abbreviations: MAAS: Mindfulness attention awareness scale; MG: maximization of goal; MS: maximization of strategy; DD: decision difficulty; DDS: decision difficulty scale; and T*: difference between the mean score of pre- and post-*yoga*.

6.4   DISCUSSION

The research findings from our selected samples suggest that women in the sample benefit more compared to men, which is in accordance with earlier studies on mindfulness training for substance abuse (Brewer et al., 2013; Katz & Toner, 2013). Furthermore, our analysis excluded explanations of important baseline differences or differences in Yoga practice hours. However, some improvement is likely to be observed if men and women started with different levels of affect at the entry point. But no entry point difference was observed in positive or negative affect. Additionally, our findings show that in a 15-week semester, female adolescents on average spend seven hours more than male adolescents. Therefore, it is clear that increased Yoga and a high dose of treatment didn't show any marked improvement in male adolescents compared to female adolescents. The research suggests that the application of gendered emotional regulation techniques caused divergent effects in both males and females. These gender-based mechanistic differences are indicated by neuroimaging research using MAAS. This technique reported that compared to women, men show lesser activation of brain regions like the amygdala and prefrontal regions associated with emotional regulation.

Furthermore, men show decreased involvement of ventral striatal regions involved in reward processing (Ochsner et al., 2002; McRae et al., 2012; De la Peña-Arteaga et al., 2021). Another similar fMRI study conducted during a working memory task revealed that negative emotion induction leads to heightened involvement of emotion-associated regions like the amygdala and orbitofrontal cortex in the case of women. Whereas men show higher activation of regions associated with cognitive control like prefrontal and superior parietal regions of the brain (Koch et al., 2007).

The research findings suggested that the mechanism of emotional regulation and response to negative situations is different in both genders (Deng et al., 2016). Adolescent males tend to externalize their emotions by distracting themselves in external activities like playing sports or watching TV, whereas girls tend to internalize their feelings by self-involving activities like writing their negative thoughts (Chaplin & Aldao, 2013; Mendez & Bozzay, 2021). Moreover, some studies emphasize the role of mindfulness intervention in reducing rumination (Heeren & Philippot, 2011; Hawley et al., 2014; Yu, 2017). Since it has been shown that the process of rumination affects a woman's tendency to internalize her emotions during stress, therefore the hypothesis that mindfulness intervention might reduce rumination effects in women can be put forth. But men show lesser rumination effects than women (Johnson & Whisman, 2013). Increased mindfulness attention through yoga to emotions and thoughts in men showed greater negative affect as compared to women (Kingery et al., 2021). The data obtained has a higher correlation with the hypothesis proposed. The correlation indicates a positive effect in women with improved self-compassion skills and mindfulness intervention that also includes specific subscales to counter emotions with non-reactivity and to boost kindness towards oneself. This observation supports components of theoretical explanation on the central role of mindfulness in reducing rumination (van Vugt et al., 2012). Moreover, the observation also supports the two-factor pathway (Bishop et al., 2004) that provides clarity in paying attention and accepting experience that all together accords to clarity of experience on one hand and improved strategies of negative emotion regulation on the other hand (Burschka et al., 2014). Conversely, men in the sample showed no improvement in overall negative affect but they showed certain improvements in measures of self-compassion. The changes obtained were correlated with an improved aspect of mindfulness which dictates the capability to recognize, describe, and demarcate one's emotions. Hence, it can be proposed that no specific improvement in affect was observed in this relationship; although heightened exposure to ignored emotions could have resulted in an improvement in mood or in negative effect. Therefore, more research should be conducted to investigate this hypothesis further.

If we associate the ability to recognize, describe, and demarcate one's emotions as an indicator of improvement of affect in men, then certain practices like open-monitoring and affect labeling can appear beneficial to men. Further, other research on a similar context has emphasized the development of an 8-week MBIs program (Gotink et al., 2016; Britton et al., 2017) that aims to train men in advanced skills in monitoring and labeling of currently occurring experiences openly. Moreover, active mindfulness training like Yoga and Tai Chi (Yu et al., 2019; Wall, 2005) might work better for men as compared to silent Yoga techniques, as men are better at accommodating external coping strategies. Further, it has also been indicated in previous research that the higher the masculinity rating in men and women, the better their response to active training practices for stress redressal, making them perfectly apt for targeted treatment (Friedman & Berger, 1991).

6.5   CONCLUSION

Early adolescence is the period of heightened vulnerability towards changing mental, physical, and social well-being of both males and females. This study proposes that both adolescent male and female students show divergent responses to Yoga training. The findings of the study suggest that female adolescents showed a higher positive response to Yoga training compared to male adolescents. The female students reflect a higher trajectory in improving their self-compassion skills and mindfulness, along with reduced negative affect. On the other hand, male students do not reflect any marked improvements in self-compassion skills and mindfulness, along with no improvement in negative affect. The results obtained from this study suggest the power and potential of mindfulness training in bridging the gender gap in psychopathological distress. Moreover, this research provides insight into gender-tailored methodologies that regulate emotional pathways. The results suggest that the effect of mindfulness intervention may not be the same in all cases. The gender-sensitive application of mindfulness interventions in men has played a paramount role in the redressal of psychopathological symptoms. Further, the results showed that the efficacy of mindfulness training in adolescent boys increased if the practice of mindfulness intervention matches with the adoption of their normally used coping style. This work highlights that greater attention must be paid to the ways in which male adolescents express their problems related to psychology. Therefore, gender must be considered as an important variable in all Yoga training programs. With heightened focus on existing gender disparities as well as existing and evolving ways to address them, definite solutions may be available in the future for the emotional, social, and mental well-being of all individuals.

KEYWORDS

- **decision difficulty scale**
- **decision making**
- **gender-sensitive application**
- **MASS**
- **mindful-based interventions**
- **PANAS**
- **pedagogy interventions**
- **yoga training**

REFERENCES

Arch, J. J., & Craske, M. G. (2006). Mechanisms of mindfulness: Emotion regulation following a focused breathing. *Behavior Research and Therapy, 44*(12), 1849–1858. https://doi.org/10.1016/j.brat.2005.12.007.

Askari, M. S., Rutherford, C. G., Mauro, P. M., Kreski, N. T., & Keyes, K. M. (2022). Structure and trends of externalizing and internalizing psychiatric symptoms and gender differences among adolescents in the US from 1991 to 2018. *Social Psychiatry and Psychiatric Epidemiology, 57*(4), 737–748. https://doi.org/10.1007/s00127-021-02189-4.

Bask, M. (2014). Externalizing and internalizing problem behavior among Swedish adolescent boys and girls. *International Journal of Social Welfare, 24*(2), 182–192. https://doi.org/10.1111/ijsw.12106.

Bluth, K., Campo, R., Pruteanu-Malinici, S., Reams, A., Mullarkey, M., & Broderick, P. (2015). A school-based mindfulness pilot study for ethnically diverse at-risk adolescents. *Mindfulness, 7*, 90–104. https://doi.org/10.1007/s12671-014-0376-1.

Bluth, K., Roberson, P. N. E., & Girdler, S. S. (2017). Adolescent sex differences in response to a mindfulness intervention: A call for research. *Journal of Child and Family Studies, 26*(7), 1900–1914. https://doi.org/10.1007/s10826-017-0696-6.

Brewer, J. A., Elwafi, H. M., & Davis, J. H. (2013). Craving to quit: Psychological models and neurobiological mechanisms of mindfulness training as treatment for addictions. *Psychology of Addictive Behaviors, 27*(2), 366–379. https://doi.org/10.1037/a0028490.

Broderick, P. C. (2005). Mindfulness and coping with dysphoric mood: Contrasts with rumination and distraction. *Cognitive Therapy and Research, 29*(5), 501–510. https://doi.org/10.1007/s10608-005-3888-0.

Brown, M. M., Arigo, D., Wolever, R. Q., Smoski, M. J., Hall, M. H., Brantley, J. G., & Greeson, J. M. (2021). Do gender, anxiety, or sleep quality predict mindfulness-based stress reduction outcomes? *Journal of Health Psychology, 26*(13), 2656–2662. https://doi.org/10.1177/1359105320931186.

Burschka, J., Keune, P. M., Hofstadt-van Oy, U., Oschmann, P., & Kuhn, P. (2014). Mindfulness-based interventions in multiple sclerosis: Beneficial effects of Tai Chi on balance, coordination, fatigue and depression. *BMC Neurology, 14*, 165. https://doi.org/10.1186/s12883-014-0165-4.

Caron, C., & Rutter, M. (1991). Comorbidity in child psychopathology: Concepts, issues and research strategies. *Journal of Child Psychology and Psychiatry, and Allied Disciplines, 32*(7), 1063–1080. https://doi.org/10.1111/j.1469-7610.1991.tb00350.x.

Carragher, N., Krueger, R., Eaton, N., & Slade, T. (2015). Disorders without borders: Current and future directions in the meta-structure of mental disorders. *Social Psychiatry and Psychiatric Epidemiology, 50*, 339–350. https://doi.org/10.1007/s00127-014-1004-z.

Carsley, D., Khoury, B., & Heath, N. L. (2018). Effectiveness of mindfulness interventions for mental health in schools: A comprehensive meta-analysis. *Mindfulness, 9*(3), 693–707. https://doi.org/10.1007/s12671-017-0839-2.

Chambers, R., Lo, B. C. Y., & Allen, N. B. (2008). The impact of intensive mindfulness training on attentional control, cognitive style, and affect. *Cognitive Therapy and Research, 32*(3), 303–322. https://doi.org/10.1007/s10608-007-9119-0.

Chang, V. Y., Palesh, O., Caldwell, R., Glasgow, N., Abramson, M., Luskin, F., Gill, M., Burke, A., & Koopman, C. (2004). The effects of a mindfulness-based stress reduction program on stress, mindfulness self-efficacy, and positive states of mind. *Stress and Health, 20*(3), 141–147. https://doi.org/10.1002/smi.1011.

Chen, K. W., Comerford, A., Shinnick, P., & Ziedonis, D. M. (2010). Introducing qigong meditation into residential addiction treatment: A pilot study where gender makes a difference. *Journal of Alternative and Complementary Medicine (New York, N.Y.), 16*(8), 875–882. https://doi.org/10.1089/acm.2009.0443.

Cotto, J. H., Davis, E., Dowling, G. J., Elcano, J. C., Staton, A. B., & Weiss, S. R. B. (2010). Gender effects on drug use, abuse, and dependence: A special analysis of results from the national survey on drug use and health. *Gender Medicine, 7*(5), 402–413. https://doi.org/10.1016/j.genm.2010.09.004.

Davis, L. W., Lysaker, P. H., Kristeller, J. L., Salyers, M. P., Kovach, A. C., & Woller, S. (2015). Effect of mindfulness on vocational rehabilitation outcomes in stable phase schizophrenia. *Psychological Services, 12*(3), 303–312. https://doi.org/10.1037/ser 0000028.

De la Peña-Arteaga, V., Berruga-Sánchez, M., Steward, T., Martínez-Zalacaín, I., Goldberg, X., Wainsztein, A., Abulafia, C., Cardoner, N., Castro, M. N., Villarreal, M., Menchón, J. M., Guinjoan, S. M., & Soriano-Mas, C. (2021). An fMRI study of cognitive reappraisal in major depressive disorder and borderline personality disorder. *European Psychiatry, 64*(1), e56. https://doi.org/10.1192/j.eurpsy.2021.2231.

Deng, Y., Chang, L., Yang, M., Huo, M., & Zhou, R. (2016). Gender differences in emotional response: Inconsistency between experience and expressivity. *PLOS ONE, 11*, e0158666. https://doi.org/10.1371/journal.pone.0158666.

Donald, J., & Atkins, P. (2016). Mindfulness and coping with stress: Do levels of perceived stress matter? *Mindfulness, 7*, 1423–1436. https://doi.org/10.1007/s12671-016-0584-y.

Essau, C. (2002). plIn N. N. Singh, T. H. Ollendick, & A. N. Singh (Eds.), *International Perspectives on Child and Adolescent Mental Health* (Vol. 2, pp. 375–394). Elsevier. https://doi.org/10.1016/S1874-5911(02)80017-3.

Felver, J. C., & Jennings, P. A. (2016). Applications of mindfulness-based interventions in school settings: An introduction. *Mindfulness, 7*(1), 1–4. https://doi.org/10.1007/s12671-015-0478-4.

Goldin, P. R., & Gross, J. J. (2010). Effects of mindfulness-based stress reduction (MBSR) on emotion regulation in social anxiety disorder. *Emotion, 10*(1), 83–91. https://doi.org/10.1037/a0018441.

Gotink, R., Meijboom, R., Smits, M., Vernooij, M., & Hunink, M. (2016). 8-week mindfulness-based stress reduction induces brain changes similar to traditional long-term meditation practice–A systematic review. *Brain and Cognition, 108*, 32–41. https://doi.org/10.1016/j.bandc.2016.07.001.

Greenberg, M., & Harris, A. (2012). Nurturing mindfulness in children and youth: Current state of research. *Child Development Perspectives, 6*(2), 161–166. https://doi.org/10.1111/j.1750-8606.2011.00215.x.

Haydicky, J., Wiener, J., Badali, P., Milligan, K., & Ducharme, J. M. (2012). Evaluation of a mindfulness-based intervention for adolescents with learning disabilities and co-occurring ADHD and anxiety. *Mindfulness, 3*(2), 151–164. https://doi.org/10.1007/s12671-012-0089-2.

Heeren, A., & Philippot, P. (2011). Changes in ruminative thinking mediate the clinical benefits of mindfulness: Preliminary findings. *Mindfulness, 2*, 8–13. https://doi.org/10.1007/s12671-010-0037-y.

Hofmann, S. G., Grossman, P., & Hinton, D. E. (2011). Loving-Kindness and Compassion Meditation: Potential for Psychological Interventions. *Clinical Psychology Review, 31*(7), 1126–1132. https://doi.org/10.1016/j.cpr.2011.07.003.

Hölzel, B., Lazar, S., Gard, T., Schuman-Olivier, Z., Vago, D., & Ott, U. (2011). How does mindfulness meditation work? Proposing mechanisms of action from a conceptual and neural perspective. *Perspectives on Psychological Science, 6*, 537–559. https://doi.org/10.1177/1745691611419671.

Johnson, D., & Whisman, M. (2013). Gender differences in rumination: A meta-analysis. *Personality and Individual Differences, 55*, 367–374. https://doi.org/10.1016/j.paid.2013.03.019.

Kabat-Zinn, J. (2005). *Full Catastrophe Living: Using the Wisdom of Your Body and Mind to Face Stress, Pain, and Illness* (15th anniversary ed.). Delta Trade Paperback/Bantam Dell.

Katz, D., & Toner, B. (2013). A Systematic Review of Gender Differences in the Effectiveness of Mindfulness-Based Treatments for Substance Use Disorders. *Mindfulness, 4.* https://doi.org/10.1007/s12671-012-0132-3.

Kessler, R. C. (2003). Epidemiology of women and depression. *Journal of Affective Disorders, 74*(1), 5–13. https://doi.org/10.1016/s0165-0327(02)00426-3.

Kessler, R. C., Berglund, P., Demler, O., Jin, R., Merikangas, K. R., & Walters, E. E. (2005). Lifetime prevalence and age-of-onset distributions of DSM-IV disorders in the National Comorbidity Survey Replication. *Archives of General Psychiatry, 62*(6), 593–602. https://doi.org/10.1001/archpsyc.62.6.593.

Khusid, M. A., & Vythilingam, M. (2016). The emerging role of mindfulness meditation as effective self-management strategy, part 1: Clinical implications for depression, post-traumatic stress disorder, and anxiety. *Military Medicine, 181*(9), 961–968. https://doi.org/10.7205/MILMED-D-14-00677.

Kingery, J., Bodenlos, J., Peltz, J., & Sindoni, M. (2021). Dispositional mindfulness predicting psychological adjustment among college students: The role of rumination and gender. *Journal of American College Health, 71*(5), 1584–1595. https://doi.org/10.1080/07448481.2021.1943411.

Klatt, M., Harpster, K., Browne, E., White, S., & Case-Smith, J. (2013). Feasibility and preliminary outcomes for Move-Into-Learning: An arts-based mindfulness classroom intervention. *The Journal of Positive Psychology, 8*(3), 233–241. https://doi.org/10.1080/17439760.2013.779011.

Koch, K., Pauly, K., Kellermann, T., Romanczuk-Seiferth, N., Reske, M., Backes, V., Stoecker, T., Shah, N., Amunts, K., Kircher, T., Schneider, F., & Habel, U. (2007). Gender differences in the cognitive control of emotion: An fMRI study. *Neuropsychologia, 45*, 2744–2754. https://doi.org/10.1016/j.neuropsychologia.2007.04.012.

Lilienfeld, S. O. (2003). Comorbidity between and within childhood externalizing and internalizing disorders: Reflections and directions. *Journal of Abnormal Child Psychology, 31*(3), 285–291. https://doi.org/10.1023/a:1023229529866.

Malhotra, S., & Shah, R. (2015). Women and mental health in India: An overview. *Indian Journal of Psychiatry, 57*(Suppl 2), S205–S211. https://doi.org/10.4103/0019-5545.161479.

Matud, M. (2004). Gender differences in stress and coping styles. *Personality and Individual Differences, 37*, 1401–1415. https://doi.org/10.1016/j.paid.2004.01.010.

Matud, M. P., Bethencourt, J. M., & Ibáñez, I. (2015). Gender differences in psychological distress in Spain. *The International Journal of Social Psychiatry, 61*(6), 560–568. https://doi.org/10.1177/0020764014564801.

McRae, K., Gross, J. J., Weber, J., Robertson, E. R., Sokol-Hessner, P., Ray, R. D., Gabrieli, J. D. E., & Ochsner, K. N. (2012). The development of emotion regulation: An fMRI study of cognitive reappraisal in children, adolescents and young adults. *Social Cognitive and Affective Neuroscience, 7*(1), 11–22. https://doi.org/10.1093/scan/nsr093.

Mendelson, T., Greenberg, M. T., Dariotis, J. K., Gould, L. F., Rhoades, B. L., & Leaf, P. J. (2010). Feasibility and preliminary outcomes of a school-based mindfulness intervention for urban youth. *Journal of Abnormal Child Psychology, 38*(7), 985–994. https://doi.org/10.1007/s10802-010-9418-x.

Mendez, B., & Bozzay, M. (2021). Internalizing and externalizing symptoms and aggression and violence in men and women. *Aggressive Behavior, 47*(4), 439–452. https://doi.org/10.1002/ab.21962.

Menezes, C., & Bizarro, L. (2015). Effects of a brief meditation training on negative affect, trait anxiety and concentrated attention. *Paidéia, 25*, 393–401. https://doi.org/ 10.1590/1982-43272562201513.

Mitchell, J. T., Zylowska, L., & Kollins, S. H. (2015). Mindfulness meditation training for attention-deficit/hyperactivity disorder in adulthood: Current empirical support, treatment overview, and future directions. *Cognitive and Behavioral Practice, 22*(2), 172–191. https://doi.org/10.1016/j.cbpra.2014.10.002.

Nelson, L., Roots, K., Dunn, T. J., Rees, A., Hull, D. D., & Van Gordon, W. (2022). Effects of a regional school-based mindfulness programme on students' levels of wellbeing and resiliency. *International Journal of Spa and Wellness, 5*(1), 1–15. https://doi.org/10.1080/24721735.2021.1909865.

Ochsner, K., Bunge, S., Gross, J., & Gabrieli, J. (2002). Rethinking feelings: An fMRI study of the cognitive regulation of emotion. *Journal of Cognitive Neuroscience, 14*, 1215–1229. https://doi.org/10.1162/089892902760807212.

Osayomi, T., & Adegboye, O. (2016). Gender and psychological distress: A geographical perspective. *Papers in Applied Geography, 3*, 1–14. https://doi.org/10.1080/23754931.2016.1249511.

Pepping, C., Walters, B., Davis, P., & O'Donovan, A. (2016). Why do people practice mindfulness? An investigation into reasons for practicing mindfulness meditation. *Mindfulness, 7*, 542–547. https://doi.org/10.1007/s12671-016-0490-3.

Poehlmann, J., Vigna, A., Weymouth, L., Gerstein, E., Burnson, C., Zabransky, M., Lee, P., & Zahn-Waxler, C. (2015). A pilot study of contemplative practices with economically disadvantaged preschoolers: Children's empathic and self-regulatory behaviors. *Mindfulness, 7*, 46–58. https://doi.org/10.1007/s12671-015-0426-3.

Rosenfield, S. (2012). Gender and dimensions of the self: Implications for internalizing and externalizing behavior. In E. Frank (Ed.), *Gender and Its Effects on Psychopathology* (pp. 23–36). American Psychiatric Publishing, Inc.

Rosenfield, S., & Mouzon, D. (2013). Gender and mental health. In *Handbook of the Sociology of Mental Health* (pp. 277–296). https://doi.org/10.1007/978-94-007-4276-5_14.

Rosenfield, S., & Smith, D. (2010). Gender and mental health: Do men and women have different amounts or types of problems? In *A Handbook for the Study of Mental Health: Social Contexts, Theories, and Systems* (pp. 256–267).

Sallis, H., Szekely, E., Neumann, A., Jolicoeur-Martineau, A., van IJzendoorn, M., Hillegers, M., Greenwood, C. M. T., Meaney, M. J., Steiner, M., Tiemeier, H., Wazana, A., Pearson, R. M., & Evans, J. (2019). General psychopathology, internalizing and externalizing in children and functional outcomes in late adolescence. *Journal of Child Psychology and Psychiatry, 60*(11), 1183–1190. https://doi.org/10.1111/jcpp.13067.

Saluja, G., Iachan, R., Scheidt, P. C., Overpeck, M. D., Sun, W., & Giedd, J. N. (2004). Prevalence of and risk factors for depressive symptoms among young adolescents. *Archives of Pediatrics & Adolescent Medicine, 158*(8), 760–765. https://doi.org/10.1001/archpedi.158.8.760.

Sciutto, M. J., Veres, D. A., Marinstein, T. L., Bailey, B. F., & Cehelyk, S. K. (2021). Effects of a school-based mindfulness program for young children. *Journal of Child and Family Studies, 30*(6), 1516–1527. https://doi.org/10.1007/s10826-021-01955-x.

Sedlmeier, P., Loße, C., & Quasten, L. (2018). Psychological effects of meditation for healthy practitioners: An update. *Mindfulness, 9,* 371–387. https://doi.org/10.1007/s12671-017-0780-4.

Segal, Z. V., Williams, J. M. G., & Teasdale, J. D. (2002). *Mindfulness-Based Cognitive Therapy for Depression: A New Approach to Preventing Relapse* (pp. xiv, 351). Guilford Press.

Singh, N. N., Lancioni, G. E., Karazsia, B. T., Winton, A. S. W., Singh, J., & Wahler, R. G. (2014). Shenpa and compassionate abiding: Mindfulness-based practices for anger and aggression by individuals with schizophrenia. *International Journal of Mental Health and Addiction, 12*(2), 138–152. https://doi.org/10.1007/s11469-013-9469-7.

Tang, Y.-Y., Hölzel, B. K., & Posner, M. I. (2015). The neuroscience of mindfulness meditation. *Nature Reviews Neuroscience, 16*(4), 213–225. https://doi.org/10.1038/nrn3916.

Teasdale, J. D., Segal, Z. V., Williams, J. M. G., Ridgeway, V. A., Soulsby, J. M., & Lau, M. A. (2000). Prevention of relapse/recurrence in major depression by mindfulness-based cognitive therapy. *Journal of Consulting and Clinical Psychology, 68*(4), 615–623. https://doi.org/10.1037/0022-006X.68.4.615.

Thoits, P. A. (1991). Gender differences in coping with emotional distress. In J. Eckenrode (Ed.), *The Social Context of Coping* (pp. 107–138). Springer US. https://doi.org/10.1007/978-1-4899-3740-7_6.

Turner, R. J., & Lloyd, D. A. (1995). Lifetime traumas and mental health: The significance of cumulative adversity. *Journal of Health and Social Behavior, 36*(4), 360–376. https://doi.org/10.2307/2137325.

van de Weijer-Bergsma, E., Langenberg, G., Brandsma, R., Oort, F. J., & Bögels, S. M. (2014). The effectiveness of a school-based mindfulness training as a program to prevent stress in elementary school children. *Mindfulness, 5*(3), 238–248. https://doi.org/10.1007/s12671-012-0171-9.

van Vugt, M. K., Hitchcock, P., Shahar, B., & Britton, W. (2012). The effects of mindfulness-based cognitive therapy on affective memory recall dynamics in depression: A mechanistic model of rumination. *Frontiers in Human Neuroscience, 6,* 257. https://doi.org/10.3389/fnhum.2012.00257.

Viertiö, S., Kiviruusu, O., Piirtola, M., Kaprio, J., Korhonen, T., Marttunen, M., & Suvisaari, J. (2019). Gender and psychological distress: Contribution of work-family balance. *European Journal of Public Health, 29*(Supplement_4), ckz187.116. https://doi.org/10.1093/eurpub/ckz187.116.

Volanen, S., Lassander, M., Hankonen, N., Santalahti, P., Hintsanen, M., Simonsen, N., Raevuori, A., Mullola, S., Vahlberg, T., But, A., & Suominen, S. (2016). Healthy learning mind—A school-based mindfulness and relaxation program: A study protocol for a cluster randomized controlled trial. *BMC Psychology, 4*(1), 35. https://doi.org/10.1186/s40359-016-0142-3.

Wall, R. (2005). Tai chi and mindfulness-based stress reduction in a Boston public middle school. *Journal of Pediatric Health Care: Official Publication of National Association of Pediatric Nurse Associates & Practitioners, 19,* 230–237. https://doi.org/10.1016/j.pedhc.2005.02.006.

Weinstein, N., Brown, K., & Ryan, R. (2009). A multi-method examination of the effects of mindfulness on stress attribution, coping, and emotional well-being. *Journal of Research in Personality, 43*, 374–385. https://doi.org/10.1016/j.jrp.2008.12.008.

Willner, C. J., Gatzke-Kopp, L. M., & Bray, B. C. (2016). The dynamics of internalizing and externalizing comorbidity across the early school years. *Development and Psychopathology, 28*(4 Pt 1), 1033–1052. https://doi.org/10.1017/S0954579416000687.

Yu, M. (2017). The effects of mindfulness on self-rumination, self-reflection, and depressive symptoms: A research proposal. *Behavioral Sciences Undergraduate Journal, 3*, 1–7. https://doi.org/10.29173/bsuj399.

Zeng, X., Chiu, C. P. K., Wang, R., Oei, T. P. S., & Leung, F. Y. K. (2015). The effect of loving-kindness meditation on positive emotions: A meta-analytic review. *Frontiers in Psychology, 6*. https://www.frontiersin.org/articles/10.3389/fpsyg.2015.01693.

CHAPTER 7

Impact of Yoga and Meditation with Mudras in Building Quality of Life

SHEELU SAGAR,[1] ROHIT RASTOGI,[2] ISHWAR V. BASAVARADDI,[3] and VIKAS GARG[4]

[1]*Amity International Business School, Amity University, Noida, Uttar Pradesh, India*

[2]*Depertment of Computer Science and Engineering, ABES Engineering College, Ghaziabad, Uttar Pradesh, India*

[3]*Morarji Desai National Institute of Yoga, Ministry of AYUSH, New Delhi, India*

[4]*Amity Business School, Amity University, Noida, Uttar Pradesh, India*

ABSTRACT

In the wake of the difficult time of the COVID-19 epidemic, the worldwide human population of the modern era has entered into a phase of transformation and optimism. Today, there is a growing demand and attention towards enhancing alternative solutions and workable practices to ensure the good and effective functioning of biological organs, and to maintain balanced physical and mental health throughout a lifetime at a very preliminary level.

Yoga and meditation have attracted the attention of the masses; however, there is a paucity of research regarding the assessment of factors of meditation and Yoga such as:

Yoga and Meditation: Past and Present Evidence. Sachi Nandan Mohanty, Rabindra Kumar Pradhan, & Sugyanta Priyadarshini (Eds.)

- Building mentally and physically strong employees who are resilient to stressful situations in their workplace.
- Through the practice of Yoga and meditation, an individual can improve mental clarity, work capacity, and significantly enhance the quality of life with mental alertness.

This manuscript provides an overview of the traditional Indian style of Mudrā Meditation collected from various books and articles written by Yoga experts and empiricists. The objective is to provide insight to modern-age mankind who are interested in keeping themselves fit, spirituality, and Mudra Meditation.

7.1 INTRODUCTION

7.1.1 PATANJALI YOGA

One of the seven most revered *Rishis*/sages of India and the founder of Yoga philosophy and practices was Maharishi Patanjali. His physical existence was more than 4,000 years ago. Maharishi Patanjali explained in his Patanjali Yoga Sutras, the classic text on Yoga, how the human physical body, physiological functions of organs, and mental health can remain in perfect condition, and the length of life can be optimized to 100 years of age (Vivekananda, 2015). The young and aged working people who engage themselves in Yoga and meditation practice are reported to show better performance at work and have lower stress levels. Such employees enjoy and experience a joyful life by having sound functioning of biological organs and mental health (Bhandari et al., 2010).

7.1.2 MUDRA SCIENCE

According to Saraswati et al. (1996), the fingers of the hand have the ability to do some amazing feats besides their common functions such as eating, holding, and writing. The coordination for every task is controlled by hands and fingers. There are hundreds of *Mudras*, symbolic gestures performed by hands and fingers in the science of Yoga and Meditation. Scientifically, the mudras are designed to enhance body energy, restore energy potential, and provide strength for wellbeing. In Hinduism, other parts of the human body like the head and eyes also symbolize different aspects of life with different poses and movements as *Mudras*. In Yoga, each posture has a unique *Mudrā*, and certain breathing techniques are also considered *Mudras* that are used to achieve the best results from within the human body (Sadhguru, 2015) (*please refer to* Table 7.1).

TABLE 7.1 Mudrās–Certain Hand Gestures

SL. No.	Mudrā	Importance
1.	*Vyaghra Mudrā*	To give good facial exercise
2.	*Simha Mudrā*	To give good facial exercise
3.	*Chin Mudrā*	Required for effective Pranayama
4.	*Chainmaya*	Required for effective Pranayama
5.	*Aadi Mudrā*	Required for effective Pranayama

7.1.3 PROTOCOLS FOR DOING MUDRA

The *Mudras* can be accomplished simply while seated in a straight-backed chair or while meditating in the lotus position. It is required to wash hands prior to *Mudra*'s practice and massage hands together 5–7 times while holding them in front of your navel to promote energy flow. Place both hands on knees in the shape of bowls, with thumbs of both the hands touching index finger, to do *Dhyana Mudras* (Sharma, 1995). For a thorough description of *Mudras*, please see Figure 7.1 through 10 below (*Gayatri Maha Vigyan*, 1996, p. 87).

Dhyan Mudra (Meditation) is helpful for brain disorders like insomnia, memory loss, and attention problems. Additionally, it benefits in spiritual growth. People with good health can engage in this *Mudra*. This *Mudra* has been depicted on numerous monuments and idols throughout India. To practice, join the tips of the thumb and index finger and chant the *Vedic mantra Gayatri* during the early morning hours as shown in Figure 7.1.

Prithvi Mudra or (Earth Mudra) can be practiced by joining the tips of the thumb and ring finger together and chanting a *Vedic mantra*. It is beneficial for people suffering from physical and mental weakness due to low immunity. For best results, the practice should be done one hour before sunrise. This aids in the treatment of physical and mental weakness. A sick person gets rejuvenated, while a healthy person becomes more cheerful and stronger than before (as seen in Figure 7.2).

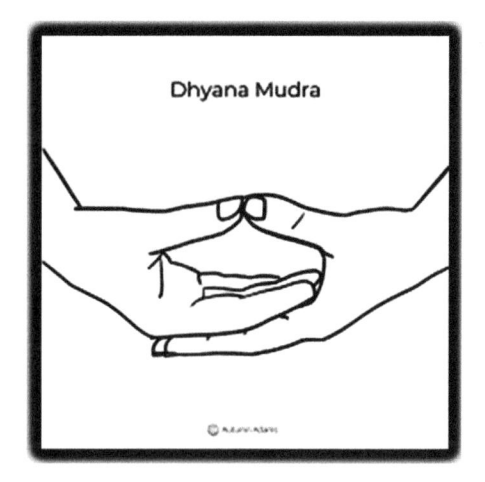

FIGURE 7.1 *Dhyan.*

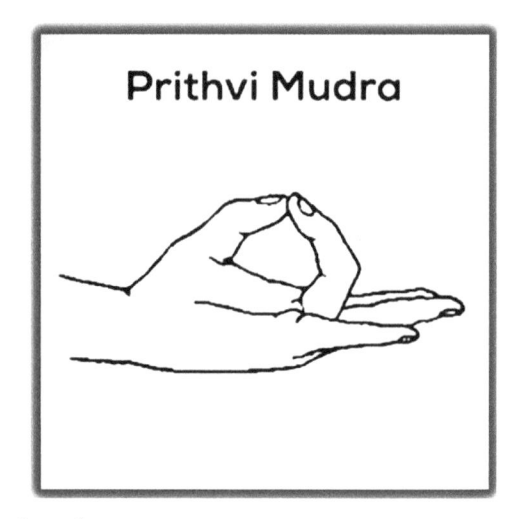

FIGURE 7.2 Earth *mudra.*

Vayu Mudra or (Air *Mudra*; as per Figure 7.3) is very useful for patients suffering from diseases like inflammation or pain in joints, arthritis, gout, loss of muscle function (paralysis), Parkinson's syndrome, and issues related with blood circulation. To practice this mudra, the patient should sit or lie in a comfortable position, press as much as possible at the base of the thumb (the mount of Venus) with the index finger, and keep the thumb on the first or index finger to lock it. This *mudra* can be practiced any time during the day, chanting of *Vedic mantra* is recommended for a better healing process. While receiving medical therapy, the practice of *Vayu Mudra* is quite beneficial and provides rapid relief from pain.

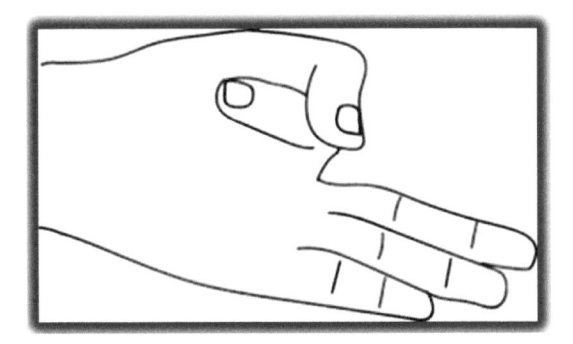

FIGURE 7.3 Air *mudra.*

Shunya Mudra (also known as Zero or Sky *Mudra*; Figure 7.4). Similar to *Vayu Mudra*, it is performed by putting the middle finger on the base of the thumb and pressing the tip of the middle finger with the thumb, as indicated in the illustration. This mudra can be practiced with chanting of *Gayatri mantra* during morning, afternoon, and evening hours for 30–45 minutes. The results are significant in the treatment of ear-related illnesses such as pain in ears, hearing loss, infection inside the ears, etc.

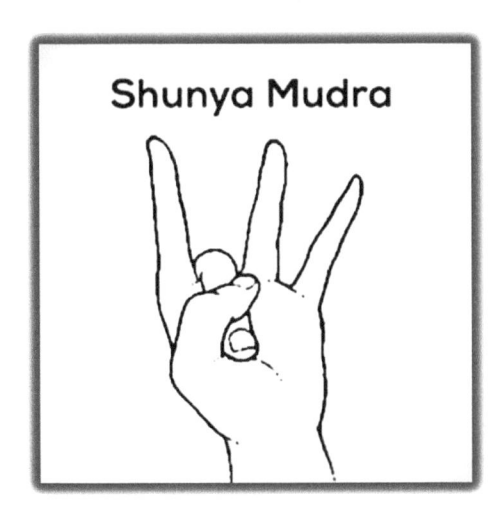

FIGURE 7.4 Sky *mudra.*

Varun Mudra (Water *Mudra*) is practiced by bringing the tips of the little finger closer to the thumb, pressing together as exhibited in Figure 7.5. The *Varun Mudra* can be practiced by patients with illnesses related to blood impurity, skin problems, and excess water retention inside the body. For the best results, *Varun Mudra* should be practiced while sitting in a relaxed position facing east, one hour before and after sunrise, while chanting the *Gayatri Mantra*. Results of this *Mudra* can be seen within two weeks as it brings luster to the skin, making it smooth and radiant.

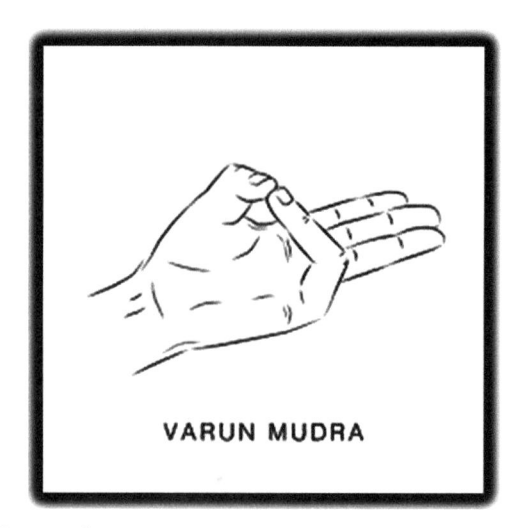

VARUN MUDRA

FIGURE 7.5 Water *mudra*.

Hridhay Mudra or (Heart *Mudra*) is useful for curing chronic respiratory diseases like asthma as well as heart issues like irregular heartbeats, angina, blockages of arteries, and heart valve disorders.

For practicing Heart *Mudra*, the index finger should be placed between the thumb's point at the base of the thumb and touching the tips of the middle finger and ring finger, as indicated in Figure 7.6. *Hridhay mudra* should be practiced with both hands while sitting in a comfortable position facing the eastern direction in the morning at sunrise. Chanting the *OM mantra* or *Gayathri mantra* gives excellent results in curing heart ailments.

Ling Mudra (Regeneration Phallic *Mudra*) (as seen in Figure 7.7): Interlock the fingers of both hands, keeping the left thumb raised (it is surrounded by the right thumb and index finger). Regular practice of *Ling*

Mudra provides very good resistance against congestion in the chest, viral infections due to seasonal changes, cures lung infections due to phlegm, etc. The body warms up when *Ling Mudra* is performed. One can practice it for 20 minutes in the morning.

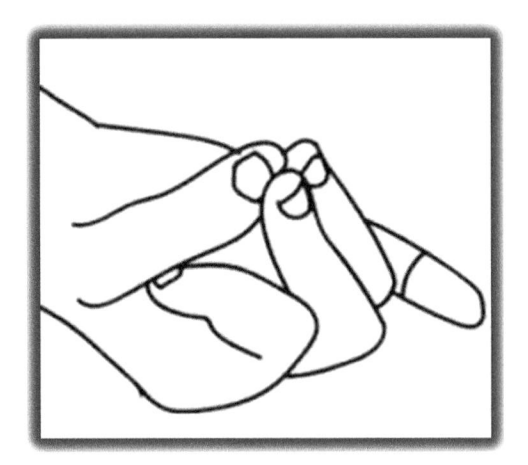

FIGURE 7.6 Heart *mudra.*

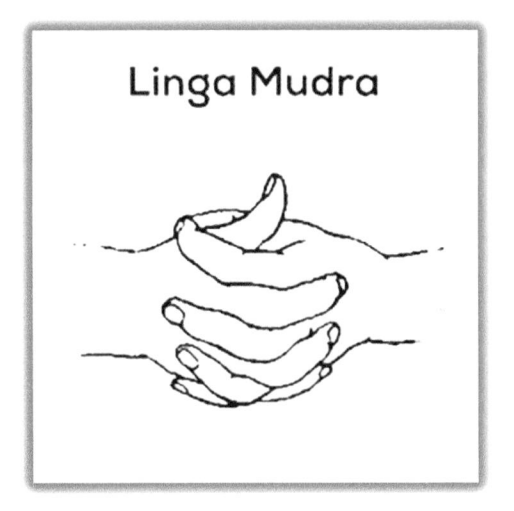

FIGURE 7.7 *Ling mudra.*

As shown in Figure 7.8, *Praan Mudra* (Life *Mudra*) is useful in the treatment of eye infections, physical and mental weakness, and a lack of vital forces in the body. To practice it, sit in a comfortable position and use both hands: keep the index and middle fingers straight while touching the tips of the little finger and ring fingers with the tip of the thumb, and chant the *Gayatri mantra*. This can be practiced every day for a minimum of 15 minutes at sunrise. This Life *Mudra* gives a glow and brightness to the skin, body, face, and eyes.

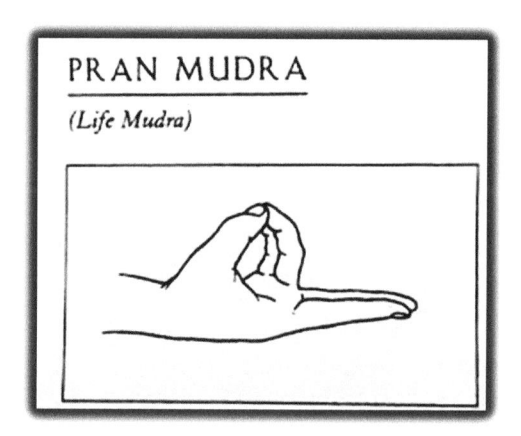

FIGURE 7.8   Life *mudra.*

(As per Figure 7.9) *Surya Mudra* (Sun *Mudra*) helps in lowering excessive levels of blood cholesterol and body fat. It should be practiced while reciting the *Gayatri Mantra* during early morning. To make this mudra, place the ring finger at the base of the thumb and gently press the thumb down, as shown in Figure 7.9. It can be practiced every day for 30 minutes for a minimum of two months to see a significant difference in the results.

As depicted in Figure 7.10, *Apan Mudra* or (Digestion *Mudra*) is made by touching the tips of the thumb, middle finger, and ring finger while keeping the other fingers straight. This can be practiced any time during the day. This mudra helps to cure constipation and enhances digestion.

7.2   OBJECTIVE

To study impact of yoga and meditation on quality of life.

7.3 METHODOLOGY

Qualitative descriptive method is followed in this study.

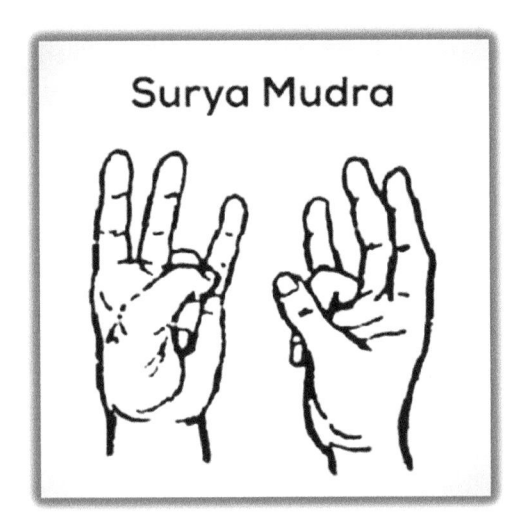

FIGURE 7.9 Sun *mudra*.

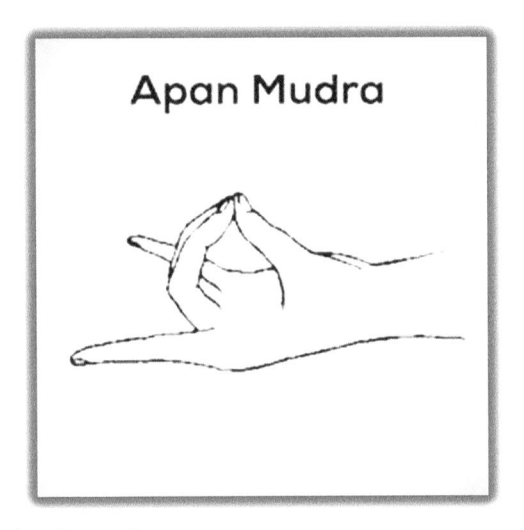

FIGURE 7.10 Digestion *mudra*.

7.4 REVIEW OF LITERATURE

7.4.1 *SCIENCE OF YOGA*

According to Broad (2012), yoga and meditation are traditional Indian practices that date back 5,000 years. Ever since then, Yoga has been adopted to lower blood pressure, reduce stress, improve coordination and flexibility of muscles, develop concentration power, promote good sleep, and aid digestion. It has also been used as an alternative therapy for various diseases including cancer, diabetes, asthma, and heart ailments (Isath et al., 2023). As per (Halappa, 2023), excessive exercise sometimes prevents athletes from continuing their sports journey due to the generation of disorders or injuries related to musculoskeletal and mental disturbances; however, Yoga practices are a safe method for sports players and prevent musculoskeletal injuries.

Yoga *mudra asanas* consist of 84 different types, including postures for standing, sitting, backbends, front bends, twists, and curves, etc. (Svatmarama, 1992). Each posture is helpful in revitalizing and reviving the muscles and organs of the human body systems. Yoga is indeed a powerful tool for human resource development and total quality management. It deals with the practical aspects of Yoga discipline in detail, in a very lucid manner. Yoga works as an element for Stress Reduction Mindfulness-Based programs, with each element being a combination of precise breathing techniques for each physical posture and finishing the program with specific meditation. They are meant to maintain perfect physical health, mental fitness, and a happy spiritual body (Pandurang et al., 2017).

Yoga has the potency to establish a socio-cultural network portrayed with purity, peace, and prosperity (Vivekananda, 2015). It was predicted by the visionary Pandit Sri Ram Sharma Acharya (Sharma, 1990) that Yoga will become a global force in the future and will contribute to rebuilding and reshaping many global events. Researcher (Barooah, 2023) states that slow muscle weakness with degeneration in the cardiac and respiratory tract is accompanied by emotional disturbance and mental unrest in the patient. However, introducing meditation and Yoga at any stage of the disease as an add-on therapy helps to prevent complications and improve the quality of life for the patient. The science of Yoga was advanced from the Eastern 'Sankhya philosophy' in ancient India (Figure 7.11).

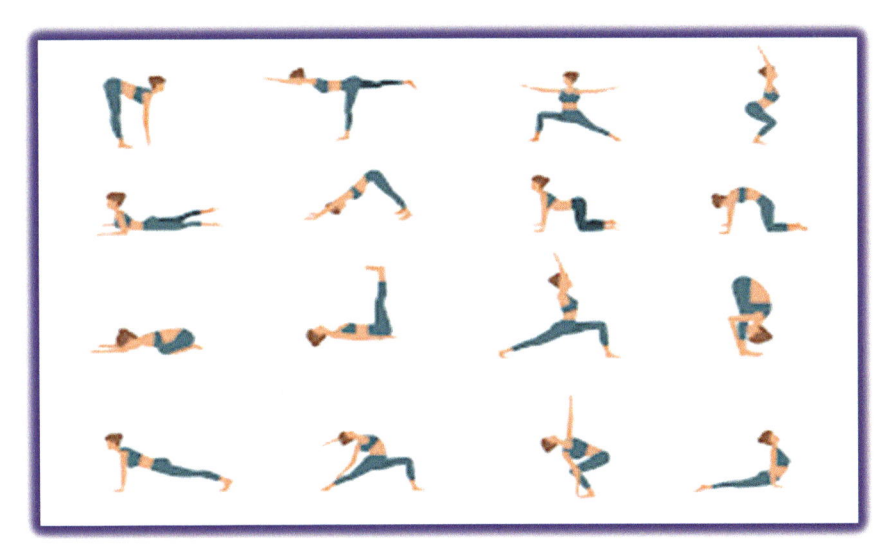

FIGURE 7.11 Common yoga poses.

Source: Reprinted from Vecteezy. Workout Vectors by Vecteezy. https://www.vecteezy.com/free-vector/workout

7.5 RESULTS AND DISCUSSIONS

7.5.1 REVOLVING ENERGIES

According to Aruchunan et al. (2023), Yogic breathing (*Pranayama*) and meditation techniques (YBMT) are the most essential elements of Yoga. Recent studies carried out by the authors have attempted to understand the effects of breathing through either the left or the right nostril and the functioning of the brain in verifying the Yoga concepts enunciated in the ancient texts as well as those described by present-day neurology. Every person is a combination of two fundamental energies. The nostrils reveal details regarding the state of the energy supplying the body and intellect, regardless of sex. According to Sagar et al. (2022), the left nostril is linked to an inward, nurturing energy that is feminine in nature. The energy in the left nostril, which is linked to the Shakti or latent power of consciousness as well as to sustenance and replenishment, is cooling like the moon. The right nostril is linked to male characteristics including impulses that move outward. The right nostril's energy is warming like the sun and is linked to

Shiva's dynamic aspect of consciousness as well as expansion and growth. According to Sagar et al. (2022), thinking connected with the left nostril tends to be intuitive and introspective, whereas thinking related to the right nostril tends to be rational and logical. The realm of these two fundamental forms of human energy encompasses all actions. Examples of activities that will thrive when the left nostril is prominent include digging the dirt, taking medications, establishing gardens, visiting shrines, entering residence, investing safely, performing arts, or chanting mantras (Rastogi et al., 2022). While one is most likely to engage in these activities when the right nasal passage is active when exercising, driving a car, prescribing medications, generating a good appetite, carrying out physically demanding tasks, arguing, motivating others, falling asleep (warmed by an inner fire), and carrying out any difficult or harsh action (Rastogi et al., 2022).

7.5.2 MEDITATION FOR PERSONAL AND SPIRITUAL GROWTH

According to Sagar et al. (2022), meditation is a means of letting go of one's preoccupations and complexes and living more fully in the present. One becomes better able to concentrate on the task at hand without distraction, emotion, and daydreaming – one becomes more effective in carrying out the tasks of everyday life. The practice of meditation with calmness, without hurry, helps to discipline the mind to develop inner strength and raise the level of concentration.

The researcher (Rahmani et al., 2023) finds that by following meditation, one not only gains spiritual development, but there are many more benefits with regular practice. To live a simple, optimum, balanced everyday life is achieved. External things do not simply influence the devotee (Sadhak) due to the development of tolerance power. A person begins to respect and maintain the dignity of other human beings, including plants and animals, by cultivating positive traits in mind, finally experiencing true freedom.

One learns to neutrally observe their thoughts, memories, emotions, and desires and becomes a detached witness to the spectacular activities taking place in their mind and personality. As one learns to watch each thought without judgment, evaluation, interest, or aversion, they become free from all ailments and enjoy the pure state of freedom.

The impact of meditation on human philosophy and saintly development of an individual is real when it is supported by its clear, positive effects and when we can readily exhibit increased comprehension and unconstrained functional capacities. The level of consciousness and understanding can be known by how well our lifestyle aligns with the current circumstances that exist, just like the quality of fruits a tree produces depends on its traits and vitality. Our regular levels of consciousness and mental states directly affect what we do and how we feel. The impact of meditation on human philosophy and saintly development of an individual is real when it is supported by its clear, positive effects and when we can readily exhibit increased comprehension and unconstrained functional capacities. The level of consciousness and understanding can be known by how well our lifestyle aligns with the current circumstances that exist, just like the quality of fruits a tree produces depends on its traits and vitality. Our regular levels of consciousness and mental states directly affect what we do and how we feel.

As the awareness for spirituality grows, life becomes more harmonious and fulfilling. Frequent demonstration of superior functional abilities as an empowered soul with a clear and firm mindset is seen. Chances of fewer false impressions, invalid beliefs, and illusions exist, and such things are dealt with more skillfully. Higher skills call for higher challenges to remain in that flow channel (Ganesan et al., 2022) states that although meditation makes the mind practice to learn to focus attention on an object or experience. If a person continues to display traits of hazy states of perception, lack of logical skill, habitual personality illnesses, constant desire for dissatisfaction, and other such limitations, then a person is not spiritually awake (Joshi et al., 2022). If results are not showing up in a positive light in everyday circumstances, then one should acknowledge the problems and the need to solve them. No wonder even if such people say they 'love God' and consider themselves to be committed to spiritual growth or holy.

For people suffering from life-threatening illnesses, meditation is a very useful therapeutic therapy. Meditation enables one to recover truly with a transcendent dimension and restores one's connection to a mysterious superpower according to their faith and religion. This cures the illness and diminishes the fear of death from the horizon of thought (Bormolini et al., 2022).

7.6 THE ENERGY CENTER OF HUMAN BODY

Sushumna Nadi is in the core of the spinal cord, the channel through which energy flows. It extends from the base of the spinal cord to the forehead center (Vigyan, 2023). *Sushumna Nadi* is considered the wheel of life, remaining unaltered despite the powerful energies swirling around it.

One of the most common health problems is low back pain. According to Singh et al. (2023); and Sethi et al. (2023), when the energy pathways in the spinal cord become imbalanced due to the wind element, described in Ayurveda and ancient texts as '*Vata Dosha*,' it can cause back pain. Releasing the blocked energy through different approaches of traditional healing systems such as meditation and Pranayama has been found to be effective in treating low back pain disorders.

The mind naturally begins to merge into the energy of the central channel as deep breathing is practiced continually during meditation. Upon reaching this level, an even and balanced flow of air begins from both nostrils (Kumar et al., 2023). Beeler et al. (2023) describe that as soon as concentration is well caught on the balanced flow of energy, the individual experiences a deep sense of joy with an illuminated mind. It is said that the feeling of joy manifests for no reason. The energy generated is useful to a great degree for discovery within, but it does not have a use for materialistic activity; rather, the inner joyfulness pervades, and interest in the activities of the world fades away from the '*Sadhak*' (one who practices). The inner mind becomes self-radiant with joy. Since the mind is in a state of inner joy, it does not bother or depend on worldly success or failure. When seen from the meditator's perspective, an even state of mind is achieved as well as detachment, and fascinating worldly affairs seem less distinguished. The mind is still, more like a spinning top that gives the appearance of being motionless to an onlooker. After some time, however, the focus returns to worldly things, and an active interest in external concerns is revived with even more passion. However, the allure of the meditative experience keeps the subdued mood constantly content and happy for no apparent reason (Shavir, 2023; Sagar et al., 2022).

7.7   AGNI SARA

Agni Sara is when continuous powerful practice of *Pranayama* stimulates to awaken the inner dormant energy. It focuses on the solar plexus nerves in the surrounding region of the sympathetic system. This methodical practice, after some time, strengthens the digestive, circulatory, and nervous system, stimulates elimination, improves health, and increases energy levels (Kalavade et al., 2023; Sagar et al., 2022). You take the position supporting the weight of your upper torso with your arm, breathe smoothly and evenly through your nostrils, keeping the inhalation and exhalation equal. When you have established a baseline breath, push your abdominal well inward as you exhale, as if you were trying to touch the spine with your navel. Continue exhaling until your abdomen is concave and your lungs are empty. Without pausing, begin inhaling while slowly relaxing the abdominal muscles. Do not push the muscles outward, simply relax them. At the end of the inhalation, begin exhaling again without pushing, repeat until you have reached a comfortable capacity (Surya et al., 2022).

7.8 WHEN TO PRACTICE

Your stomach must be empty when you perform *Agni Sara*, and as such, the best time is early morning just before meals. It takes about five minutes. You can do it at work if you can find a private space; just choose the time before you go for lunch and take those moments for yourself. Experience and find the best time. Start with 5 to 10 repetitions and work gradually up to 20 to 30 at each session. The first stage of *Agni Sara* involves squeezing and releasing the abdominal muscles, as described above. The second step involves the application of root lock. This requires contracting the anal and urinary sphincter muscles and holding the contraction. As per Juniartha et al. (2023), the muscles used for the root lock can be strengthened by the practice of *Aswin Mudra* – slowly and smoothly contracting the anal and urinary muscles (the muscles used for controlling defecation and urine) along with the muscles of the buttocks. Hold the maximum concentration for three to five seconds and then release it smoothly (Rastogi et al., 2021).

7.9 AN OVERVIEW OF PRAYERS

Prayer or *Prarthana* helps in inculcating a positive attitude in our approach towards life. The happenings in life never permit smooth sailing. At such difficult times, it is only the power of prayers which can help us not to lose sight of our goal. According to Dunner et al. (1996), elderly women with hip surgery, having strong religious faith got back on their feet faster than non-believers. *Prarthana* develops conviction, and conviction helps us not to lose our mental balance in tense moments when we are about to achieve our goal. It gives us the strength to snatch victory from the jaws of defeat (Sagar et al., 2022). According to Anwari et al. (2023), variable intensity with daily five times prayers has a significant positive relationship with the variable of stress level. The study by Gist, Ferdik et al. (2023) showed that individuals with resilient power are able to cope better with trauma and other adverse circumstances in life. The author team found that correctional officers are exposed to stressors in their workplace causing harm to them mentally. Hence, they were given treatment with prayer and meditation; the outcome of the experiment showed improvement in their mental health. Turcan (2023) argues that during prayer, names used do not actually name the essence of God or his presence as an ontic. Stern & Kohn (2023) claimed that prayer and schools have an uncomfortable history together. Prayer in school was a useful 'test' to understand different aspects of schooling. The authors did empirical research on prayer among students at school for developing particularly new terms for spirituality and theories.

According to Rastogi et al. (2021), prayers help to open hearts to the superconscious, and one begins to feel freer and happier, which speeds up recovery from a diseased state. Prayers are, in essence, about how to enjoy living, not how to avoid dying. It is an effective way of managing stress and leading a better quality of life. Prayers banish isolation and promote inner healing in more ways than one. Like meditation, prayer also reduces stress by calming the mind, lowers blood pressure, and reduces the hormone cortisol causing stress. Resting heart rate and respiration rates are also reduced. When we want something from life, the first thing that happens is that we become aware of the need. Then, we desire it. When we desire it, we start looking for it. Then, we communicate our desire to others – those who can give it to us or those who can help us get it. We ask for it and keep asking for it. Prathana and Prayer both have the first three letters in common. Prayer means intensely, something which is intensely desirable. Therefore, we pray for it and call it Prathana or prayer. How does it work? When we intensely desire something, we are also prepared to work for it. When we do prayer daily, it keeps our desire alive. It keeps us abreast of our goals every day, every time, so that we do not miss any opportunity that will take us closer to our goal, which comes our way. It generates alertness.

7.10 *MUDRĀ*: THE CONTROL PANEL

Deshlahra et al. (2023) says that Yoga involves the use of various finger and hand gestures (*Mudra*), which are typically performed while reclining in the poses of *Padmasana* or *Vajrasana*. *Pranayama* is the term for the yogic breathing process. Different organs and bodily components are stimulated and activated by each mudra creation. *Mudras* have an impact on the flow of energy and can assist in altering a person's mood when combined with breathing exercises. Harmonizing the physical body with mind and emotions can be well accomplished with the practice of asana, Pranayama, mudra, bandha, and meditation.

There are specific asanas for young practitioners to establish celibacy by controlling one of the most powerful urges bestowed on mankind and sublimating it for enlightenment. The following asanas are known to bestow self-control, celibacy, and tranquility as the sensual motivation in thought and action is checked to a great extent:

- *Siddhasna* (accomplished sitting posture);
- *Svastikasana* (auspicious posture);
- *Simhasana* (lion posture);
- *Virasana* (martial posture);
- *Guptasana* (concealed posture);
- *Sarvangasana* (inverted posture);
- *Matsyendrasna* (full spine twist posture);
- Gupta *Gorakshasana* (back-lying Gorksha's posture);
- *Utkatasana* (squatting posture);
- *Kukkutasna* (cock posture);
- *Vrkshasana* (tree posture);
- *Salabhasan* (locust posture); and
- Yoga *mudra* (yoga-gesture posture).

These *asanas* help in the upward channelization of the sexual energy and its sublimation. For more details, you may like to study Authentic Yoga–The Ancient Science and Philosophy of *Gheranda Samhita*, by Swami Samarpananda Saraswati, Munger, India, published by the Bihar School of Yoga, 1999.

7.11   BEGINNING PRACTICE OF MEDITATION AND YOGA

Zok et al. (2023) states that dynamic forms of Yoga combined with mindfulness techniques can be applied effectively over a 12-week period to reduce a significant amount of sleep problems and stress in cancer patients. It also contributes to improving their well-being; however, a basic protocol must be followed:

Breathe in and out through your diaphragm, feeling the sides of your lower ribcage stretch and tighten as you inhale and exhale while sitting upright with your eyes closed. Your stomach should be relaxed and naturally move as you breathe. Breathe 5 to 10 times, pretending and experiencing that your whole body is getting purified with the effects of each breath.

Focus your attention on the sensation of breath touching your active nostril and concentrate on the sound of the breath moving in and out as if it were only coming from the active side. Continue to focus as you sense your breath moving along this mainstream until it becomes steady with an audible sound with each inhale and exhale. The sound of 'So' is inhaling air and 'Haam' is exhaling air.

Let your ideas come and go without focusing on or giving them any attention and energy. Focus attention on the breath in the passive nostril after focusing on the breath in the active nostril until you can maintain your concentration without being distracted, allowing your nervous system to calm down. Stay here longer than on the active side. The nostril might open if the focus is maintained. Try to combine these two streams at the end to form a single, central stream. When inhaling, imagine that your breath is flowing all the way up to the '*Agya Chakra*,' which is located between the eyebrows. Breathe in and out along the mainstream before you begin to unwind your mind. This practice serves as an introduction to forming Sushumna breathing.

Sit for as long as you wish, gradually focusing only on the music and the breath, and letting your body, breathing, and mind become relaxed. Using the *so-ham mantra* is an effective way to instantly feel calm and energized.

7.12   NOVELTIES

Through this chapter, all authors have attempted to provide awareness of the impact of Yoga and meditation, along with the practice of *mudra* and *Pranayama*, on human health. The authors' desire to learn how to enhance the quality of life may be regarded as novel during the COVID-19 pandemic, when the general population is eager to adopt alternative interventions for sound physical and mental health.

7.13 RECOMMENDATIONS

It is recommended for:

1. **Emotional and Spiritual Restoration:**
   i. The regular practice of relaxation, Asanas, aerobics, and meditation supports calmness, clarity, and self-awareness, and reduces confusion and anxiety. This may well be the most valuable of all possible approaches for strengthening your immune system and ensuring good health and a sense of well-being.

2. **Immunity of the Mind:**
   i. The human body is governed by the immense creative power that lies at our source. Yoga helps us to locate the control switch that manipulates the body's immense intelligence and counteracts aging. Long before you grow old, you can prevent such losses by consciously activating your mind and remaining youthful. Meditation is the classic technique for mastering the technology of taking your awareness into the region of timelessness at will and perfecting every moment.
   ii. The next level is deep meditation (*Dhyana*). In this state of uninterrupted concentration, where one no longer requires the external stimuli of the earlier phases, one learns to forget oneself. *Samadhi*, the ultimate state of self-awareness in which the act of meditation and the objects of the meditation merge, may be attained by the yogi. *Samadhi*, according to those who have attained it, is the happiest experience of their lives.

7.14 FUTURE RESEARCH DIRECTIONS AND LIMITATIONS

Future research should have a stronger interventional research design. Yoga, meditation, *Pranayama*, and *Mudra* are now being practiced everywhere across the globe; however, they are being practiced without the necessary understanding and awareness.

7.15 CONCLUSION

Yoga and Meditation, as an ancient Indian cultural heritage, show the way of a 'welfare formula' for 21st-century youths. It helps to create a wonderful body (the temple of the mind). *Pranayama* and *Mudra* help to transform a common man into a superhuman being.

KEYWORDS

- *dhyana*
- **meditation**
- *mudra*
- *pranayama*
- **quality of life**
- **welfare formula**
- **yoga**

REFERENCES

Anwari, M., Agustini, M., & Wibowo, A. (2023). The relationship between the intensity of the five times of prayer to the stress of the elderly in Pekauman Village. *Jurnal Eduhealth, 14*(1), 42–50.

Aruchunan, M., & Nivethitha, L. (2023). Yogic breathing and meditation techniques on lung functions in healthy individuals: A pilot study. *Journal of Indian System of Medicine, 11*(1), 21.

Barooah, R. (2023). Role of applied physiology in management of muscular dystrophy by yoga and meditation. https://doi.org/10.5772/intechopen.109607.

Beeler, D. M., & Jonker, J. L. (2023). Reiki practice and the body as mediator for religiosity. In A. P. Araujo, & K. W. Irwin (Eds.), *The Routledge Handbook of Religion and the Body*, pp. 351–360, Publisher Routeldge.

Bhavanani, A. (2017). Role of yoga in prevention and management of lifestyle disorders. *Yoga Mimamsa, 49*(2), 42–47.

Bormolini, G., Ghinassi, A., Pagni, C., Milanese, S., & de Ponzuelo, M. M. (2022). The source of life: Meditation and spirituality in healthcare for a comprehensive approach to the COVID-19 syndemic. *Pastoral Psychology, 71*(2), 187–200.

Broad, W. J. (2012). *The science of yoga: The Risks and the Rewards*. Simon and Schuster.

Deshlahra, P., & Singh, M. K. (2023). Effect of yogic intervention on the vital capacity of school going children. *International Journal of Physical Education, Sports and Health, 10*(1), 53–56.

Dunner, K., & Goosen, G. (1996). Secondary students and changing attitudes to prayer. *Word in Life: A Catechetical Review, 44*(2), 8–10.

Ganesan, S., Beyer, E., Moffat, B., Van Dam, N. T., Lorenzetti, V., & Zalesky, A. (2022). Focused attention meditation in healthy adults: A systematic review and meta-analysis of cross-sectional functional MRI studies. *Neuroscience & Biobehavioral Reviews, 141*, 104846. https://doi.org/10.1016/j.neubiorev.2022.104846.

Gist, J. T., Ferdik, F., & Smith, H. P. (2023). A qualitative inquiry into the sources of resilience found among maximum security correctional officers. *Criminal Justice Policy Review, 34*(3), 088740342211437. https://doi.org/10.1177/08874034221143750.

Halappa, N. G. (2023). Integration of yoga within exercise and sports science as a preventive and management strategy for musculoskeletal injuries/disorders and mental disorders–A review. *Journal of Bodywork and Movement Therapies, 34*, 34–40.

Isath, A., Kanwal, A., Virk, H. U. H., Bandyopadhyay, D., Wang, Z., Kumar, A., & Krittanawong, C. (2023). The effect of yoga on cardiovascular disease risk factors: A meta-analysis. *Current Problems in Cardiology, 48*, 101593. https://doi.org/10.1016/j.cpcardiol.2023.101593.

Joshi, S. P., Wong, A. K. I., Brucker, A., Ardito, T. A., Chow, S. C., Vaishnavi, S., & Lee, P. J. (2022). Efficacy of transcendental meditation to reduce stress among health care workers: A randomized clinical trial. *JAMA Network Open, 5*(9), e2231917. https://doi.org/10.1001/jamanetworkopen.2022.31917.

Juniartha, M. G., & Anjani, N. K. (2023). Mudrā yoga dalam teks Hatha Yoga Pradipika dan Gerandha Saṁhitā. *Jurnal Yoga dan Kesehatan, 6*(1), 109–126.

Kalavade, V. A., Prakash Mane, D., & Ghate, U. (2023). A clinical observational study on prakriti analysis and its application in Ayurveda. *Journal of Pharmaceutical Negative Results*, 2215–2222.

Kumar, A., & Bharti, P. K. (2023). A study of 'monistic idealism' in Śaivism and Buddhism on reality, consciousness, and liberation. *International Journal of Multidisciplinary Educational Research, 12*(5), 12–17. http://ijmer.in.doi./2023/12.03.82

Pandurangi, A. K., Keshavan, M. S., Ganapathy, V., & Gangadhar, B. N. (2017). Yoga: Past and present. *American Journal of Psychiatry, 174*(1), 16–17. https://doi.org/10.1176/appi.ajp.2016.16080853.

Patanjali Yoga Sutra by Swami Vivekananda. (2015). https://www.amazon.in/Patanjalis-Yoga-Sutras-Swami-Vivekananda/dp/9389567351.

Rahmani, A. F., & Busro, B. (2023). Meditation as a path to inner calm in the life of Buddhists. *Subhasita: Journal of Buddhist and Religious Studies, 1*(1), 1–16.

Rastogi, R., Chaturvedi, D. K., Saxena, M., Sagar, S., Gupta, M., Choudhary, R., & Sharma, U. (2022). Measuring happiness index and electronic gadgets radiations on AI IoT systems: Return to Indian scriptures and science for mental fitness during global threats. *International Journal of Social Ecology and Sustainable Development (IJSESD), 13*(1), 1–37.

Rastogi, R., Sagar, S., Singh, B., Tandon, N., Rajeshwari, T., Garg, P., & Sharma, M. (2022). Statistical analysis of air quality by emission of different woods: Facing the threats of global pandemic with healthcare 4.0. *International Journal of Indian Culture and Business Management, 26*(2), 166–203.

Rastogi, R., Sagar, S., Tandon, N., Singh, B., & Rajeshwari, T. (2022). Computational statistics on stress patients with happiness and radiation indices by Vedic Homa therapy: A knowledge-based approach to get insights in a global pandemic. In *Approaches and Applications of Deep Learning in Virtual Medical Care* (pp. 99–126). IGI Global.

Rastogi, R., Saxena, M., Chaturvedi, D. K., Gupta, M., Rastogi, A. R., Rastogi, M., & Sagar, S. (2021). Kirlian experimental analysis and IoT: Part 2. *International Journal of Reliable and Quality E-Healthcare (IJRQEH), 10*(2), 44–60.

Sadhguru. (2015). Hatha yoga guide: Science, benefits and insights. Retrieved from: isha. sadhguru.org; http://isha.sadhguru.org/blog/yoga-meditation/demystifying-yoga/hatha-yoga-benefits/ (accessed on 5 July 2024).

Sagar, S., Garg, V., & Rastogi, R. (2022). Computational analysis of the impact of yoga on QoL and body flexibility. *International Journal of Reliable and Quality E-Healthcare (IJRQEH), 11*(1), 1–20.

Sagar, S., Garg, V., & Rastogi, R. (2022). Effects of yoga on the cardio-respiratory system: Socio-technical effect to reduce the impact of the pandemic on Indian employees. *International Journal of Social Ecology and Sustainable Development (IJSESD), 13*(1), 1–19.

Sagar, S., Garg, V., & Rastogi, R. (2022). Employee wellness without stress and strain: Application of yoga and meditation in management with an Industry 5.0 perspective. In *Handbook of Research on Innovative Management Using AI in Industry 5.0* (pp. 204–221). IGI Global.

Sagar, S., Rastogi, R., Garg, V., & Basavaraddi, I. V. (2022). Impact of meditation on quality of life of employees. *International Journal of Reliable and Quality E-Healthcare (IJRQEH), 11*(1), 1–16.

Saraswati, S. S., & Hiti, J. K. (1996). *Asana Pranayama Mudra Bandha* (pp. 978–8186336144). Bihar, India: Yoga Publications Trust.

Sethi, M. K., Devathia, V. K., Sai, D. K., Bishnoi, S., Bajiya, R. K., & Lal, B. (2023). Safety and efficient pain management through alternative therapy (Yoga & Naturopathy). *International Journal of Yoga and Allied Science, 12,* 88–96.

Shavir, R. C. (2023). The spiritual communication of Muallaf. In *Proceedings of the 3rd Borobudur International Symposium on Humanities and Social Science 2021 (BIS-HSS 2021)* (pp. 136–143). Atlantis Press SARL. https://doi.org/10.2991/978-2-494069-49-7_25.

Singh, A. K., Buttagat, V., & Divya, B. R. (2023). Exploring the bioenergy pathways affecting the low back pain–A review. *Journal of Applied Consciousness Studies, 11*(1), 67.

Singh, D. K., & Sakshi, Manohar, J. (2022). Applied aspect of Shadchakras and its importance: a review article, *International Journal of AYUSH; 11*(6), 115–121.

Stern, J., & Kohn, E. (2023). Prayer in schools: In search of a new paradigm. In *Reimagining the Landscape of Religious Education: Challenges and Opportunities* (pp. 237–252). Cham: Springer International Publishing.

Surya, K. P., Sujith, A., Kumar, A. M., & Lohith, B. A. (2022). Ayurvedic approach in the management of Henoch–Schönlein Purpura (HSP): A single case study. *International Journal of Health Sciences, 6*(S4), 11633–11640.

Turcan, N. (2023). The phenomenology of prayer and the relationship between phenomenology and theology. *Religions, 14*(1), 104.

Ved Murti Pt. Sri Ram Sharma Acharya. (1995). *Gayatri Maha Vigyan* (1(1), pp. 255–256). Available at http://literature.awgp.org (accessed on 5 July 2024).

Zok, A., Matecka, M., Zapala, J., Izycki, D., & Baum, E. (2023). The effect of Vinyasa yoga practice on the well-being of breast-cancer patients during COVID-19 pandemic. *International Journal of Environmental Research and Public Health, 20*(4), 3770.

CHAPTER 8

Managing Polycystic Ovarian Syndrome Through Suryanamaskar

YASHVI PANJRATH,[1] ANJALEE,[2] and VIJENDRA NATH PATHAK[1]

[1]*Department of Psychology, School of Social Science and Language, Lovely Professional University, Punjab, India*

[2]*Department of Psychology, Gurukula Kangari University, Haridwar, Uttarakhand, India*

ABSTRACT

Polycystic ovarian syndrome (PCOS) is becoming a common issue in women, and yoga has been shown to be successful in reducing and managing its symptoms and complications, which include irregular menses, hormonal imbalances, hirsutism, and mood disturbances. Yoga has been considered successful in complementary medicine systems. The present study aims to identify the impact of yoga, specifically Surya namaskar, in managing the symptoms of PCOS and also to identify its effect on anxiety induced by PCOS. This study explores the relationship between these factors and identifies gaps in the literature. PCOS has been found to cause anxiety and depression. While *Surya namaskar* has been found to be effective in managing the physiological symptoms of PCOS, there is still a lack of studies that solely focus on the impact of Surya namaskar on PCOS-induced anxiety.

Yoga and Meditation: Past and Present Evidence. Sachi Nandan Mohanty, Rabindra Kumar Pradhan, & Sugyanta Priyadarshini (Eds.)

8.1   INTRODUCTION

8.1.1   POLYCYSTIC OVARY SYNDROME (PCOS)

Polycystic ovary syndrome or PCOS is a medical condition which has been found to affect 7–20% of women (Day et al., 2018). The most common feature includes increased testosterone levels or 'Hypoandrogenism.' It involves irregularity in menstrual cycles and multiple cysts in the ovaries. There is ambiguity about the diagnosis of PCOS even in today's times, making its management all the more complex. Stein and Leventhal first recognized this disorder in 1935. Under ultrasound, a polycystic ovary is defined as 12 or more follicles in the 2–9 mm range (Balen et al., 2009). In the 1960s, PCOS was known as Stein-Leventhal Syndrome and was later renamed as polycystic ovarian syndrome (Rosenfield, 1997). Not all women with PCOS have polycystic ovaries (Balen, 2009). The spectrum of PCOS ranges from moderate to severe, while some women only have a few symptoms, others may have a wide array of symptoms. This complication not only makes diagnosis a challenge but also its treatment.

PCOS is a syndrome which involves hormonal imbalance in women of reproductive age. In some cases, the ovaries of the woman may become enlarged and develop many harmless fluid-filled sacs called follicles. These follicles are underdeveloped sacs which are meant for developing eggs. Irregular or absent periods are common signs of the condition. It also includes excessive pain during the menstrual cycle or heavy flow, breakouts like acne due to elevated testosterone levels, pain in the pelvic area, excessive male hormones or androgen that can cause hirsutism which is the growth of hair on the face or chest. Women with PCOS also experience thinning of hair or hair loss like male pattern baldness. PCOS is also a cause of infertility and also increases the risk of other health conditions like diabetes. It is also associated with weight gain especially in the abdominal area due to a condition called insulin resistance which is an increase in insulin levels. This causes an increase in male hormones in women. Insulin helps the body process glucose and use it for energy; however, due to insulin resistance causing high glucose levels in the blood leading to weight gain or obesity. While the above-mentioned are the symptoms of PCOS, not every woman experiences all these symptoms, and the condition may vary from individual to individual.

8.1.2 PCOS AND MENTAL HEALTH

Women with PCOS often experience elevated stress levels and symptoms of anxiety and depression. Since PCOS is related to distressing symptoms like obesity and facial hair, these women often experience an increased level of stress. This creates a vicious cycle as stress further causes an increase in visceral fat and inflammation (Farrell & Antoni, 2010). Research has found that anxiety and depression are more common among people with PCOS. In a 2016 research review by Blay et al., it was found that people with PCOS were nearly 3 times as likely to report anxiety as those without the condition. People with PCOS have been found to experience social anxiety, generalized anxiety, and panic attacks due to the physical manifestations of PCOS. The cause, however, still remains unclear but it could possibly be due to the symptoms of PCOS, or hormonal imbalances associated with the disorder.

8.2 SURYA NAMASKAR

Surya Namaskara is the Hindu term for the Sun God's invocation. The Sun, also known as *Surya*, is the most powerful and ultimate source of energy on this world. The '*Rigveda*' (old literature), which is considered to be one of the earliest Vedas, contains primarily passages in honor of the Sun. Cults of Sun worship were prevalent in India, and evidence in the Sun temples' shape (e.g., the well-known *Konark* and *Odisha Sun Temples)* has led to emulation and adoration of the deity. Scientists have discovered that allowing the sun's rays to enter the body through the practice of *Surya Namaskar* in the morning is extremely beneficial to one's health. As stated in the '*Puranas,*' the sun created the universe by placing a ray in the sun's beams, thereby creating the cosmos. The importance of water, air, and light has been emphasized.

When we look at our closest star, we may see only a brilliant yellow ball of light since the sun is our primary energy and light source. Hindus have worshipped the Sun as *Surya*, the spiritual and physical center of our globe, and also as the origin of all life for thousands of years (Sarita et al., 2021).

Surya namaskar is a set of 12 asanas that include breathing awareness, physical postures, and mantras. *Surya namaskar* is a form of Yoga that originated in India. "*Pranamasana* (prayer posture), *Hastthothanasana* (raised arm stance), *Padhasthasana* (hand to foot pose), *Aswasanchala-sana* (equestrian pose), *Dandasana* (stick pose), *Asthangamaskara* (salute with eight pieces or points), *Bhujanasana* (cobra pose), and *Paravatasana* (mountain pose) are the 12 asanas. *Surya namaskar* inoculates us against disease on all levels: physically, psychologically, and spiritually" (Manoj Kumar Sharma, 2014) (Figure 8.1).

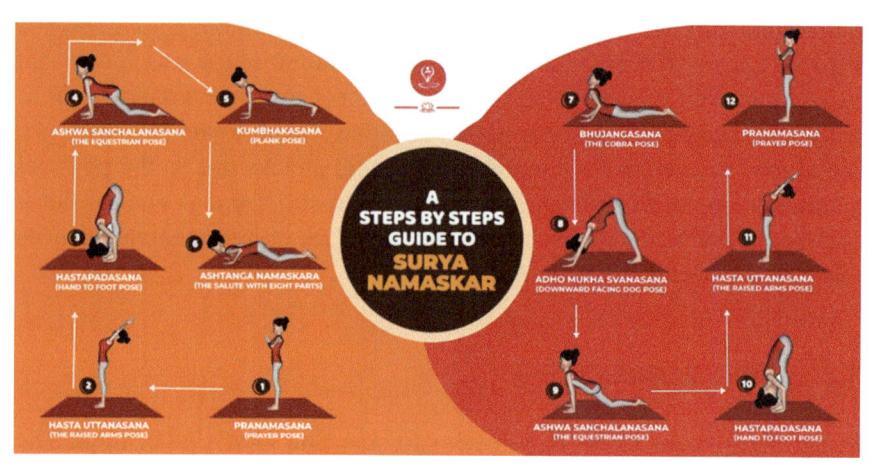

FIGURE 8.1   Around 12 asanas of sun salutation.

Source: 7pranyama. https://7pranyama.com/step-step-guide-surya-namaskar-sun-salutation/

Step *Surya Namaskar* of a 12-step gentle workout routine is *Surya Namaskar*. It's always asserted that it improves proportionate size and physical fitness of the practitioner. Performing this exercise, which is dynamic, helps to build strong joints and muscles. Obesity is becoming more prevalent among youngsters and people in their mid-20s today. The eight basic asanas include the mountain pose, upward salute, standing forward bend, low lunge, plank pose, four-limbed staff pose, upward-facing dog pose, downward-facing dog pose.

The shift from posture to posture is done with the help of inhalation or exhaling of breath. Studies have demonstrated the physical and mental benefits of regularly performing *Surya Namaskar*. In a study carried out by Kursi et al. (2018); Yashvi & Vijendra (2023), slow breathing, which is an essential aspect of Sun Salutation, has been found to have a significant effect on the respiratory, cardiovascular, and autonomic nervous system.

During this posture breathing regime, followed by each step, has been found to improve blood circulation. Practicing *Surya Namaskar* has also been found to lower blood sugar levels by stimulating pancreatic cells (Dunaif, 1997).

Yoga has been found to be beneficial in dealing with obesity, stress, and hormonal imbalance (Harrison et al., 2010). It has also been demonstrated that 12 consecutive weeks of practicing Yoga significantly improve glucose levels, lipid profile, and insulin sensitivity in women with PCOS.

Performing Sun Salutation at least 5 times a day can aid in weight loss, improve lipid profile, and regulate menstrual cycles.

Performing Surya Namaskar not only brings physical benefits but is also essential for mental health. A study by Godse et al. (2015) concluded that Surya Namaskar was beneficial and brought about physical relaxation, mental peace, reduced somatic stress, worry, and negative emotions. Thus, this yogic practice has been found to provide both physical and mental benefits.

PCOS or polycystic ovarian syndrome, is a disorder marked by infertility, obesity, male-like characteristics in females (such as baldness, facial hair, acne), and obesity. This can lead to body dissatisfaction, social isolation, anxiety, and depression. The self-perception of women with PCOS is not well researched, creating a gap in the current literature and highlighting the need to investigate the psychosocial dimensions of PCOS and develop interventions to manage it.

The aim of the present study is to identify the impact of Yoga specifically Suryanamaskar in managing the symptoms of PCOS and also identify the effect of the same on anxiety induced as a result of PCOS. Pranayama is the key to living a more fulfilling life. The practice of *Suryanamaskar* on a regular basis immunizes the entire body. This action increases metabolic rate, resulting in the production of heat and the elimination of toxins from the body. *Surya namaskar* (Sun Salutation) increases mental serenity and reduces stress and anxiety levels. According to Niranjananada (1997), with a Surya namaskar practice, the level of stress of students going to college can be decreased to an impressive degree. According to Viveka Sharma (2003), the practice of Surya namaskara with mantras for a month reduces anxiety in test subjects. She starts with 5 repetitions each day and gradually increases to 10 repetitions per day. The difference between post and pre findings of the Surya namaskar on anxiety is statistically significant at 0.01. As a result, the Suryanamaskar has been shown to significantly reduce stress.

Archana, in 2018, found that the *Surya Namaskar* is important for the treatment of menstrual cycle irregularities. According to Vahid Ghaffararilaleh et al. (2018), women with premenstrual syndrome who practice *Surya Namaskar* had better sleep. Amit Vaibhav and colleagues, in 2016, went into great length in their article regarding the techniques and benefits of performing *Surya Namaskar* for good health. The research conducted by Anand Sharad Godse et al., in 2015, demonstrated that the practice of *Surya Namaskar* can help college students relax and reduce stress.

Surya Namaskar is a holistic exercise that provides an everyday dosage of Vitamin D, mobility training, intellectual boost, cardiovascular tuning, psychological health, glucose metabolism, and spinal adjustments. Shakeela & Sugumar, in 2020, according to the findings of their research, found that abnormal BMI is a contributing element to Premenstrual Syndrome. When done in conjunction with walking, Surya Namaskar can help you lose the weight you've accumulated from a sedentary lifestyle while also providing relief from menstrual difficulties. Exercise may save the lives of teenage girls and provide a long-term solution to their PMS issues, according to the results of the research.

Surya Namaskara is a time-saving technique that is useful to everyone, including the general public, patients, and sportspeople. It is also a beneficial habit for those who have a limited amount of time to dedicate to their health. They have their origins in the ancient practice of *Surya* worshipping Hindus who lived thousands of years ago. Today's athletes are incorporating Yoga, *Pranayama*, and sun salutations into their training to improve their overall performance. This is because Yoga, Pranayama, and sun salutations improve flexibility, balance, cardiovascular efficiency, and the strength of anatomical and physiological organs while simultaneously lowering stress levels, tension, anxiety, and depression.

Sharma et al. (2008) found out the impact of Yoga on the subjective well-being of patients who have diabetes as well as healthy individuals, coronary artery disease, and hypertension, among other conditions. The study shows that a Yoga-based training program is beneficial in stress management, maintaining a healthy lifestyle, and disease prevention. The study describes the function played by *Surya Namaskar* in the maintenance of human health and well-being. It is essential for the maintenance of physical, mental, and spiritual well-being. By performing *Suryanamaskara*, you will be able to improve your musculoskeletal system as well as your internal organs. It improves our ability to concentrate and remain calm, as well as trains our neuromuscular system. Spiritual well-being has a positive impact on the human mind and aids in the development of stability, balance, and adjustment in one's life. *Surya Namaskara* is an important tool in the reduction of stress and anxiety. *Suryanamaskara* is a dynamic and complete Yoga practice that has many benefits. However, it is important to practice Suryanamaskara according to Punam (2019).

Yoga has been shown to generate consistent and favorable physiological changes in participants. Yoga practice on a regular basis can help to improve a variety of physiological and psychological functions. The *Surya Namaskar* is supposed to improve overall health and fitness. It improves the condition of the lungs and the cardiovascular system. *Surya Namaskar* is a fundamental mix of *asana* and *Pranayama* that anybody and everyone can practice on a daily basis. Yoga helps us develop positive characteristics and maintain our health. It also helps to develop concentration, self-confidence, and self-discipline. *Surya Namaskar* is a complete practice in and of itself, incorporating *asana, Pranayama*, and *mantra. Surya Namaskar* is an element of the yogic approach which can be included in daily life with ease for immediate as well as positive results. According to the findings of the study, *Surya Namaskar* should be done by everyone, on a daily basis, in order to reap the benefits (Kathane, 2013).

Polycystic ovarian syndrome (PCOS) is becoming more prevalent among women of reproductive age, and Yoga has been shown to be successful in reducing its symptoms and complications, which include irregular menses, hormonal imbalances, hirsutism, and mood disturbances. Yoga has been considered successful in complementary medicine systems. Yogasana is a technique that can be used to relieve tension and weariness. Practices such as *Shavasana, Bharadvajasana, Makarasana, Padmasana, Baddhakonasana, Surya Namaskara, Dhanurasana, Chakki Chalanasana* (Shalini et al., 2018), *Bhadrasana,* and *Padmasana* boost blood circulation by applying pressure on the reproductive organs.

One of the most significant and safest treatments is changing one's lifestyle, which has long been regarded as the first step in treatment. Lifestyle change therapy includes behavioral changes (reduction of psychosocial stressors), exercise therapies, and nutritional improvements (Amiri et al., 2020). Individuals with metabolic syndrome can benefit from physical activity and dietary improvements, which help reduce the prevalence of hormonal disorders and obesity in this population (Mishra et al., 2015). Physical activity combined with weight loss has been shown to lower insulin and testosterone levels, improving the symptoms of people with type 2 diabetes (Gibson-Helm et al., 2014). In overweight and obese women with polycystic ovarian syndrome, it has been well documented that a weight loss of 5–14% achieved through physical activity and dietary restriction can result in improvements in reproductive function and hormonal features (Swaraj et al., 2014).

Yoga is one of the suggested workouts for this condition, and it has been shown to help patients feel better. It is a critical part in the improvement of mental as well as physical ailments, particularly in the area of emotional health. It is crucial to observe that practicing Yoga does not necessitate any flexibility or physical fitness on your part (Menezes et al., 2020). In addition to helping to build muscular strength and flexibility, respiratory, and physical Yoga exercises can additionally aid in improving oxygen delivery and blood circulation to all reproductive tissues and cells in the body (Ouyang et al., 2020). Furthermore, Yoga's relaxation and reassuring thoughts help to improve the autonomic nervous system (ANS), which helps to decrease blood pressure (BP) and triglycerides, moderate emotional responses, and regulate respiration (Kumar et al., 2015). Through the regulation of the endocrine system, stress reduction, and the balance of neuronal hormones, Yoga helps to improve reproductive function. Yoga also has the additional benefit of decreasing serum cortisol through enhancing cortisol excretion, which can assist in reducing the symptoms of PCOS.

The effects of fencing, swimming, Yoga sessions, and physical conditioning were evaluated by Berger & Owen (1988), who discovered that only one of the groups, the group receiving Yoga treatment, showed a statistically significant short-term reduction in state anxiety. Yoga can lower anxiety in students, but only in male students according to Ray et al. (2001). Participants in Yoga, swimming, and the Feldenkrais method, as well as a control group, were shown to have lower anxiety levels than those in the study by Netz & Lidor (2003). On the other hand, Blumenthal et al. (1989) found that in a study of senior individuals, Yoga participants did worse on anxiety measures compared to those in a group doing aerobic exercise and were not better compared to the other treatment plans. The outcomes for people with certain anxiety disorders or anxiety can't be predicted based on this research, so it's essential to consider the data that is currently available. Palomba et al. (2008) studied PCOS for 24 weeks and discovered that ovulation improved much more in the group who exercised than it did in the group who ate less well. Despite the fact that their BMI did not change much, women with PCOS who took part in an 8-to 12-week fitness training intervention reported a substantial reduction in insulin resistance, as reported by Brown et al. (2009).

Women with PCOS, according to Kirthika & colleagues (2019), should engage in 30 minutes of resistance training and/or moderate-intensity aerobic exercise at least five days every week in order to minimize long-term problems of the disease. Michael et al. (2015) examined the impact of moderate to intense physical exercise on depression in 35 young women who have PCOS (aged 12–21). While parental depression evaluations were linked to the duration of activity, the young women's self-reported depression scores were not. They saw that those who took part exercised every day for around 10 minutes.

Stress, anxiety, and depression levels can be reduced by practicing Yoga (Salmon et al., 2009) through influencing neurophysiological and biochemical systems, such as controlling the stress response and autonomic nervous system. When it comes to dealing with stress, anxiety, and depression, Chandra (2021) discovered that the practice of Yoga can be both a complement to other therapies and a stand-alone treatment. According to Streeter et al., regular Yoga practice can help alleviate symptoms of depression and anxiety, which are linked to low GABA levels. After studying 300 women and men, Telles et al. (2009) found that both the physical practice of Yoga as well as its philosophical underpinnings reduce anxiety, although the physical practice of Yoga reduces anxiety more than the theoretical parts of Yoga. A study by Smith et al. found that relaxation techniques like Yoga were equally helpful at reducing stress and anxiety. Gupta et al. found that after 10 days of a pressure control program, levels of state and trait anxiety dropped considerably.

Surya namaskara is a great procedure to have a good workout in a shorter period of time. It lowers cholesterol levels and maintains a healthy hormonal balance because it increases circulation. Stress and anxiety can be reduced by practicing Suryanamaskara. Research has shown that *Suryanamaskara* has a beneficial effect on both mental and physical health and helps in reducing stress, depression, and anxiety in practitioners (Dave et al., 2021).

Suryanamaskara increases blood circulation throughout the body. When actively inhaling and exhaling, it keeps the lungs ventilated and blood oxygenated at all times. It is an excellent approach to assist the body in detoxing, and excessive carbon dioxide and other harmful gases are eliminated. Regular practice of asanas may assist women who have PCOS in maintaining regularity in menstrual cycles, and if practiced every day, it makes delivery easier. Calming and anti-anxiety effects on memory and the nervous system are aided by the practice of *Surya Namaskar*. It stabilizes the thyroid and endocrine glands, resulting in a feeling of full relaxation and tranquility, and reduces anxiety (SrujanaAili, 2021). *Surya Namaskar* is beneficial because it boosts metabolism, decreases stress and anxiety, and helps in checking obesity (Savita et al., 2021). Women who have PCOS and participated in a Yoga training program resulted in having low levels of depression. Based on the findings, experts believe that Yoga can assist PCOS women in coping with depression (Jaimala et al., 2017).

PCOS risk can be reduced by tailoring yoga and fitness to schoolgirls' schedules and involving school instructors, according to a study. An appreciable reduction of risk was seen in the experimental group after treatments, indicating the value of such measures. These findings provide a platform for lifestyle treatments in adolescent girls at risk for PCOS who are enrolled in school. Adolescent females who attend school and make lifestyle changes may be an effective technique for reducing PCOS risk in the Indian population (Selvaraj et al., 2020).

Researchers advocate yoga as a complementary therapy for teenage PCOS patients to assist in slowing the disease's progression (Godse et al., 2015). It has been shown that *Surya namaskar* is beneficial for promoting dispositions including mental calmness, ease/peace, rejuvenation, strength, awareness, and joy. The stress dispositions of the *Surya namaskar* group (somatic tension, concern, and negative mood) were less than the control group. However, Alka Natu (2009) conducted a study on 32 PCOS-afflicted sub-fertile women to demonstrate the benefits of yoga exercises. For a period of 12 weeks, yogic practices comprised *shuddikriyas, asanas, Surya namaskar, Pranayama, dharna, mantra yoga, naad yoga*, and *dhyan*, all of which incorporated dynamic loosening activities. After ovulation induction, women who practiced meditation and yoga had significantly more follicles, lower levels of serum triglycerides, lower insulin levels, a lower LH/FSH ratio, and lower depression ratings.

One of the most common reasons people engage in mind-body therapies like Yoga is to combat anxiety (Stussman et al., 2015); Yoga practitioners report lower stress levels and increased relaxation as a result of their practice (Barnes et al., 2008). It is reported that mindfulness is low in individuals with other emotional disorders and GAD, indicating a need for ways to improve mindfulness (Curtiss & Klemanski, 2014).

Yoga can be considered supplementary medicine because it is effective for reducing stress, anxiety, and depression. By reducing the use of pharmaceuticals and other medications, it has the potential to lower medical costs per treatment (Masoumeh, 2018). Barsing et al. (2015) noted that Sun-salutation causes several beneficial physiological changes in the body. Aerobic activity during sun-salutation is good for the lungs and oxygen. Blood pressure is reduced, and cardiovascular functions are improved. It has a calming influence on the mind, required for mood elevation. Body size and form are improved as a result of the musculoskeletal activity, which is beneficial to fitness and confidence. It helps individuals with diabetes, sleeplessness, anxiety, and depression, and prevents cardiac and pulmonary disorders. Therefore, it works both as a preventative and a therapy.

Bhargav (2013), Yoga is a holistic mind-body healing practice that has been shown to reduce stress and sympathetic tone in the body. Yoga has been proven to be more effective than physical activity in reducing the Gallway and Modified Ferriman scores for hirsutism and improving menstrual frequency in patients with PCOS in a recently completed 12-week randomized controlled experiment. In addition to addressing PCOS symptoms, Yoga may also help prevent long-term issues like cardiovascular disease, diabetes, and other disorders. Yoga is also more cost-effective and long-lasting because it is a holistic strategy, rather than a narrow one. This means that as a primary intervention or as an addition to regular medical therapy, Yoga may be suggested for the treatment of PCOS.

Yoga and exercise tailored to the schedules of schoolgirls, engaging schoolteachers, were found to have a positive influence on lowering the risk of PCOS. A significant reduction in risk was observed in the experimental group following interventions, which supports the value of such measures. Lifestyle interventions will be beneficial for adolescent schoolgirls at risk of PCOS. Healthy lifestyle improvements among adolescent females attending school in India may be an effective method for reducing the risk of PCOS (Anitha et al., 2020).

Harrison et al. (2011) conducted a study in which they found that physical activity can help women with PCOS manage their symptoms such as irregular periods, insulin resistance, hypertension, and a high lipid profile. The study showed that the Yoga program and physical activity led to significant improvements in lipid profile and glucose metabolism in people with PCOS. Yoga was found to be more successful as compared to traditional physical exercise at increasing lipid, glucose, and insulin sensitivity.

PCOS is the most frequent health disease in women of reproductive age. It is caused by hormonal imbalance induced by bad behaviors, a hectic and stressful lifestyle, and a stressful environment. Women with PCOS have high levels of insulin resistance, are overweight, and have elevated androgen levels. Weight loss is the most important preventive and therapeutic measure in the fight against this condition, and it can be achieved by making lifestyle adjustments. Yoga interventions and nutritious food (PathyaAhar) mentioned in Ayurvedic literature are crucial for maintaining an individual's health and regulating the functions of the endocrine system. *Pranayama* (breathing techniques) can be beneficial in alleviating PCOS symptoms, keeping the individual motivated to combat the condition and deep-seated mental stress. These lifestyle modifications have been shown to improve reproductive rates and enhance the overall quality of life of patients with PCOS (Thakur et al., 2018).

8.3 CONCLUSION

One in five Indian women suffer from PCOS (The Hindu, 2019). With such an alarmingly high prevalence of this condition, there is still ambiguity about PCOS diagnosis even in today's times, making its management all the more complex. PCOS can be managed and reduced through the practice of *Surya Namaskar*. By focusing on breathing and relaxation, *Surya Namaskar* helps individuals with PCOS manage their stress levels, which can in turn lead to improved mental well-being. It is important to note that while *Surya Namaskar* can be beneficial for women with PCOS, it is important to consult with a healthcare professional before beginning any exercise routine. Additionally, it is important to practice *Surya Namaskar* under the guidance of a qualified Yoga instructor to ensure proper form and technique. Studies reveal that doing Surya Namaskar for 10 to 15 minutes for 12 consecutive weeks can help improve lipid profile, regulate menstrual cycles, and lower the waist-to-hip ratio, improving irregularities.

KEYWORDS

- **anxiety**
- **lipid profile**
- **menstrual cycles**
- **mental health**
- **polycystic ovarian syndrome**
- *Surya namaskar*
- **therapeutic measure**

REFERENCES

Alha, S., Kumar, M., Dave, H. H., & Kumar, B. (2021). Role of Surya-Namaskara in polycystic ovarian syndrome: A conceptual study. *International Research Journal of Ayurveda & Yoga, 4*(7), 117–120. https://doi.org/10.47223/IRJAY.2021.4716.

Alka, Natu, Neela, Tamhane, Shaila Bhate, Kanchan, Samel, Ghantali, & Mitra Mandal. (2009). Effect of yogic practices on infertility related to PCOD. Best Research Paper in the International Yoga Conference—SYASA, Bangaluru 2009.

Barsing, D. B., & Mishra, B. R. (2015). Sunsalutation and health. *International Journal of Development Research, 5*(1), 2875–2879.

Behan, C. (2020). The benefits of meditation and mindfulness practices during times of crisis such as COVID-19. *Irish Journal of Psychological Medicine, 37*(4), 256–258. https://doi.org/10.1017/ipm.2020.38.

Bhargav, H. (2013). Yoga for polycystic ovarian syndrome. *Alternative and Complementary Therapies, 19*(2), 101–106. https://doi.org/10.1089/act.2013.19205.

Bharshankar, J. R., Bharshankar, R. N., Deshpande, V. N., Kaore, S. B., & Gosavi, G. B. (2003). Effect of yoga on cardiovascular system in subjects above 40 years. *Indian Journal of Physiology and Pharmacology, 47*, 202–206.

Bhasin, M. K., D. J., Chang, B. H., Joseph, M. G., Denninger, J. W., Fricchione, G. L., Benson, H., & Libermann, T. A. (2013). Relaxation response induces temporal transcriptome changes in energy metabolism, insulin secretion and inflammatory pathways. *PLoS One, 8*(5), e62817.

Blumenthal, J. A., Emery, C. F., & Madden, D. J., et al. (1989). Cardiovascular and behavioral effects of aerobic exercise training in healthy older men and women. *Journal of Gerontology, 44*, M147–157.

Brand, S., Holsboer-Trachsler, E., Naranjo, J. R., & Schmidt, S. (2012). Influence of mindfulness practice on cortisol and sleep in long-term and short-term meditators. *Neuropsychobiology, 65*(3), 109–118.

Cramer, H., Ward, L., Steel, A., Lauche, R., Dobos, G., & Zhang, Y. (2016). Prevalence, patterns, and predictors of yoga use: Results of a U.S. nationally representative survey. *American Journal of Preventive Medicine, 50*(2), 230–235. https://doi.org/10.1016/j.amepre.2015.07.037.

De Michelis, E. (2005). *A History of Modern Yoga: Patanjali and Western Esotericism.* London, UK: Continuum International Publishing Group.

Desikachar, K., Bragdon, L., & Bossart, C. (2005). The yoga of healing: Exploring yoga's holistic model for health and well-being. *International Journal of Yoga Therapy, 15*, 17–39.

Godse, A. S., et al. (2015). Effects of suryanamaskar on relaxation among college students with high stress in Pune, India. *International Journal of Yoga, 8*(1), 15–21. https://doi.org/10.4103/0973-6131.146049.

Gupta, N., Kera, S., Vempati, R. P., Sharma, R., & Bijlani, R. L. (2006). Effect of yoga-based lifestyle intervention on state and trait anxiety. *U.S. National Library of Medicine, 50*(1), 7–41.

Harrison, C. L., Lombard, C. B., Moran, L. J., & Teede, H. J. (2011). Exercise therapy in polycystic ovarian syndrome: A systemic review. *Human Reproduction, 17*(2), 171–183.

Himelein, M. J., & Thatcher, S. S. (2006a). Depression and body image among women with polycystic ovary syndrome. *Journal of Health Psychology, 11*(4), 613–625.

Himelein, M. J., & Thatcher, S. S. (2006b). Polycystic ovary syndrome and mental health: A review. *Obstetrical & Gynecological Survey, 61*(11), 723–732.

Huber-Buchholz, M. M., Carey, D. G. P., & Norman, R. J. (1999). Restoration of reproductive potential by lifestyle modification in obese polycystic ovary syndrome: Role of insulin sensitivity and luteinizing hormone. *The Journal of Clinical Endocrinology & Metabolism, 84*(4), 1470–1474.

Kishore, D. M., Manjunath, N. K., Metri, K., Babu, N., & Basavaraj, A. (2020). Depression, anxiety and stress among nurses working in a tertiary care center in Southern India. *Asian Journal of Medicine and Health, 18*(9), 147–152.

Kumar, K. (2011). Yoga Nidra and its impact on students' wellbeing. *Yoga Mimamsa, Kaivalyadham, Lonavala, 36*, 11.

Mohseni, M., et al. (2021). Yoga effects on anthropometric indices and polycystic ovary syndrome symptoms in women undergoing infertility treatment: A randomized controlled clinical trial. *2021,* 5564824. https://doi.org/10.1155/2021/5564824.

Nagendra, H. R. (2020). Yoga for COVID-19. *International Journal of Yoga, 13*, 87–88.

National Center for Complementary and Integrative Health. (2015). Mind and body practices. https://nccih.nih.gov/health/mindbody (accessed on 5 July 2024).

Nidhi, R., Padmalatha, V., Nagarathna, R., & Amritanshu, R. (2013). Effects of a holistic yoga program on endocrine parameters in adolescents with polycystic ovarian syndrome: A randomized controlled trial. *Journal of Alternative and Complementary Medicine, 19*(2), 153–160. https://doi.org/10.1089/acm.2011.0868.

Nidhi, R., Padmalatha, V., Nagarathna, R., & Ram, A. (2012). Effect of a yoga program on glucose metabolism and blood lipid levels in adolescent girls with polycystic ovary syndrome. *International Journal of Gynecology & Obstetrics, 118*(1), 37–41. https://doi.org/10.1016/j.ijgo.2012.01.027.

Nidhi, R., Padmalatha, V., Nagarathna, R., & Ram, A. (2013). Effect of yoga program on quality of life in adolescent polycystic ovarian syndrome: A randomized control trial. *Applied Research in Quality of Life, 8*(3), 373–383.

Palomba, S., Giallauria, F., Falbo, A., Russo, T., Oppedisano, R., Tolino, A., & Orio, F. (2008). Structured exercise training programme versus hypocaloric hyperproteic diet in obese polycystic ovary syndrome patients with anovulatory infertility: A 24-week pilot study. *Human Reproduction, 23*, 642–650.

Panjrath, Y., & Pathak, V. N. (2022). A systematic review on the impact of Surya Namaskar and loving-kindness meditation in treating social body anxiety and body dissatisfaction in women with polycystic ovarian syndrome. *Journal of Pharmaceutical Negative Results, 13*, 10146–10151. https://doi.org/10.47750/pnr.2022.13.S09.1188.

Patel, V., et al. (2020). Regular mindful yoga practice as a method to improve androgen levels in women with polycystic ovary syndrome: A randomized, controlled trial. *The Journal of the American Osteopathic Association, 120*(5). https://doi.org/10.7556/jaoa.2020.050.

Raja-Khan, N., Stener-Victorin, E., Wu, X., & Legro, R. S. (2011). The physiological basis of complementary and alternative medicines for polycystic ovary syndrome. *American Journal of Physiology-Endocrinology and Metabolism, 301*(1), E1–E10.

Rajni, N. (2016). Effect of Surya Namaskar on weight loss in obese persons. *International Journal of Science and Consciousness, 2*(1), 1–5.

Sahni, P. S., Singh, K., Sharma, N., & Garg, R. (2021). Yoga an effective strategy for self-management of stress-related problems and wellbeing during COVID-19 lockdown: A cross-sectional study. *PLoS ONE, 16*(2), e0245214. https://doi.org/10.1371/journal.pone.0245214.

Salmon, P., Lush, E., Jablonski, M., & Sephton, S. E. (2009). Yoga and mindfulness: Clinical aspects of an ancient mind/body practice. *Cognitive and Behavioral Practice, 16*(1), 59–72. https://doi.org/10.1016/j.cbpra.2008.07.002.

Savita, P. Patil, Bijendra Singh, Jyoti Bisht, Shipra Gupta, & Rupa Khanna. (2021). Yoga for holistic treatment of polycystic ovarian syndrome. *Journal of Medical Pharmaceutical & Allied Sciences, 10*(2), 120–125. https://doi.org/10.22270/jmpas.2021.V10S2.2035.

Selvaraj, V., et al. (2020). Impact of yoga and exercises on polycystic ovarian syndrome risk among adolescent schoolgirls in South India. *Health Science Reports, 3*(4), e212. https://doi.org/10.1002/hsr2.212.

Sengupta, P. (2012). Health impacts of yoga and pranayama: A state-of-the-art review. *International Journal of Preventive Medicine, 3*(7), 444–458.

Shalini, B., Mirunaleni, P., Suresh, K., Sundharam, M. M., & Banumathi, V. (2019). The effect of Siddha Internal Medicine with Asanam & Varmam on Sinaipaineerkatti (PCOS)-a case series. *World J Pharm Res, 8*(2), 1122–1129.

Sharma, M. P. K., Mishra, H., & Balodhi, J. P. (1990). Therapeutic effects of Vipassana meditation in tension headache. *Journal of Personality and Clinical Studies, 6*(2), 201–206.

Shohani, M., & Badfar, G. (2018). The effect of yoga on stress, anxiety, and depression in women. *International Journal of Preventive Medicine, 9*, 21. https://www.ncbi.nlm.nih.gov/labs/pmc/articles/PMC5843960/ (accessed on 5 July 2024).

Shukla, M. (2019). Holistic nature of Surya Namaskar for the millennials, reviewing and investigating its scientific rationale. *Journal of Yoga & Physio, 7*(4), 555718. https://doi.org/10.19080/JYP.2019.07.555718.

Smith, C., Hancock, H., Mortimer, J. B., & Eckert, K. (2006). A randomized comparative trial of yoga and relaxation to reduce stress and anxiety. *Complementary Therapies in Medicine, 15*(2), 77–83.

Sode, J. A., & Bhardwaj, M. A. (2017). Effect of yoga on level of depression among females suffering from polycystic ovarian syndrome (PCOS). *International Journal on Arts, Management and Humanities, 6*(2), 178–181.

Srujana, A. (2021). Role of Yogasana in prevention of polycystic ovarian syndrome. *Journal of Ayurveda and Integrative Medical Sciences, 1*, 166–171.

Streeter, C. C., Jensen, J. E., Perlmutter, R. M., Cabral, H. J., Tian, H., Terhune, D. B., & Renshaw, P. F. (2007). Yoga asana sessions increase brain GABA levels. *The Journal of Alternative and Complementary Medicine, 13*(4), 419–426.

Stussman, B. J., Black, L. I., Barnes, P. M., Clarke, T. C., & Nahin, R. L. (2015). Wellness-related use of common complementary health approaches among adults: United States, 2012. *National Health Statistics Reports, 85*, 1–12.

Telles, S., Gaur, V., & Balkrishna, A. (2009). Effect of yoga practice session and yoga theory session on state anxiety. *U.S. National Library of Medicine, 109*(3), 30–924.

Turakitwanakan, W., Mekseepralard, C., & Busarakumtragul, P. (2013). Effects of mindfulness meditation on serum cortisol of medical students. *Journal of the Medical Association of Thailand, 96*, S90–S95.

Venkatesh, L. P., & Vandhana, S. (2022). Insights on Surya namaskar from its origin to application towards health. *Journal of Ayurveda and Integrative Medicine, 13*(2), 100530. https://doi.org/10.1016/j.jaim.2021.10.002.

Waelde, L. C., Uddo, M., Marquett, R., Ropelato, M., Freightman, S., Pardo, A., & Salazar, J. (2008). A pilot study of meditation for mental health workers following hurricane Katrina. *Journal of Traumatic Stress, 21*, 497–500. https://doi.org/10.1002/jts.20365.

Witchel, S. F., Oberfield, S., Rosenfield, R. L., Codner, E., Bonny, A., Ibáñez, L., et al. (2015). The diagnosis of polycystic ovary syndrome during adolescence. *Hormone Research in Paediatrics, 83*(6), 376–389.

Woodyard, C. (2011). Exploring the therapeutic effects of yoga and its ability to increase quality of life. *International Journal of Yoga, 4*, 49–54.

Yunesian, M., Aslani, A., & Vash, J. H. et al. (2008). Effects of Transcendental Meditation on mental health: A before-after study. *Clinical Practice and Epidemiology in Mental Health, 4*, 25. https://doi.org/10.1186/1745-0179-4-25.

Zheng, M., Yao, J., & Narayanan, J. (2020). Mindfulness buffers the impact of COVID-19 outbreak information on sleep duration. *PsyArXiv*. https://doi.org/10.31234/osf.io/wuh94.

CHAPTER 9

Statistically Examining the Effect of Herbal and Spiritual Environment on Various Dimensions of Adolescents' Fitness Post-COVID Effects

ROHIT RASTOGI,[1] MAMTA SAXENA,[2] PRANAV SHARMA,[3]
YATI VARSHNEY,[1] VAIBHAV AGGARWAL,[4] and RICHA SINGH[5]

[1] *Department of Computer Science and Engineering, ABES Engineering College, Ghaziabad, Uttar Pradesh, India*

[2] *Ex-DG, MoS-PI, Government of India, New Delhi, India*

[3] *Dayalbagh Educational Institute, Agra, Uttar Pradesh, India*

[4] *Department of Electronics and Communication Engineering, ABES Engineering College, Ghaziabad, Uttar Pradesh, India*

[5] *Ramjas College, Delhi University, India*

ABSTRACT

In the past few years, humanity has faced many challenges due to the outbreak of the coronavirus pandemic. But even in such difficulties, the world can't stop growing, so we humans have adopted various lifestyle changes like working from home, online education, etc., in order to get our jobs done. However, these changes have affected us physically and mentally in many ways, and the major impact of these changes is seen on adolescents (age group of 10 to 18 years), resulting in them being

Yoga and Meditation: Past and Present Evidence. Sachi Nandan Mohanty, Rabindra Kumar Pradhan, & Sugyanta Priyadarshini (Eds.)

diagnosed with many physical and mental health ailments like obesity, lack of mobility, stress, mental trauma, etc., due to less exposure to the outside environment and a sudden increase in social media. All these aspects are hindering the overall growth needed in that particular age group.

Therefore, this study is based on the impact of some techniques based on Indian Vedic Science to rejuvenate the physical and mental health of adolescents or to counter the post-COVID effects. These techniques basically include the consumption of an herbal Vedic formulation named *Saraswati Panchak* and protocols of yoga and *Yajna* to be followed for a period of 3 months. Two groups, namely the control group (not following the Vedic protocol) and the experimental group (following the Vedic protocol), are assessed for various aspects like IQ, courage, mathematical ability, etc., on various scales, and a comparative study is conducted followed by data analysis using various tools like Python and Tableau.

> **Motivation:** The COVID-19 pandemic has had a profound impact on the well-being of adolescents, affecting not only their physical health but also their mental and emotional states. By examining the effect of herbal and spiritual environments on their fitness, we hope to shed light on how we can support and empower young people to heal and thrive during these challenging times. This research is not just about presenting data, it's about giving hope and creating a brighter future for the next generation.

> **Scope of the Study:** Adolescence is the bridge between innocent childhood and ambitious chaotic adulthood, and the sudden changes in our bodies physically and mentally as part of growing up often leave teenagers in a very confusing situation with a messy mind. The anxiety and curiosity due to hormonal and physical changes are compounded by social insecurities. Surveys report an increase in rates of psychological disorders, suicides, and addictions among teenagers. The effect of the psychic distress caused as an additional effect of COVID-19, due to social isolation and grief from deaths and the challenges of being confined to a house, directly impacted the developing neuroanatomy. Alterations in the frontal limbic system of the brains of children suffering from PTSD were also reported in a few cases. In such a scenario, this research study offers hope for the future. The attempt to use a scientific approach to prove the efficacy of Yajna and herbs as

remedies for the traumas of adolescence, and as a way to ensure emotional, physical, mental, and social stability among teenagers, provides an opportunity to explore ancient wisdom through the lens of modern technologies. The research paves the way for the integration of ancient science and modern innovation to create a better world. It also emphasizes the need to use science not only as a way to make life easier, but also as a light to cure the darkness of this world.

➢ **Topic Organizations:** The chapter sheds light on the post-COVID lifestyle and how it affected the particular age group of teenagers, the mental confusion they had to suffer from. The team later illuminates the impact of Indian Vedic science and its different aspects, including Yajna as a solution to all the problems of adolescence. It further explains the role of artificial intelligence, machine learning, and modern technologies in the social scientific studies like the one represented by this chapter. This is succeeded by the briefing of already established literary work. The methodologies are further explained along with a flow chart. In the results sections, individual graphs of all the subjects are demonstrated to show the outcome of the experiment conducted. The conclusion from this was obtained reporting the astounding effect of Yajna and Saraswat Panchak on the subjects.

➢ **Ethical Committee and Funding:** The experiments don't include any human-related experiments, so no ethical constraints have been violated. Though the subjects performing the study were humans and air quality directly affects them, the study doesn't violate any health-related measures. The project is not funded by any agency.

➢ **Role of Authors:** Dr. Rohit Rastogi acted as the team leader and coordinated among all co-authors. He prepared the topic introduction and background study, and also contributed to experiments. He also prepared the structure of the manuscript and ensured the quality of the content along with all co-authors. Dr. Mamta Saxena conducted the protocol of Ayurveda medicines and Yajna on teenagers. Ms. Yati did the data analysis. Mr. Pranav did the experimental analysis and provided concluding remarks. Ms. Richa compiled the literature survey along with graphical representations. Mr. Vaibhav contributed to the results and discussions along with concluding remarks.

9.1   INTRODUCTION

The ancient Indian Vedic science methodologies are well established by years of practice among the Indian population and are being practiced continuously. These practices can positively elevate human fitness levels, whether they are mental or physical. The herbal and spiritual approach of these practices is highly beneficial if used in today's scenario of post-COVID effects. The post-COVID effects on mental and physical health are a topic of concern nowadays, and these problems can be effectively managed by the Indian Vedic science-based practices for rejuvenating overall fitness.

9.1.1   *POST-COVID LIFESTYLE AND CHALLENGES TO ADOLESCENTS*

During the timeline of the coronavirus pandemic, adolescents faced many lifestyle changes in a short span. As a result, many psychological and physiological changes occurred subconsciously, making it difficult for them to realign with normal lifestyle after COVID. Symptoms of these changes can be observed as many children in this age group experiencing anxiety, depression, and short temper due to the lack of social exposure during the pandemic. They have developed physical and mental inertia, making it difficult for them to return to the playground and make new friends.

It is observed that during the pandemic, they have developed the Fear of Missing Out (FOMO), which is causing them to restrict themselves from socializing. They have also developed a fear of losing their close ones during the pandemic, leading to some form of mental trauma during that time. Additionally, due to the lack of physical activity, they have developed some serious lifestyle health issues such as obesity, high blood pressure, and diabetes at a younger age, which in the long run will pose a serious threat to their lives (as per Figure 9.1) (Ashwin et al., 2022).

Figure 9.1 is a pictorial representation of the condition of an adolescent's mind during the pandemic. It is showing COVID-19 affecting the central nervous system and resulting in various psychological negative changes in the youngsters' minds like FOMO, lack of willpower, lack of motivation, and various other suppressing conditions.

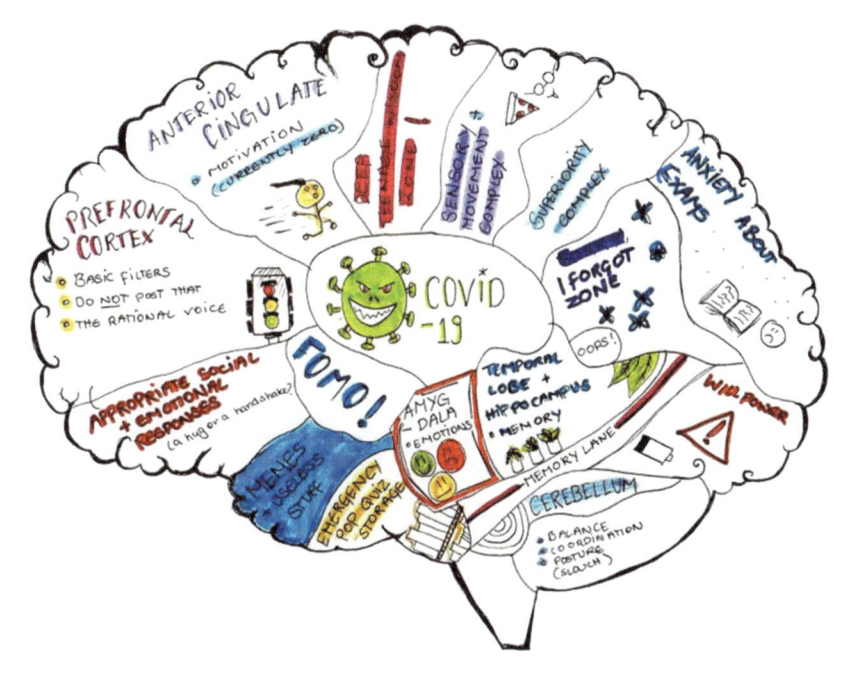

FIGURE 9.1 Insights into an adolescent mind through the pandemic.

Source: Reprinted from Ashwin et al., 2022. https://creativecommons.org/licenses/by/4.0/

9.1.2 INDIAN VEDIC CULTURE AND ITS POSITIVE IMPACT ON ONE'S COMPLETE FITNESS

Indian Vedic Culture, as its name suggests, has its origin from the ancient Indian scriptures known as *Vedas*. These *Vedas* are the compilation of the research studies of various ancient scholars of the Indian subcontinent. These scriptures also mention the ideal fitness regime of an individual and practices required to maintain a healthy lifestyle. According to Vedic science, we humans are a combination of mind, body, and soul. When we talk about fitness in Vedic terms, it is the balancing and nurturing of these three aspects of an individual. Yoga and *asanas* (different body postures) are mentioned for the well-being of the physical body, while *Pranayama* and meditation are mentioned for soothing the nervous system. Various spiritual practices like *Yajna* (a fire ritual with Vedic chants) are there for improving the soul, which results in the overall improvement of mental and physical health.

With these practices, many herbal combinations are prescribed for various ailments (*doshas*) to provide micro- and macro-nutrients to the body for naturally increasing the resistance of the body towards the ailments. Some examples of these combinations are *Triphala, Saraswati Panchak*, etc. The Indian Vedic Science ideologies are based on the fact that the human body is a combination of five elements, namely Earth, Wind, Fire, Water, and Space, and these elements represent nature. To cure any imbalance, either mental or physical, we have to follow protocols in an herbal and spiritual environment in the vicinity of Mother Nature (as per Figure 9.2) (Mondal et al., 2013).

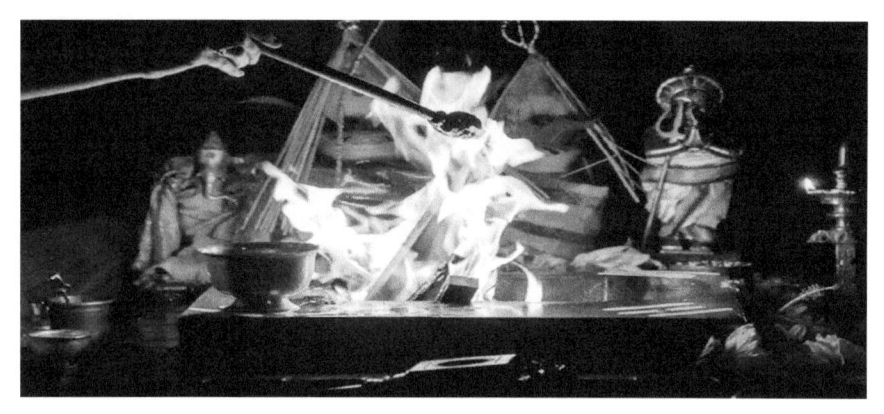

FIGURE 9.2   Representation image of yajna.

Source: Reprinted from Sanatan Prabhat. https://sanatanprabhat.org/english/40859.html.

The given picture is a pictorial representation of a *Yajna* (an ancient Indian Vedic fire ritual) in which offerings are given to the fire. Various medicinal herbs and essential oils are offered in the fire to purify the surroundings and also as a source of spiritual growth.

9.1.3   MENTAL TRAUMA AND NEEDS OF YOUNG KIDS IN FAST ENVIRONMENT

During the pandemic period, young kids have gone through many stressful situations like the fear of losing their close ones, fear of getting infected, and some of them also get quarantined for many days in single rooms during the pandemic. All these situations lead them to a state of psychological trauma.

They were restricted from going outside and also had to do their studies in online mode, resulting in increased screen time, which exposed them to harmful blue light that causes damage to retinal cells and also disturbs sleep cycles, leading to mental stress. Due to these fast changes in their environment, young kids are facing difficulties in aligning themselves to these changes. But these changes are required for continuous growth. So, it is necessary for the kids to practice some protocols that make them capable of facing these changes and methods through which they can maintain a healthy mental and physical lifestyle in this fast environment. Ancient Vedic techniques are methodologies that are easy to understand and can be practiced even at home without the need for expensive equipment. Yoga and meditation can be practiced at home to elevate the mental health of a person, and *Yajna* can be practiced at home to elevate the quality of the atmosphere at home. These practices are proving to be very beneficial in this period of busy lifestyles (Cikanavicius, 2019).

An Ancient Indian practice of meditation and physical postures called Yoga, is very helpful in balancing the physical and mental health of the body and providing an overall fitness to an individual. Thus, it helps in reducing mental stress.

9.1.4 AI, ML, AND DATA SCIENCE APPLICATIONS IN SOCIAL AND BEHAVIORAL STUDIES

Artificial Intelligence (AI), Machine Learning (ML), and Data Science are rapidly transforming the field of social and behavioral studies. These technologies are being used to analyze large datasets and uncover new insights about human behavior and social patterns. AI and ML are being used to develop sophisticated models that can predict how individuals and groups will behave in different situations. Data Science is being used to analyze large datasets, such as social media data, to understand how people interact and form communities online. AI and ML are also being used to identify patterns in social media data that can be used to inform public policy decisions. In healthcare, AI and ML are being used to analyze medical data and develop personalized treatment plans for patients. AI and ML are also being used to improve mental health treatments by analyzing patterns in patient data and identifying new treatment approaches. Data Science is being used to understand how people's behavior changes over time, which can inform public policy decisions (Human Behavior Analysis).

AI and ML are being used to identify patterns in economic data and predict economic trends, which can help businesses make better decisions. In education, AI and ML are being used to personalize learning experiences and improve student outcomes. AI and ML are also being used to analyze data from social experiments and determine the causes and effects of different social phenomena. In criminal justice, AI and ML are being used to analyze crime data and identify patterns that can inform policing strategies and reduce crime rates. Data Science is also being used to understand how people's behavior changes over time, which can inform public policy decisions. AI and ML are being used to predict how people will behave in different situations, which can help businesses and organizations make better decisions. Data Science is also being used to analyze data from social experiments and determine the causes and effects of different social phenomena. AI and ML are being used to identify patterns in economic data and predict economic trends, which can help businesses make better decisions. In summary, AI, ML, and Data Science are powerful tools that can be used to improve our understanding of human behavior and social patterns, which can inform public policy decisions and improve people's lives (as per Figure 9.3) (what-is-behavioral-data-science-and-how-to-get-into-it).

Figure 9.3 depicts a flowchart representing data generations and handling using AI and Machine learning. At first data is generated and then it is cleaned or rearranged using data rearrangement. Few set algorithms are then applied to it. The data is then in this way prepared, processed, tested, and trained. At the end we get a final model which is capable of predicting new data set points based on previous data fed to it.

9.1.5 IOT AND SENSORS-BASED MEASUREMENTS OF HUMAN QUALITATIVE SYMPTOMS

IoT and sensor-based measurements are revolutionizing the way we collect data on human qualitative symptoms, such as pain, fatigue, and mood. IoT devices, such as wearables, can track and transmit data on various physiological and behavioral indicators, providing a more detailed and accurate picture of human health. Sensors can be used to measure

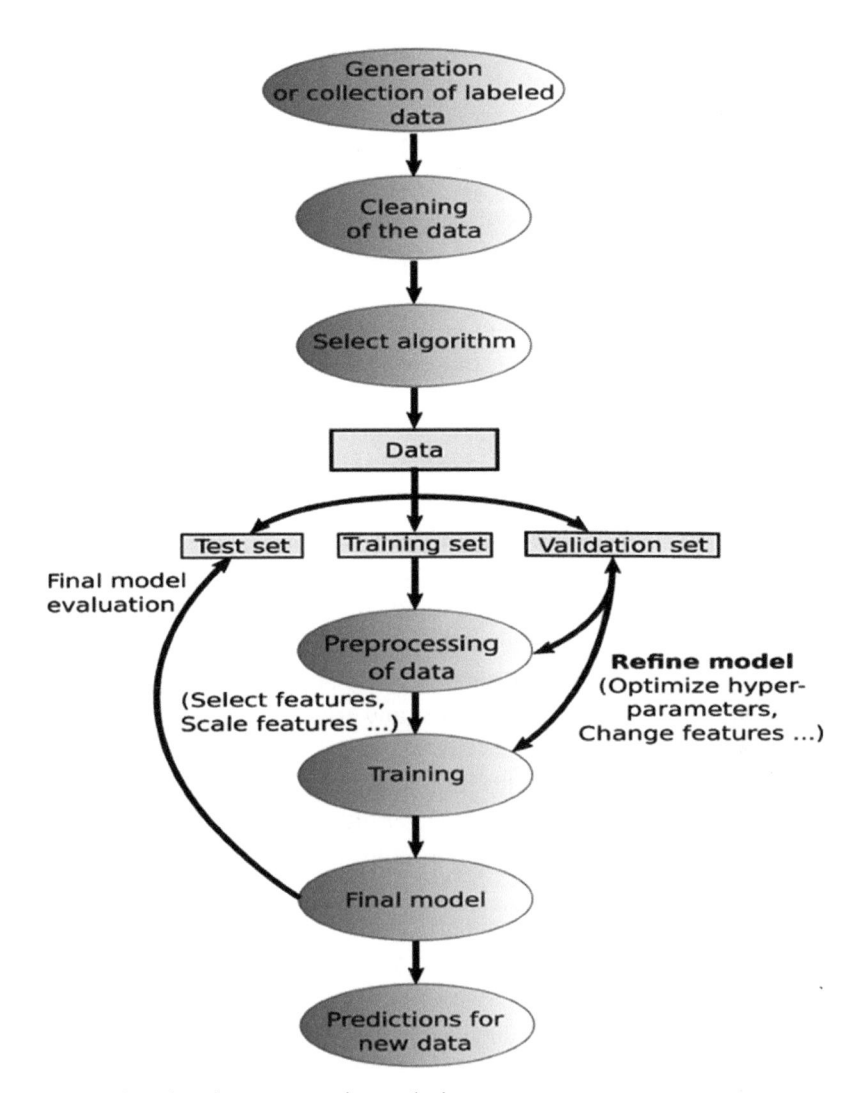

FIGURE 9.3 Flowchart representing analysis pattern.

Source: Reprinted from Schmidt et al., 2019. http://creativecommons.org/licenses/by/4.0/

a wide range of symptoms, including heart rate, skin temperature, and movement patterns, providing a more comprehensive understanding of human health. IoT and sensor-based measurements can be used to track symptoms over time, allowing doctors and researchers to identify patterns and trends in patient health. This technology can also be used to monitor patients remotely, enabling doctors to provide care and support to patients in their own homes. IoT and sensor-based measurements can be used to improve the accuracy of diagnoses and treatment plans, as well as to monitor the effectiveness of treatment over time. This technology can also be used to identify risk factors for certain diseases, such as heart disease or diabetes, allowing patients to take preventative measures. IoT and sensor-based measurements can be integrated into electronic health records, allowing doctors to easily access and analyze patient data. This technology can also be used to improve communication between patients and doctors, enabling patients to provide real-time feedback on their symptoms (Castro et al., 2017).

IoT and sensor-based measurements can be used to improve the quality of life for patients with chronic conditions, such as arthritis or fibromyalgia, by providing them with more information about their symptoms. This technology can also be used to improve the quality of life for elderly people by allowing them to live independently for longer. IoT and sensor-based measurements have the potential to improve patient outcomes by providing more accurate and detailed information about human qualitative symptoms. Additionally, this technology can be used to reduce healthcare costs by allowing doctors to identify and treat problems early on. IoT and sensor-based measurements are a powerful tool for advancing our understanding of human health and improving patient outcomes. This technology is a promising solution to various healthcare challenges, such as remote care, early diagnosis, and monitoring of treatment effectiveness (Pradhan et al., 2021).

The image depicts the various processes included from physiological data measurement of the human body to final result generation and understanding. At first, data is measured using some sensors and various measuring systems. Then it undergoes data preprocessing, and the meaning of the data is obtained. It is then received by medical staff or researchers for various uses.

9.1.6 *KNOWLEDGE PYRAMID, KNOWLEDGE MANAGEMENT, AND ITS IMPACT ON SOCIAL LIFE*

The Knowledge Pyramid is a framework that describes the different levels of knowledge and how they relate to each other. At the base of the pyramid are data and information, which are raw and unorganized. As we move up the pyramid, we reach knowledge, which is information that has been processed and understood. At the top of the pyramid is wisdom, which is the ability to apply knowledge in a practical and meaningful way. Knowledge management is the process of acquiring, organizing, and sharing knowledge within an organization or community. This can involve creating databases, implementing knowledge-sharing systems, and providing training and development opportunities. The impact of knowledge management on social life is far-reaching. It allows people to access and share information more easily, leading to improved decision-making, better collaboration, and increased innovation. It also enables individuals to learn and grow, fostering a culture of continuous learning and improvement. Knowledge management promotes a sense of community and belonging as people share and learn from each other. It helps bridge cultural and language barriers, making it easier for people from different backgrounds to communicate and collaborate. In addition, it can help organizations achieve their goals and objectives more effectively by utilizing the collective intelligence of the group. In today's fast-paced and constantly changing world, knowledge management has become an essential tool for staying competitive and relevant. It is vital for individuals, organizations, and communities to regularly assess and improve their knowledge management systems to stay ahead of the curve. Effective knowledge management can lead to better social outcomes and improve the quality of life for all (Castro et al., 2017; Damgaard, 2023; What is the Data, Information, Knowledge, Wisdom (DIKW) Pyramid? 2023).

9.1.7 EXTRACTION OF USEFUL INFORMATION FROM HUMAN PHYSICAL AND MENTAL PARAMETERS

The extraction of useful information from human physical and mental parameters is a crucial aspect of healthcare and wellness. With advances in technology, it is now possible to use sensors and other devices to gather data about a person's physiology and psychology. This data can then be analyzed to gain insights into a person's physical and mental health. By tracking vital signs such as heart rate, blood pressure, and temperature, doctors can detect early signs of illness or disease. Additionally, by monitoring sleep patterns, physical activity, and stress levels, healthcare professionals can identify potential risk factors for certain conditions. The extraction of information from mental parameters such as emotional state, mood, and cognitive function can also provide valuable insights into a person's mental well-being.

By using techniques such as brain imaging and cognitive testing, researchers can study the brain and its functions in greater detail. This can lead to a better understanding of conditions such as depression, anxiety, and dementia. Additionally, by using machine learning algorithms, it is possible to analyze large amounts of data and identify patterns that might otherwise be missed. This can help healthcare professionals make more accurate diagnoses and develop more effective treatment plans. The extraction of useful information from human physical and mental parameters can lead to better health outcomes and improved quality of life for individuals. It is an ongoing and rapidly developing area of research with many exciting possibilities for the future (Russ et al., 2019).

Data science has a multidimensional role in healthcare for it helps not only in detection, data collection, surveys, but also helps in developing ways for the cure and support people to live well with mental health conditions.

9.1.8   HOMA THERAPY ALONG WITH HERBAL USAGE AS AN ESTABLISHED INDIAN SCIENCE TO CURE DISEASES AND TRAUMA

Originated from the holy texts of knowledge and wisdom, the *Vedas-Homa* therapy has been a part of human civilization since the very early times. *Homa* therapy can be defined as a science that uses the energy of the universe to establish order between its biotic and abiotic components. Essentially, it is based on the natural principle of give and take where we heal the environment and its components through *Yajna* and *Havan* and in return the healed environment heals our mind, body, and soul. Various scientific research have been performed to bring to light the effect of *Yajna* and *Havan* on the individual aspects of the environment and human health. But the marvelous fact about Homa therapy is not its healing power but rather its efficiency to keep us disease-free, as it has been said in the *Charak Samhita* as well.

> *"PRAYOJANAM CHASYA–SWASTHASYA SWASTHA RAKSHANAM AATURASYA VIKARPRASHAMANAM CHA" (CH.SM.SU. 30/26)*

Which states the objective of Ayurveda, the ancient traditional medicinal science of healing, as not only to make the unhealthy person disease-free but also to maintain the good health of an already healthy person. Ayurveda in detail deals with different herbal formulations which are capable of fighting deadly diseases like cancer. As it has been established, food is our first medicine. Ayurveda guides us on how we can actually implement the same. And *Homa* therapy is a way to ensure that the food we intake stays healthy as well. The times of pandemic have forced us to accept the lost treasure of Ayurveda and Yagyopathy as our only source of light in the times of darkness (Koach et al., 2004).

Agnihotra is a comprehensive science and practice that integrates the benefits of both biotic and non-biotic parts of Mother Earth. It is not only beneficial for the body but also a potential brain tonic. It increases brain efficiency by releasing stress and maintaining the appropriate chemical balance of the nervous system.

Turmeric, which is also an important food component in almost all Indian dishes, possesses magical qualities including its anti-inflammatory, anti-obesity, anti-diabetic, antioxidant, anti-cancer effects, etc.

9.1.9 MANTRA AND YAJNA: A POWERFUL WEAPON FOR SUSTAINABLE DEVELOPMENT

Ayurveda describes a phenomenon called *Janpad* on *Dhwansa*, which is a condition where a large human habitation faces a situation of a pandemic due to contamination of panchtatva, i.e., *jal* (water), *agni* (fire), *aakash* (space), *vayu* (air), *bhoomi* (earth), resulting in the loss of human lives. Sustainable development is the only way to prevent the forecasted condition of *Janpad* on *Dhwansa* from actually occurring. Sustainable development follows the idea of attaining human developmental goals without hindering nature and its functioning. *Yajna* and *mantra* are the ways to achieve that (Rastogi et al., 2021).

Originating from the ancient treasures of Vedas, the *Yajna* techniques follow the belief of nature being the divinity of all. *Shanti mantra* prays for the goodness of all the components of nature, both living and nonliving. All the ingredients of *Yajna* – the woods, Samagri, and ghee–not only purify nature but also replenish it with nutrients and positivize it. Science has observed the positive impact of yajna and mantra on the human nervous system, thus promising not only better lives but also better efficiency (Rafaj et al., 2018).

Yajna is a comprehensive technique of purification of mind, body, soul, and surroundings. This not only rejuvenates our mind and soul but also the environment. This is no longer a religious belief but a proven science. The various wondrous effects of *Yajna* include its ability to improve AQI, purify water, replenishment of nutrients in soil, and create a positive environment. Also, it purifies blood, reduces stress, and helps in diabetes and blood pressure.

9.2   LITERATURE REVIEW

Literature reviews are very important for any study, as they are the basis of existing ideas. The literature review provides insight into already established information related to the study being conducted, and sheds light on topics that may have been overlooked among other issues. It connects the dots to map the extent of work that has already been done on a particular topic. In this case, the team has summarized the literary works of different authors and journals to bring to light information regarding herbal medication, mental illness, adolescence growth, and more.

Xiang and his team conducted a study examining the associations between lifestyle changes such as screen time and physical activity, which occurred during or before the COVID-19 pandemic, with mental health. The study involved 2,423 children in Shanghai, China. Their lifestyle behaviors and psychological conditions (depression, anxiety, and stress) were noted and assessed through a self-reported questionnaire in January and March 2020. This study was conducted in two waves, and the impact of lifestyle activities on mental health was documented.

Then the results showed that adolescents with less screen time before/ during the pandemic have a much lower risk of psychological disorders than the ones with prolonged screen time and persistent screen time. Also, individuals with high physical activity were on the safer side. The final conclusions of the study were that an increase in screen time and a decrease in physical activity during the COVID-19 pandemic drastically increased the chances of developing psychological disorders. In order to prevent this, effective steps must be taken by improving physical activity and controlling leisure screen time (Xiang et al., 2022).

Gururaja (2011) and his team conducted a study to find out the effect of Yoga on mental health of the individuals. They also compared the effect of the same on both the elders and younger age group people. For this, a study was done in Japan on 25 individuals of different age groups. This study was approved by the Kawasaki University of Medical Welfare. Individuals of both genders were taken into account and were divided into two groups. There were 10 participants in one group (65–75 years of age) and 15 participants in another group (20–30 years of age). These participants were subjected to 90 minutes of Yoga protocol once or twice a week, and their Salivary Amylase activity was noted before and after the Yoga session. To assess the change in state anxiety and trait anxiety, the State Trait Anxiety Inventory (STAI) was given before the first Yoga class and after one month of the protocol. Results were obtained, showing a reduction in salivary amylase activity from 111.2 ± 42.7 to 83.48 ± 39.5 kU/L for seniors and 60.74 ± 31.8 to 42.39 ± 24 kU/L for the younger age group. State anxiety and trait anxiety scores were also found to be reduced, and these changes were statistically significant with $P<0.05$. These results indicate that the decrease in salivary amylase activity is due to the reduction in sympathetic response. Also, the reduction in state and trait anxiety concludes that Yoga is beneficial in the short term as well as long term for managing anxiety and stress (Gururaja et al., 2011).

Rathi (2019) in her study revealed the effect of *Yagya* on Environment purification and mental and Physical health of an individual in a more scientific way. A group of scientists and the Uttar Pradesh Pollution Control Board performed various experiments during Ashvamedha Yagya in Gorakhpur, Uttar Pradesh. Sensitive instruments like the high-volume Envirotech APM-45 were used to analyze the water and air samples of the surroundings. The results showed a decrease in the levels of nitrous oxide and sulfur oxide in the air samples of the surroundings, and a significant reduction in bacteria counts in the water samples. It was later discovered that the ash from the Yagya contained certain minerals, making it a good fertilizer. This claim was supported by the Deputy Director of the Agriculture Department. All these findings support the claim that the *Yagya* reduces air pollution and improves overall environmental quality when performed using the proper herbal content and methodology prescribed in ancient Indian Vedic texts (Rathi et al., 2019).

Khedkar (2018) defined the transition from childhood to adulthood. This age of adolescence is full of turbulence. Making up almost 1/5th of India's population, teens aging from 12–19 years come under this category. The study explores the role of pitta dosha in the human body as a significant factor for several transformations that are part of adolescence. Also, the role of *kapha doshas* is found relevant during this time. The five types of *kaphas–avlambaka, kledak, bodhak, shleshak, tarpaka*—present in different regions of the body, i.e., chest, stomach, tongue, joints, and head respectively, govern different physiological processes of the body. Similarly, *alochaka, bhrajakta, sadhaka, pachaka,* and *ranjakta* are the five kinds of pitta doshas that should be in correct balance for healthy sustainability. The study also discusses the Manas rogue to which teen-agers are more prone. These include anxiety, depression, etc., caused due to disturbances in sattva. A correct lifestyle, balanced diet, and good behavior can help avoid mental ailments. *Brahmi, Ashwagandha, Guduchi, Yashtimadhu,* and *Vacha* are described as marvelous nervine tonics and a great choice for the treatment of mental illnesses (Khedkar et al., 2018).

Singh (2020) and the team informed that the WHO links mental health with the ability to manage day-to-day stresses. One third of the world's population can be categorized as mentally ill in one way or another, suffering from diseases like depression, anxiety, and schizo-phrenia. Mental illness directly impacts other aspects of health, including the socio-economic dimension. Among adolescents, suicide is a major issue caused by mental infirmity. The formulation of the herbal weapon *Saraswati Panchak* by Pandit Shri Ram Sharma was not only a boon to humankind but also a requirement in today's time to combat the monster of mental ailments.

Saraswati Panchak comprises five redoubtable drugs, namely *Brahmi, Shankhpushpi, Vach, Gorakhmundi,* and *Shatavari.* These are medhya rasayanas (nootropic herbs) and enhance memory as well as cognitive skills by directly instigating nerve growth, increasing oxygen supply to the brain, and altering the amount of neurotransmitters, enzymes, and hormones involved in neural functioning. The chapter studies the applica-tion of these herbs as tablets and as *Havan Samagri.*

Ancient texts like *Atharva Veda, Charak Samhita, Sushrut Samhita,* etc., also described the qualities of these drugs as *medhya rasayana* and effective cures for mental illnesses. Brahmi, apart from being a brain tonic, is also effective in treating skin diseases, insanity, asthma, epilepsy, and digestive ailments. Additionally, it improves concentration and memory, repairs damaged neurons, and has anti-aging effects on them.

Shankhpushpi, apart from being a nervine tonic, is also a hypotensive drug, tranquilizer, and laxative. It can modulate hippocampal plasticity.

Vach is very effective against insomnia, mental retardation, skin diseases, hemorrhoids, dysentery, hepatic disorders, kidney problems, depression, and respiratory disorders. It shows acetylcholine enzyme inhibition effect, thus proving its direct effect on memory and cognitive behavior.

Gorakhmundi is found to be useful against elephantiasis, anemia, pain in the vagina and uterus, piles, biliousness, epileptic convulsions, looseness of the breasts, hemicranias, leukoderma, dysentery, vomiting, and urinary discharges.

Satavari is a storehouse of vitamins A, B1, B2, C, E, P, Mg, Ca, Fe, and folic acid. It shows inhibiting effects on Monoamine oxidase (MAO-A and MAO-B) activity and proves to be an excellent antidepressant.

For the preparation of the formulation, crude forms of the above-mentioned drugs were identified, collected, and stored at ambient conditions. Pharmacognosy of the extracted matter was performed and analyzed through different methods.

And thus, another gem was added to the treasure of herbal medication (Singh, 2020). COVID-19 affected not only physical health but mental health as well. The onset of COVID also increased cases of mental illnesses among humans. There was a rise in the number of people suffering from depression, anxiety, insomnia, mood swings, and suicidal tendencies. The lockdown added more to these mental disturbances.

The Rahman and team studied the sample size of 350 people all around Bangladesh from different age groups using artificial intelligence and questionnaires to observe the changes individuals had to face in different sectors of life during lockdown and COVID.

During the study, apart from surrounding conditions, the daily internet usage by an individual was also studied and recorded to further observe the relationship between mental ailments and the internet and social media.

The study did not just focus on recording the number of people affected by any kind of medical ailment but also tried to uncover their reasons for the same. Diversity among regions, age groups, genders, and professions was attempted to be maintained while selecting the subjects. It was observed that the number of affected females was greater than males. Also, decreased productivity, reduced social gatherings, loss of jobs, etc., played a role in the same (Rahman et al., 2021).

Loades (2020) and his team defined a rapid systematic review that explores the impact of social isolation and loneliness on the mental health of children and adolescents in the context of COVID-19. The authors searched several databases to identify relevant studies and used predetermined criteria to evaluate their quality. The results of this review showed that social isolation and loneliness have a significant negative impact on the mental health of children and adolescents during the COVID-19 pandemic. The authors found evidence of increased levels of anxiety, depression, stress, and emotional distress in children and adolescents due to the pandemic and associated social isolation measures.

The methodology of this review is thorough, and the authors have made a strong effort to identify and critically evaluate relevant studies. The results of the review provide important insights into the mental health implications of social isolation and loneliness in children and adolescents during the COVID-19 pandemic. The findings of this review can inform public health policy and support the development of interventions aimed at mitigating the negative impact of social isolation on the mental health of children and adolescents.

In conclusion, this rapid systematic review provides valuable insights into the impact of social isolation and loneliness on the mental health of children and adolescents during the COVID-19 pandemic. The results of the review highlight the need for further research in this area, as well as the importance of implementing interventions to support the mental health of children and adolescents during times of social isolation and increased stress. Overall, the chapter is well-written and provides important information for those working in the fields of public health and mental health (Loades et al., 2020).

Liu et al. (2015) explained in their work a comprehensive and in-depth examination of the use of herbal medicine in the treatment of anxiety, depression, and insomnia. The authors conduct a thorough literature review of the available evidence and evaluate the efficacy of different herbal remedies for these conditions. The objective of the review is to provide a comprehensive overview of the use of herbal medicine in the treatment of mental health conditions, with a focus on anxiety, depression, and insomnia. The results of the review indicate that some herbal remedies, such as valerian, kava, and passionflower, have shown promise in treating anxiety, depression, and insomnia. The authors provide a detailed discussion of the mechanism of action of each herbal remedy and the results of clinical trials that have been conducted to evaluate their efficacy. Additionally, the authors discuss the potential side effects and safety concerns associated with the use of herbal medicine for mental health conditions. The methodology of the review is well-conducted, and the authors have made a comprehensive effort to critically evaluate the available evidence.

The results of the review are presented in a clear and concise manner, making it easy for readers to understand the key findings. The authors also provide recommendations for future research to further explore the efficacy of herbal medicine in treating anxiety, depression, and insomnia. One of the strengths of this chapter is the discussion of the limitations of the available evidence. The authors acknowledge the challenges associated with conducting clinical trials of herbal medicine and the need for further research to fully understand the potential benefits and risks associated with the use of these remedies. Additionally, the authors provide an overview of the current regulatory framework for herbal medicine and discuss the importance of ensuring the safety and quality of these products. In conclusion, this chapter provides a valuable and comprehensive overview of the use of herbal medicine in the treatment of anxiety, depression, and insomnia. The authors have made a thorough effort to critically evaluate the available evidence and provide a clear and concise summary of the results. The chapter provides important information for those seeking alternative treatments for mental health conditions and highlights the need for further research to fully understand the potential benefits and risks associated with the use of herbal medicine. Overall, the chapter is well-written, well-researched, and provides a valuable contribution to the field of mental health and alternative medicine (Liu et al., 2015).

Trivedi (2020) expounded the aim of his research chapter to examine the effect of Yagya therapy on the level of emotional maturity. *Yagya* therapy is a traditional Hindu practice that involves burning specific herbs and making offerings to the divine in order to promote physical, mental, and spiritual well-being. In this study, Dr. Trivedi aims to determine whether *Yagya* therapy has any impact on the emotional maturity of individuals who participate in the therapy. The methodology of the study is well-designed and appropriate for the research question being addressed. Dr. Trivedi used a controlled experimental design in which participants were randomly assigned to either a *Yagya* therapy group or a control group. The emotional maturity of participants was assessed before and after the intervention, and the results were analyzed to determine whether *Yagya* therapy had any effect on emotional maturity. The results of the study indicate that *Yagya* therapy had a significant impact on the emotional maturity of participants. Specifically, participants in the *Yagya* therapy group showed a significant improvement in their emotional maturity scores compared to participants in the control group. The authors provide a detailed discussion of the results and suggest that *Yagya* therapy may be an effective intervention for improving emotional maturity. One of the strengths of this chapter is the use of a rigorous methodology to examine the effect of *Yagya* therapy. The controlled experimental design allows for a more accurate determination of causality, and the results of the study are convincing. Additionally, the discussion of the results is well-organized and easy to understand, making it accessible to a broad audience.

In conclusion, this chapter provides valuable insights into the impact of *Yagya* therapy on emotional maturity. The results of the study suggest that *Yagya* therapy may be an effective intervention for improving emotional maturity, and the methodology used in the study is rigorous and well-designed. This chapter will be of interest to those who are interested in alternative therapies for mental and emotional well-being, as well as those who are interested in the role of cultural and spiritual practices in promoting well-being. Overall, this is a well-written, well-researched chapter that provides valuable contributions to the field of mental and emotional health (Trivedi, 2020). The research summary and gist has been identified as per Table 9.1.

9.3 METHODOLOGY AND SETUP OF EXPERIMENT

This experiment was conducted after the second wave of the COVID-19 pandemic and lockdown 2.0 in India. It was performed using Havan Samagri and burnt in a Hawan Kunda. Dr. Mamata Saxena, a renowned scientist and former Director General of the Ministry of Statistics and PI (MoS-PI), conducted this experiment at her residence on Lodhi Road, New Delhi, India. Due to the ongoing lockdown 2.0, a public ceremony was not possible.

After COVID-19, human lives have witnessed many disastrous changes. The emergence of a large number of health problems, especially mental health-related ailments, has become a concern for people world-wide. Among the affected population, the number of adolescent groups is the highest. Therefore, Dr. Mamata Saxena, an acclaimed scientist and former Director General of the Ministry of Statistics and PI (MoS-PI), conducted an experiment at her lab located on Lodhi Road, New Delhi, India. The experiment was conducted to study the effect of Yajna and the medicinal herb *Saraswati Panchak* on the subjects.

The subjects were in the age group of 13 to 19 (teenagers). The experiment studied the impact of an orderly lifestyle including daily practice of yajna and consumption of Saraswati Panchak, encompassing the five potent herbs: *Brahmi* (*Bacopa monnieri*), *Shankhpushpi* (*Convolvulus pluri-caulis*), *Vach* (*Acorus calamus*), *Gorakhmundi* (*Sphaeranthus indicus*), and *Satavari* (*Asparagus racemosus*), on the subjects. For this, different test aspects were taken into consideration to study their all-round outcome. These include eight parameters:

- Their understanding ability, i.e., the power of comprehending;
- Their altruistic behavior, i.e., tendency to help;
- Mathematical ability;
- Memory power;
- Honesty;
- Sense of responsibility;
- Courageousness;
- Intelligence.

The study was started by dividing the population of 24 subjects into two groups – experimental group and control group, each consisting of 12 subjects. The study was performed for 37 days from 25-05-22 to 01-07-22, and readings before and after the experiments (i.e., pre-experimental readings and post-experimental readings) of each subject were recorded. The subjects of the experimental group performed *Yajna* daily, along with *Pranayama* and Yoga. Their diet was balanced, nutritious, restricted, and scheduled timely. They were also made to consume the herbal combination of *Saraswati Panchak*. They had daily math and science. *Yajna* was performed with particular protocols using woods of mango tree, pure ghee, and *Samagri* along with the recital of mantras like *Gayathri mantra, shanti path, guru mantra, Surya Gayathri mantra*, etc. The control group was exempted from all such conditions.

At regular intervals, tests were taken of the experimental group to observe the differences in the parameters discussed above. After the conduction of the study successfully, the results were analyzed using Python and Tableau to record the changes observed in both groups, which are represented graphically in Figure 9.4.

9.3.1   FLOW CHART

The flowchart discusses the methodology of the present study briefly. Before the onset of the study, the subjects were divided into controlled and experimental groups. The experimental group was made to perform *Yajna*, intake a balanced diet, administer *Sarswati Panchak*, the herbal formulation, and follow a fixed routine. The study of different parameters was then recorded, analyzed, and finally represented graphically (as per Figure 9.4).

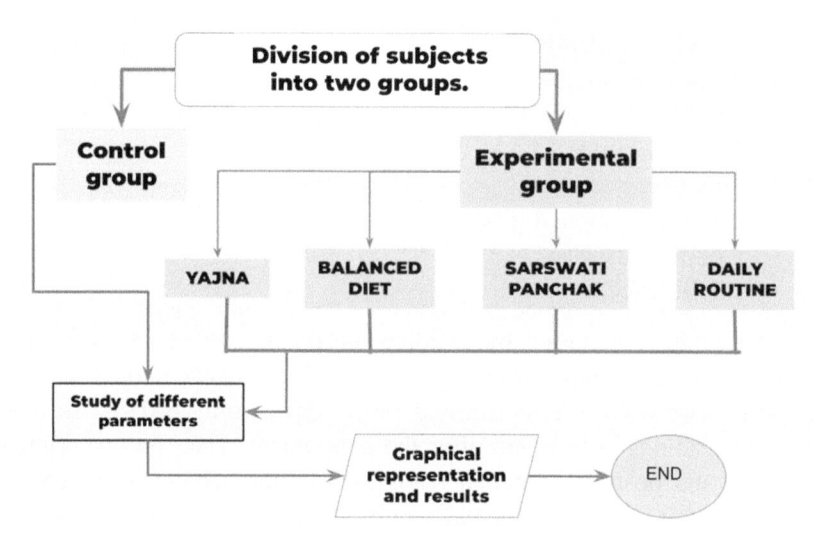

FIGURE 9.4   Flow chart of *Saraswati Panchak* experiment.

9.4   RESULTS AND DISCUSSIONS

The researcher performed paired t-tests (two-tailed) on the control group students' records. There were 15 students who took part in this test. This study performs the analysis in ways to analyze it properly.

Based on their performance, they are graded with some points from 0 to 10. These grades were provided by the faculty. There are previous scores and after scores of the students. The properties which are used to measure their performance in all dimensions. These are:

- Understanding power;
- Propensity to help;
- Math comprehension skills;
- Ability to remember;
- Honesty;
- Responsibility;
- Bravery;
- Wisdom.

9.4.1 ANALYSIS BASED ON PROPERTIES USING PAIRED T-TEST (TWO TAILED)

The analysis is done by calculating the performance of control group students according to each property.

9.4.1.1 UNDERSTANDING POWER

This property helps students to interact and understand things on their own. This analysis shows that students have developed the understanding power on their own.

9.4.1.1.1 REPRESENTATION OF THE TEST SCORES

As shown in Figure 9.5, it is clear that there is a big difference between the performances of the students according to their understanding power. The blue dot represents the previous test score, which is shown at the low level of the graph. The orange dot represents the post-test score of the students, which is shown at the high level (*please refer to* Table A) (as per Figure 9.5).

TABLE A

| Student's Name | Understanding Power | |
	Pre	Post
Prem	2	4
Raja	3	6
Krishna	3	6
Prince	2	5
Sidhu	1	4
Pooja	3	6
Anamika	2	4
Khushi	1	5
Khusboo	2	6
Karan	2	4
Pradeep	2	5
Mukund	3	6
Rajkumar	2	4
Jyoti	3	5
Govinda	4	5

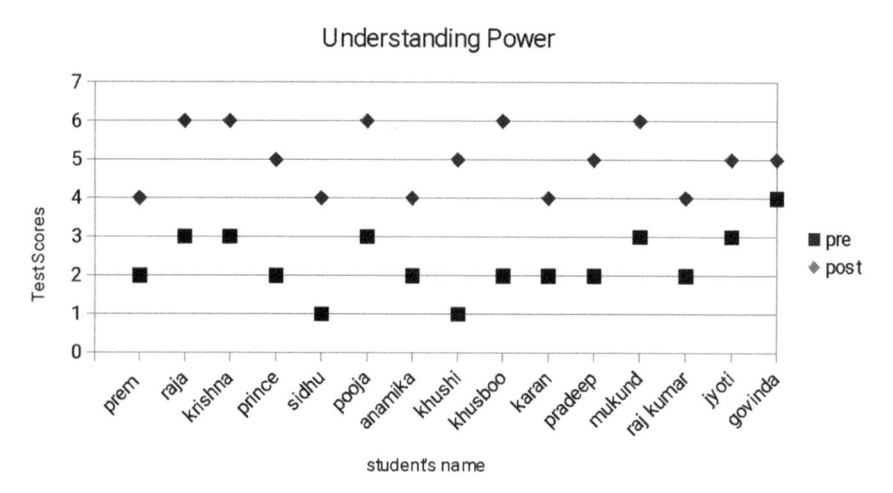

FIGURE 9.5   Representation of the test scores of the students according to their understanding power.

TABLE 9.1 The Background Summary

SL. No.	Title and Author's Name	Introduction	Methodology	Data Set and Algorithms	Future Scope and Conclusion
1.	Association of changes of lifestyle behaviors before and during the COVID-19 pandemic with mental health: a longitudinal study in children and adolescents (Xinag et al., 2022).	Examine the combined association of physical activity and screen time with mental health during the pandemic.	A two-wave longitudinal study was performed.	2,423 children were observed, Self-reported questionnaire, series of variable logistic regressions.	Concluded that having long persistent screen time before or during COVID is associated with impaired mental health.
2.	Effect of yoga on mental health: Comparative study between young and senior subjects in Japan (Guru Raja et al., 2011).	Japan has large number of elder population and Yoga can be beneficial to them. Hence there is a need for study the effects of Yoga on mental health of senior and younger citizen.	90 minutes Yoga protocol once or twice a week is followed by the individual and their Salivary amylase activity was assessed before and after Yoga.	25 normal healthy volunteers of both sexes, Concorometer for salivary amylase activity test, state trait anxiety inventory (STAI).	Yoga is helpful for both younger and elder ones for mental health. This study can be further extended by increasing data sets and using advance tools.
3.	Effects of Yagya on environment purification and human health: A review (Rathi et al., 2019)	Atmospheric pollution is a major hazard to the health of living beings. In this condition, Yagya is proved to be effective in purifying the surroundings. Hence, Reducing the air pollution.	Various experiments were performed during Ashvamedha Yagya and Air and water Quality parameters were measured before and after the yagya and results were observed.	100 ml samples of each air and water were collected and analyzed by highly sensitive instruments like High Volume Envirotech APM-45, etc.	Yagya if performed regularly performed will purify the surrounding air and water and create a medicinal atmosphere and also prevents the growth of microorganisms.

TABLE 9.1 *(Continued)*

SL. No.	Title and Author's Name	Introduction	Methodology	Data Set and Algorithms	Future Scope and Conclusion
4.	Role of ayurveda in adolescent age (Khedkar et al., 2018).	Adolescence as per Ayurveda and role of pitta dosha.	Different doshas affecting human body.	NA	Instigate the process of establishing correlation between modern science and ancient terminologies.
5.	Saraswati Panchak – A novel herbal combination for mental health (Singh, 2020).	Lime lights the increasing cases of mental illnesses and effectiveness of herbs in curing them.	Literature review and clinical study of drugs comprising Saraswati Panchak	Statistical tests, SPS tool.	Gives idea of restudying of ancient texts to invent other potent formulations to combat the increasing number of ailments.
6.	Impact of COVID-19 on mental health: A quantitative analysis of anxiety and depression based on regular life and internet use (Rahman et al., 2021).	COVID adversely impacted both the physical and mental health.	Literary review of studies discussing mental health. Data collection and analysis for affected population during the pandemic.	Statistical algorithms	Forces one to see the destructive role of AI and the internet. And how social aspect is a very important aspect of individual's health.
7.	Herbal medicine for anxiety, depression, and insomnia. *Curr. Neuropharmacol.* (Liu et al., 2015).	Impact of cognitive-behavioral therapy on the reduction of anxiety and depression symptoms in children with autism spectrum disorder.	Randomized controlled trial (RCT) methodology with two groups: one receiving cognitive-behavioral therapy and the other receiving treatment as usual.	Data set was comprised of 80 children aged 8–14 with autism spectrum disorder, and the algorithms used in the study were not specified.	Need for larger sample sizes and further exploration of specific mechanisms of change. The study concluded that cognitive-behavioral therapy can be an effective treatment for anxiety and depression symptoms in children with autism spectrum disorder.

TABLE 9.1 *(Continued)*

SL. No.	Title and Author's Name	Introduction	Methodology	Data Set and Algorithms	Future Scope and Conclusion
8.	To study the effect of Yagya therapy on the level of emotional maturity (Trivedi et al., 2020)	Use of virtual reality technology in the treatment of post-traumatic stress disorder (PTSD).	Randomized controlled trial (RCT) methodology with two groups: one receiving traditional exposure therapy and the other receiving virtual reality exposure therapy.	The data set was comprised of 42 participants diagnosed with PTSD, and the algorithms used in the study were not specified.	The study concluded that virtual reality exposure therapy is a feasible and effective treatment for PTSD. Further research is needed to investigate its long-term effects and potential use in combination with other treatments.
9.	Rapid systematic review: The impact of social isolation and loneliness on the mental health of children and adolescents in the context of COVID-19 (Lades et al., 2015)	The impact of Yagya therapy on the level of emotional maturity.	The methodology used in the study was not specified.	The data set and algorithms used in the study were not specified.	Mechanisms of Action: Future studies could explore the specific mechanisms through which Yagya therapy impacts emotional maturity, including possible physiological or psychological.

9.4.1.1.2   PAIRED SAMPLE T-TEST ANALYSIS

Table 9.2 shows the calculated values of the paired t-test. Results indicate that there is a significant large difference between previous (M = 2.3, S.D. = 0.8) and post (M = 5, S.D. = 0.8), t(14) = 12.6, p<0.001, where M abbreviates mean and S.D. means standard deviation, t(14) means the value of t at the degree of freedom 14 (as per Figure 9.5) (as per Table 9.2).

TABLE 9.2   Resultant Table of the Paired t-Test

Alpha	0.05	
	Pre-Scores	**Post-Scores**
Mean	2.3	5
S.D.	0.8	0.8
T-value	12.6491	–
P-value	4.743e-9	–
Sample size	15	–
Degree of freedom	14	–
Average of difference	2.6667	–
S.D. of difference	0.8165	–

9.4.1.1.3   REPRESENTATION AND DESCRIPTION OF THE DISTRIBUTION OF THE T-TEST

1. **H0 Hypothesis:** Since, H0 is rejected. The sample difference between the averages of the post and previous is big enough to be statistically significant (as per Figure 9.6).
2. **P-Value:** The p-value equals 4.743e-9, (P(x<=12.6491) = 1), means the chance of rejecting the correct H0 is small.
3. **Test Statistic:** The t value equals 12.6491, which is not in the acceptance.

$$t = \bar{x}\text{differences} - \mu_0/S\text{differences}/\sqrt{n}$$
$$S.E. = S \text{ differences}/\sqrt{n} = 0.8165/\sqrt{15} = 0.2108$$
$$t = 2.6667 - 0/0.2108 = 12.6491$$

4. **Effect Size:** The effect size between the average and expected average is large, 3.27.

$$Cohen's\ D = |\bar{x}\ d - \mu_o|/Sd$$
$$= |2.6667 - 0|/0.8165$$
$$= 3.266$$

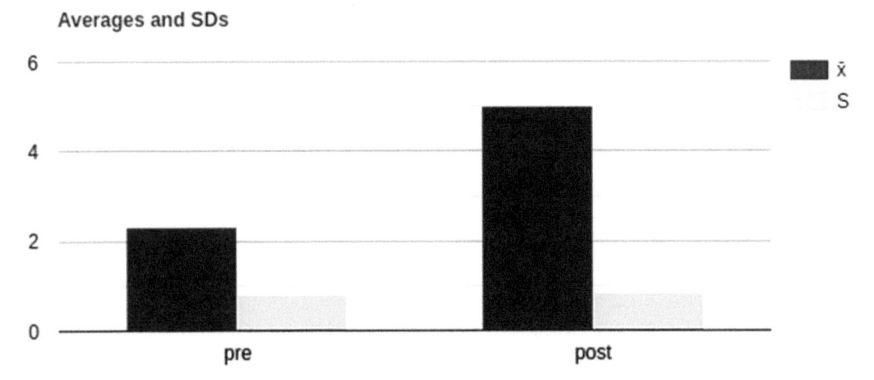

FIGURE 9.6 Average and standard derivation of the students according to understanding power.

9.4.1.2 PROPENSITY TO HELP

This is the property to help each other. This develops the togetherness between the students to interact with each other and help each other.

9.4.1.2.1 Representation of the Test Scores

As shown in Figure 9.7, it is clear that there is a big difference between the performances of the students according to their helping power. The blue dot represents the previous test score, which is shown at the low level of the graph. The orange dot represents the post-test score of the students, which is shown at the high level (*please refer to* Table B) (as per Figure 9.7).

TABLE B

	Propensity to Help	
Student's Name	**Pre**	**Post**
Prem	1	3
Raja	3	5
Krishna	2	6
Prince	1	3
Sidhu	1	3
Pooja	3	6
Anamika	2	5
Khushi	4	6
Khusboo	4	6
Karan	2	3
Pradeep	2	4
Mukund	1	3
Rajkumar	1	5
Jyoti	3	6
Govinda	1	2

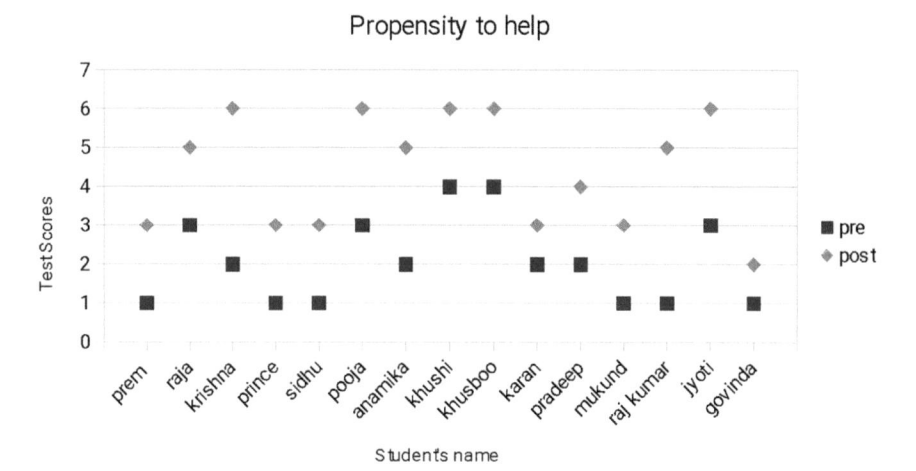

FIGURE 9.7   Representation of the test scores of the students according to their propensity to help.

9.4.1.2.2 Paired Sample t-Test Analysis

Table 9.3 shows the calculated values of the paired t-test. Results indicated that there is a significant large difference between previous (M = 2.1, S.D. = 1.1) and post (M = 4.4, S.D. = 1.5), t(14) = 10, p < 0.001, where M abbreviates mean and S.D. means standard deviation, t(14) means the value of t at the degree of freedom 14 (as per Table 9.3).

TABLE 9.3   Resultant Table of the Paired T-Test

Alpha	0.05	
	Pre-Scores	**Post-Scores**
Mean	2.1	4.4
S.D.	1.1	1.5
T-value	10.044	–
P-value	8.846e-8	–
Sample size	15	–
Degree of freedom	14	–
Average of difference	2.3333	–
S.D. of difference	0.8997	–

9.4.1.2.3 Representation and Description of the Distribution of the T-Test

1. **H0 Hypothesis:** Since, H0 is rejected. The sample difference between the averages of the post and previous is big enough to be statistically significant (as per Figure 9.8).
2. **P-Value:** The p-value equals 8.846e-8, (P(x<=10.044) =1), means the chance of rejecting the correct H0 is small.
3. **Test Statistic:** The t value equals 10.044, which is not in the acceptance.

$$t = \bar{x}\text{differences} - \mu_0/\text{Sdifferences}/\sqrt{n}$$
$$\text{S.E.} = S\text{ differences}/\sqrt{n} = 0.8997/\sqrt{15} = 0.2323$$
$$t = 2.3333 - 0/0.2323 = 10.044$$

4. **Effect Size:** The effect size between the average and expected average is large, 2.59.

$$\text{Cohen's D} = |\bar{x}d - \mu_o|/Sd$$
$$\text{Cohen's D} = |2.3333 - 0|/0.8997 = 2.5934$$

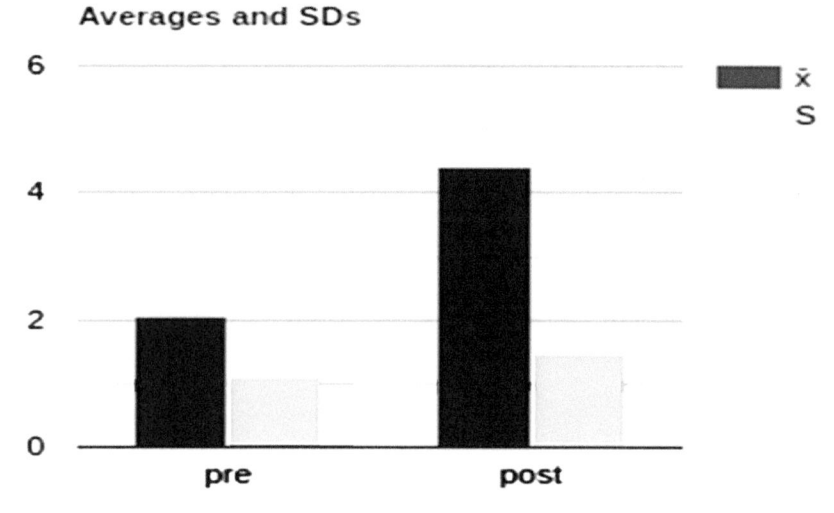

Averages and SDs

FIGURE 9.8 Average and standard derivation of the students according to propensity to help property.

9.4.1.3 *MATH COMPREHENSION SKILLS*

In the experiment session, math classes are provided to the student. This property shows the performance of the students in the math test.

9.4.1.3.1 *Representation of the Test Scores*

As shown in Figure 9.9, it is clear that there is a significant difference in the performance of the students based on their math skills. The blue dot represents the previous test score, which is shown at a low level on the graph. The orange dot represents the post-test score of the students, which is shown at a higher level (*please refer to* Table C).

TABLE C

	Math Comprehension Skills	
Student's Name	**Pre**	**Post**
Prem	1	3
Raja	3	6
Krishna	2	5
Prince	1	4
Sidhu	2	7.7
Pooja	4	6
Anamika	3	6
Khushi	3	6
Khusboo	3	5
Karan	2	3
Pradeep	2	4
Mukund	2	5
Rajkumar	1	5
Jyoti	4	6
Govinda	3	6

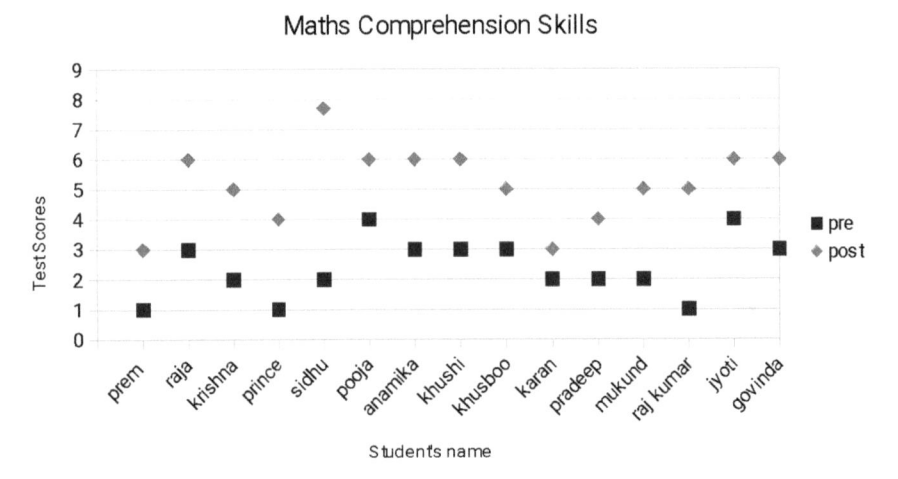

FIGURE 9.9 Representation of the test scores of the students according to their math skills.

9.4.1.3.2   Paired Sample T-Test Analysis

Table 9.4 shows the calculated values of the paired t-test. Results indicate that there is a significant large difference between previous (M = 2.4, S.D. = 1) and post (M = 5.2, S.D. = 1.3), t(14) = 9.9, p < 0.001, where M abbreviates mean and S.D. means standard deviation. t(14) represents the value of t at the degree of freedom 14 (as per Table 9.4).

TABLE 9.4   Resultant Table of the Paired T-Test

Alpha	0.05	
	Pre-Scores	**Post-Scores**
Mean	2.4	5.2
S.D.	1	1.3
T-value	9.8986	–
P-value	1.06e-7	–
Sample size	15	–
Degree of freedom	14	–
Average of difference	2.78	–
S.D. of difference	1.0877	–

9.4.1.3.3   Representation and Description of the Distribution of the T-Test

1. **H0 Hypothesis:** Since, H0 is rejected. The sample difference between the averages of the post and previous is big enough to be statistically significant (as per Figure 9.10).
2. **P-Value:** The p-value equals 1.06e-7, (P(x<=9.8986) = 1), means the chance of rejecting the correct H0 is small.
3. **Test Statistic:** The t value equals 9.8986, which is not in the acceptance.

$$t = \bar{x} \text{differences} - \mu_o / S\text{differences}/\sqrt{n}$$
$$S.E. = S \text{ differences}/\sqrt{n} = 1.0877/\sqrt{15} = 0.2808$$
$$t = 2.78 - 0/0.2808 = 9.8986$$

4. **Effect Size:** The effect size between the average and expected average is large, 2.56.

$$\text{Cohen's D} = |\bar{x}d - \mu_o|/\text{Sd}$$
$$\text{Cohen's D} = |2.78 - 0|/1.0877 = 2.5558$$

Averages and SDs

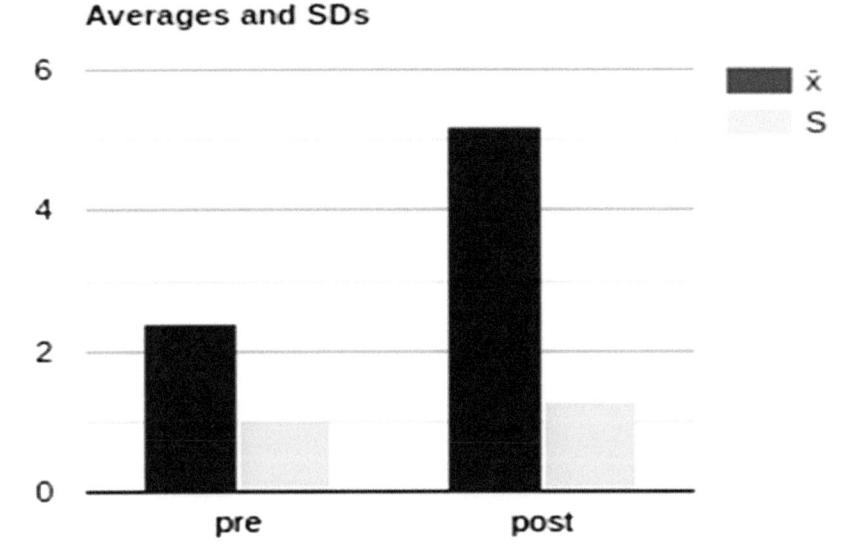

FIGURE 9.10 Average and standard derivation of the students according to maths comprehension skills.

9.4.1.4 *ABILITY TO REMEMBER*

This property helps to remember things and concepts easily. This plays a vital role in mental health.

9.4.1.4.1 *Representation of the Test Scores*

As shown in Figure 9.11, it is clear that there is a small difference in the performance of the students based on their memory quality. The blue dot represents the previous test score, which is shown at a low level on the graph. The orange dot represents the post-test score of the students, which is shown at a higher level (*please refer to* Table D).

TABLE D

	Ability to Remember	
Student's Name	**Pre**	**Post**
Prem	3	2.2
Raja	2	6.4
Krishna	3	4.5
Prince	2	3.6
Sidhu	2	4
Pooja	4	8
Anamika	3	4
Khushi	2	2.2
Khusboo	2	3.2
Karan	2	3
Pradeep	2	3
Mukund	2	5.9
Rajkumar	2	6
Jyoti	1	3.2
Govinda	0	3.2

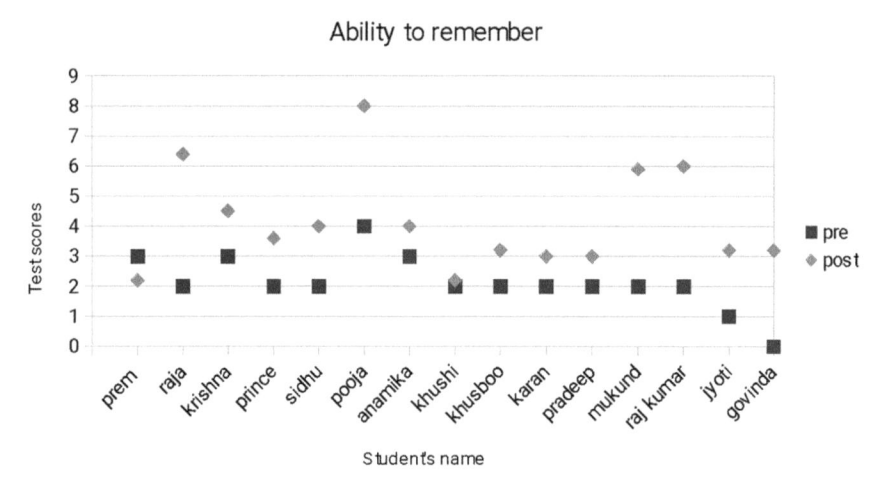

FIGURE 9.11   Representation of the test scores of the students according to their ability to remember.

9.4.1.4.2 Paired Sample T-Test Analysis

Table 9.5 shows the calculated values of the paired t-test. Results indicated that there is a significant large difference between previous (M = 2.1, S.D. = 0.9) and post (M = 4.2, S.D. = 1.7), t(14) = 5, p < 0.001, where M abbreviates mean and S.D. means standard deviation, t(14) means the value of t at the degree of freedom 9.14 (as per Table 9.5).

TABLE 9.5   Resultant Table of the Paired T-Test

Alpha	0.05	
	Pre-Scores	**Post-Scores**
Mean	2.1	4.2
S.D.	0.9	0.9
T-value	5.039	–
P-value	0.0001809	–
Sample size	15	–
Degree of freedom	14	–
Average of difference	2.0267	–
S.D. of difference	1.5577	–

9.4.1.4.3 Representation and Description of the Distribution of the T-Test

1. **H0 Hypothesis:** Since, H0 is rejected. The sample difference between the averages of the post and previous is big enough to be statistically significant.
2. **P-Value:** The p-value equals 0.0001809, (P(x<=5.039)=1), means the chance of rejecting the correct H0 is small (as per Figure 9.12).
3. **Test Statistic:** The t value equals 5.039, which is not in the acceptance.

$$t = \bar{x}\text{differences} - \mu_o/S\text{differences}/\sqrt{n}$$
$$\text{S.E.} = S \text{ differences}/\sqrt{n} = 1.5577/\sqrt{15} = 0.4022$$
$$t = 2.0267 - 0/0.4022 = 5.039$$

4. **Effect Size:** The effect size between the average and expected average is large, 1.3.

$$\text{Cohen's D} = |\bar{x}d - \mu_0|/Sd$$
$$\text{Cohen's D} = |2.0267 - 0|/1.5577 = 1.3011$$

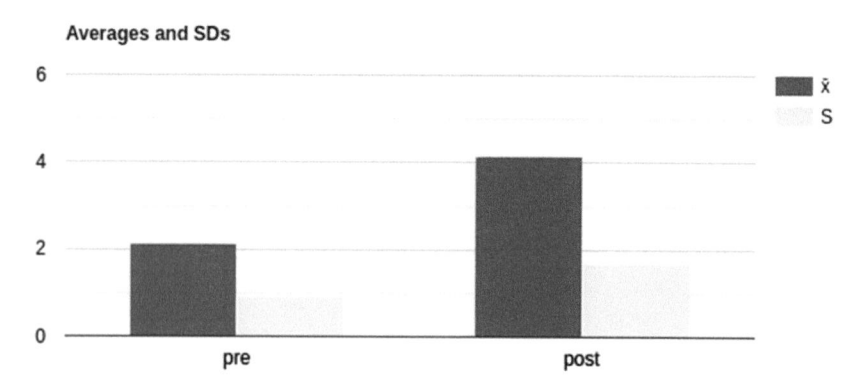

FIGURE 9.12 Average and standard derivation of the students according to ability to remember.

9.4.1.5 HONESTY

This property plays a vital role in mental health. Honesty makes the mental state calm. This should be necessary for every student.

9.4.1.5.1 *Representation of the Test Scores*

As shown in Figure 9.13, it is clear that there is a small difference between the performances of the students based on their honesty. The blue dot represents the previous test score, which is shown at the lower level of the graph. The orange dot represents the post-test score of the students, which is shown at the higher level (*please refer to* Table E).

9.4.1.5.2 *Paired Sample T-Test Analysis*

Table 9.6 shows the calculated values of the paired t-test. Results indicated that there is a significant large difference between previous (M = 3,

TABLE E

Student's Name	Pre	Post
	Honesty	
Prem	3	6
Raja	3	5
Krishna	3	6
Prince	2	5
Sidhu	3	5
Pooja	3	6
Anamika	3	6
Khushi	4	7
Khusboo	3	7
Karan	3	4
Pradeep	3	5
Mukund	3	5
Rajkumar	3	6
Jyoti	4	6
Govinda	2	4

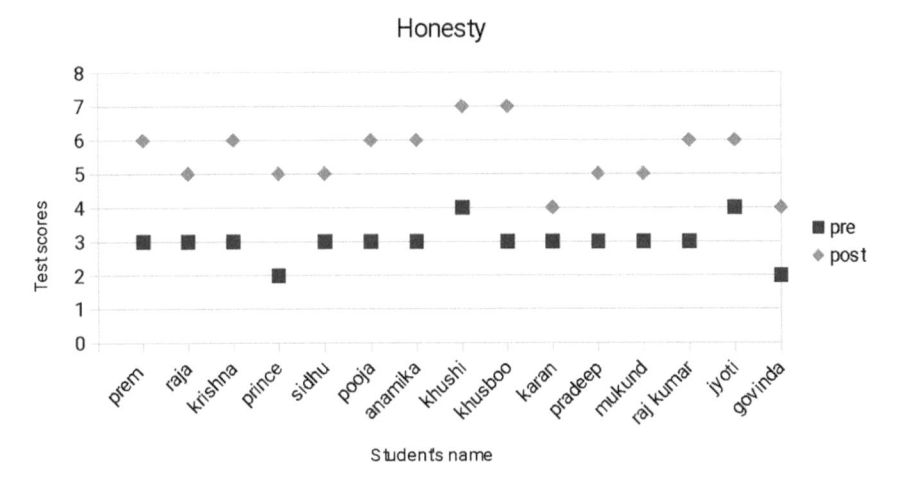

FIGURE 9.13   Representation of the test scores of the students according to their honesty.

S.D. =0.5) and post (M = 5.5, S.D.= 0.9), t(14) = 13.2, p < 0.001, where M abbreviates mean and S.D. means standard deviation, t(14) means the value of t at the degree of freedom 14 (as per Table 9.6).

TABLE 9.6 Resultant Table of the Paired T-Test

Alpha	0.05	
	Pre-Scores	**Post-Scores**
Mean	3	5.5
S.D.	0.5	0.9
T-value	13.2014	–
P-value	2.723e-9	–
Sample size	15	–
Degree of freedom	14	–
Average of difference	2.5333	–
S.D. of difference	0.7432	–

9.4.1.5.3   *Representation and Description of the Distribution of the T-Test*

1. **H0 Hypothesis:** Since, H0 is rejected. The sample difference between the averages of the post and previous is big enough to be statistically significant (as per Figure 9.14).
2. **P-Value:** The p-value equals 2.723e-9, (P(x<=13.2014) = 1), means the chance of rejecting the correct H0 is small.
3. **Test Statistic:** The t value equals 13.2014, which is not in the acceptance.

$$t = \bar{x} \text{differences} - \mu_o / \text{Sdifferences}/\sqrt{n}$$
$$\text{S.E.} = S \text{ differences}/\sqrt{n} = 0.7432\sqrt{15} = 0.1919$$
$$t = 2.5333 - 0/0.1919 = 13.2014$$

4. **Effect Size:** The effect size between the average and expected average is large, 3.41.

$$\text{Cohen's D} = |\bar{x}d - \mu_o|/Sd$$
$$\text{Cohen's D} = |2.5333 - 0|/0.7432 = 3.4086$$

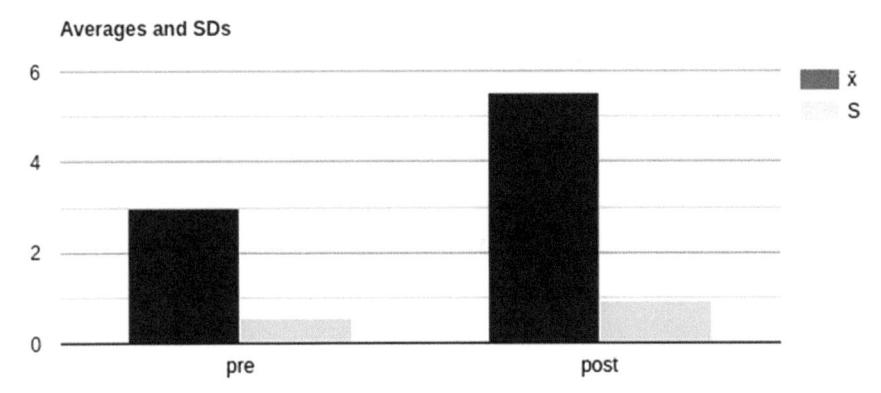

FIGURE 9.14   Average and standard derivation of the students according to their honesty.

9.4.1.6   RESPONSIBILITY

This property shows responsiveness of the students. This helps to reduce mental illness from the brain which helps students to improve their learning capacity.

9.4.1.6.1   Representation of the Test Scores

As shown in Figure 9.23, there is a clear difference in the performances of the students based on their responsibility. The blue dot represents the previous test score, which is shown at a low level on the graph. The orange dot represents the post-test score of the students, which is shown at a high level (*please refer to* Table F) (as per Figures 9.13 and 9.16).

9.4.1.6.2   Paired Sample T-Test Analysis

Table 9.7 shows the calculated values of the paired t-test. Results indicate that there is a significant large difference between previous (M = 2.9, S.D. = 0.6) and post (M = 5.3, S.D. = 1), t(14) = 11.1, p < 0.001, where M abbreviates mean and S.D. means standard deviation. t(14) represents the value of t at the degree of freedom 14 (as per Table 9.7).

TABLE F

Responsibility		
Student's Name	**Pre**	**Post**
Prem	2	5
Raja	3	6
Krishna	3	5
Prince	3	4
Sidhu	2	4
Pooja	3	6
Anamika	3	6
Khushi	4	7
Khusboo	3	7
Karan	3	4
Pradeep	2	4
Mukund	3	5
Rajkumar	3	5
Jyoti	4	6
Govinda	3	5

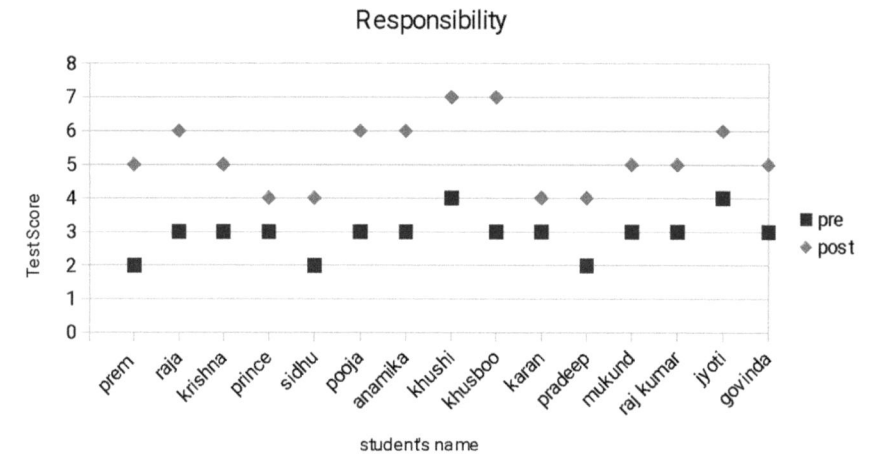

FIGURE 9.15 Representation of the test scores of the students according to their responsibility.

TABLE 9.7 Resultant Table of the Paired T-Test

Alpha	0.05	
	Pre-Scores	**Post-Scores**
Mean	2.9	5.3
S.D.	0.6	1
T-value	11.068	–
P-value	2.621e-8	–
Sample size	15	–
Degree of freedom	14	–
Average of difference	2.3333	–
S.D. of difference	0.8165	–

9.4.1.6.3 Representation and Description of the Distribution of the T-Test

1. **H0 Hypothesis:** Since, H0 is rejected. The sample difference between the averages of the post and previous is big enough to be statistically significant.
2. **P-Value:** The p-value equals 2.621e-8 (P(x<=11.068) =1), means the chance of rejecting the correct H0 is small.
3. **Test Statistic:** The t value equals 11.068, which is not in the acceptance.

$$t = \bar{x} \text{ differences} - \mu_0/\text{Sdifferences}/\sqrt{n}$$
$$S.E. = S \text{ differences}/\sqrt{n} = 0.8165\sqrt{15} = 0.2108$$
$$t = 2.3333 - 0/0.2108 = 11.068$$

4. **Effect Size:** The effect size between the average and expected average is large, 2.86.

$$\text{Cohen's D} = |\bar{x}d - \mu_0|/Sd$$
$$\text{Cohen's D} = |2.3333 - 0|/0.8165 = 2.8577$$

9.4.1.7 BRAVERY

Bravery increases the interaction and involvement of the students towards the activities. This helps them to take action on their own.

Averages and SDs

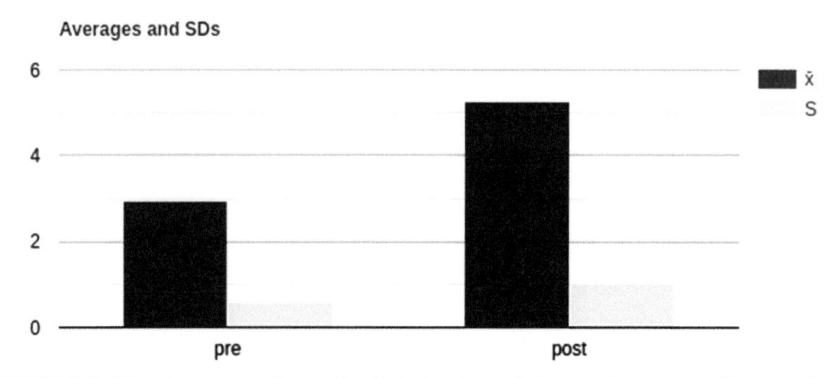

FIGURE 9.16   Average and standard derivation of the students according to their responsibility.

9.4.1.7.1 *Representation of the Test Scores*

As shown in Figure 9.25, it is clear that there is a large difference between the performances of the students according to their bravery. The blue dot represents the previous test score, which is shown at the low level of the graph. The orange dot represents the post-test score of the students, which is shown at the high level (*please refer to* Table G) (as per Figure 9.25).

TABLE G

Bravery		
Student's Name	**Pre**	**Post**
Prem	3	5
Raja	2	5
Krishna	2	5
Prince	2	4
Sidhu	2	4
Pooja	2	5
Anamika	3	5
Khushi	4	5
Khusboo	3	5
Karan	2	3
Pradeep	2	3
Mukund	1	4
Rajkumar	2	6
Jyoti	5	6
Govinda	3	5

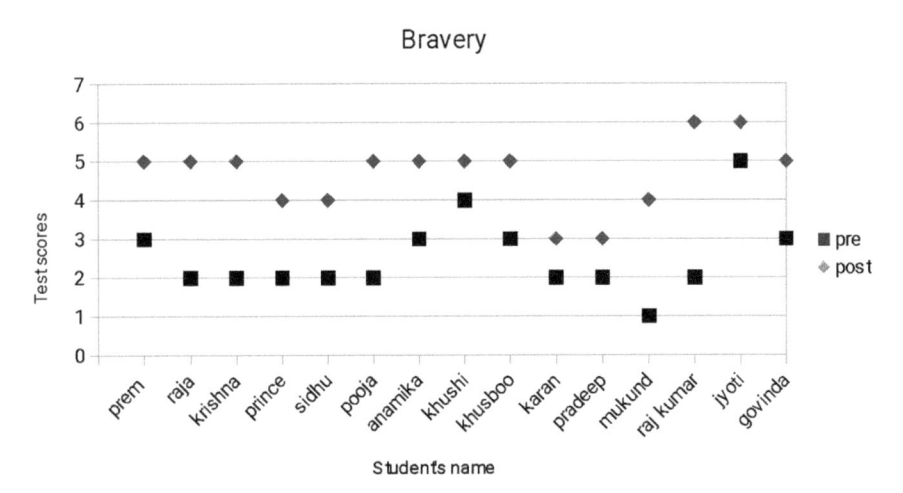

FIGURE 9.17 Representation of the test scores of the students according to their bravery.

9.4.1.7.2 Paired Sample T-Test Analysis

Table 9.8 shows the calculated values of the paired t-test. Results indicate that there is a significant large difference between previous (M = 2.5, S.D. = 1) and post (M = 4.7, S.D. = 0.9), t(14) = 9, p < 0.001, where M abbreviates mean and S.D. means standard deviation. t(14) represents the value of t at the degree of freedom 14 (as per Table 9.8).

TABLE 9.8 Resultant Table of the Paired T-Test

Alpha	0.05	
	Pre-Scores	**Post-Scores**
Mean	2.5	4.7
S.D.	1	0.9
T-value	9.0252	–
P-value	3.276e-7	–
Sample size	15	–
Degree of freedom	14	–
Average of difference	2.1333	–
S.D. of difference	0.9155	–

9.4.1.7.3   Representation and Description of the Distribution of the T-Test

1. **H0 Hypothesis:** Since, H0 is rejected. The sample difference between the averages of the post and previous is big enough to be statistically significant (as per Figure 9.26).
2. **P-Value:** The p-value equals 3.276e-7 (P(x<=9.0252) = 1), means the chance of rejecting the correct H0 is small.
3. **Test Statistic:** The t value equals 9.0252, which is not in the acceptance.

$$t = \bar{x}\text{differences} - \mu_o/\text{Sdifferences}/\sqrt{n}$$
$$\text{S.E.} = \text{S differences}/\sqrt{n} = 0.9155\sqrt{15} = 0.2364$$
$$t = 2.1333 - 0/0.2364 = 9.0252$$

4. **Effect Size:** The effect size between the average and expected average is large, 2.33.

$$\text{Cohen's D} = |\bar{x}d - \mu_o|/Sd$$
$$\text{Cohen's D} = |2.1333 - 0|/0.9155 = 2.3303$$

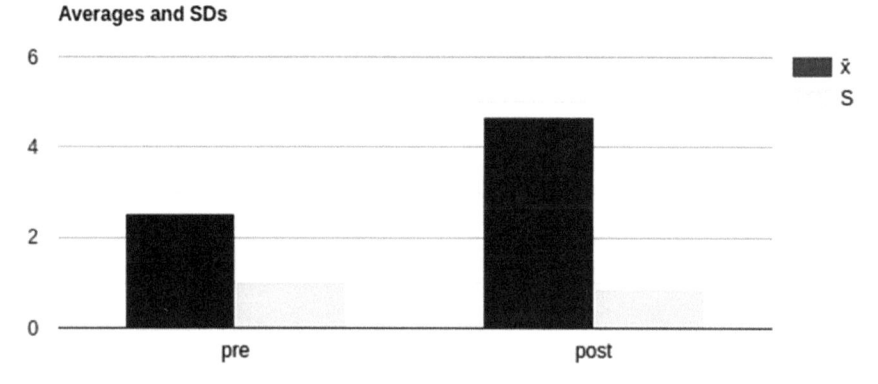

FIGURE 9.18   Average and standard derivation of the students according to their bravery.

9.4.1.8   WISDOM

Wisdom is necessary for students to make their decision. This provides a consideration and deliberative values to take judgments.

9.4.1.8.1 Representation of the Test Scores

As shown in Figure 9.27, it is clear that there is a large difference between the performances of the students according to their wisdom. The blue dot represents the previous test score, which is shown at the low level of the graph. The orange dot represents the post-test score of the students, which is shown at the high level (*please refer to* Table H) (as per Figure 9.27).

TABLE H

Student's Name	Wisdom	
	Pre	Post
Prem	2	5
Raja	3	5
Krishna	2	6
Prince	2	4
Sidhu	2	4
Pooja	3	6
Anamika	2	5
Khushi	4	6
Khusboo	2	7
Karan	2	3
Pradeep	2	4
Mukund	2	6
Rajkumar	3	5
Jyoti	4	5
Govinda	3	6

9.4.1.8.2 Paired Sample T-Test Analysis

Table 9.9 shows the calculated values of the paired t-test. Results indicated that there is a significant large difference between previous (M = 2.5, S.D. = 0.7) and post (M = 5.1, S.D. = 1.1), t(14) = 9, p < 0.001, where M abbreviates mean and S.D. means standard deviation, t(14) means the value of t at the degree of freedom 14 (as per Table 9.9).

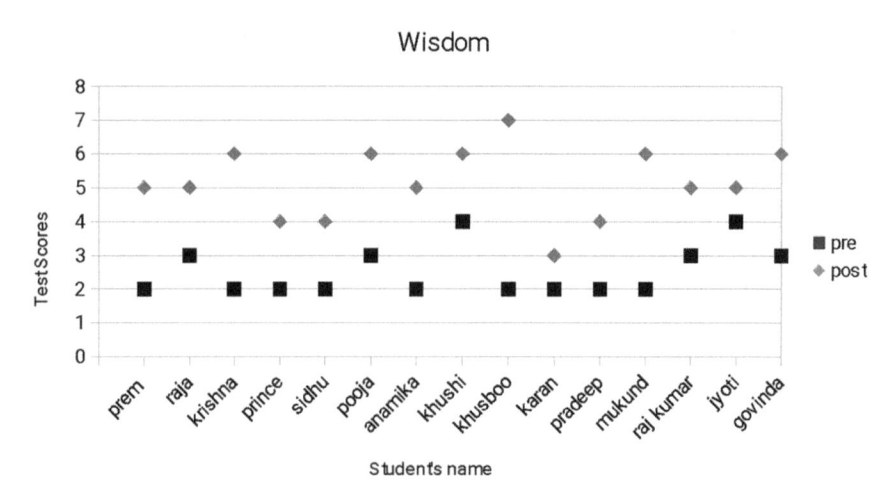

FIGURE 9.19   Representation of the test scores of the students according to their wisdom.

TABLE 9.9   Resultant Table of the Paired T-Test

Alpha	0.05	
	Pre-Scores	**Post-Scores**
Mean	2.5	5.1
S.D.	0.7	1.1
T-value	8.981	–
P-value	3.476e-7	–
Sample size	15	–
Degree of freedom	14	–
Average of difference	2.6	–
S.D. of difference	1.1212	–

9.4.1.8.3   Representation and Description of the Distribution of the T-Test

1. **H0 Hypothesis:** Since, H0 is rejected. The sample difference between the averages of the post and previous is big enough to be statistically significant.
2. **P-Value:** The p-value equals 3.476e-7(P(x<=8.981)=1), meaning the chance of rejecting the correct H0 is small.

3. **Test Statistic:** The t value equals 8.981, which is not in the acceptance.

$$t = \bar{x}\text{differences} - \mu_0/\text{Sdifferences}/\sqrt{n}$$
$$\text{S.E.} = \text{S differences}/\sqrt{n} = 1.1212\sqrt{15} = 0.2895$$
$$t = 2.6 - 0/0.2895 = 8.981$$

4. **Effect Size:** The effect size between the average and expected average is large, 2.32.

$$\text{Cohen's D} = |\bar{x}d - \mu_0|/\text{Sd}$$
$$\text{Cohen's D} = |2.6 - 0|/1.1212 = 2.3189$$

Hence, it is clearly said by the analysis that each property has a large difference after the experiments in the students (as per Figure 9.28).

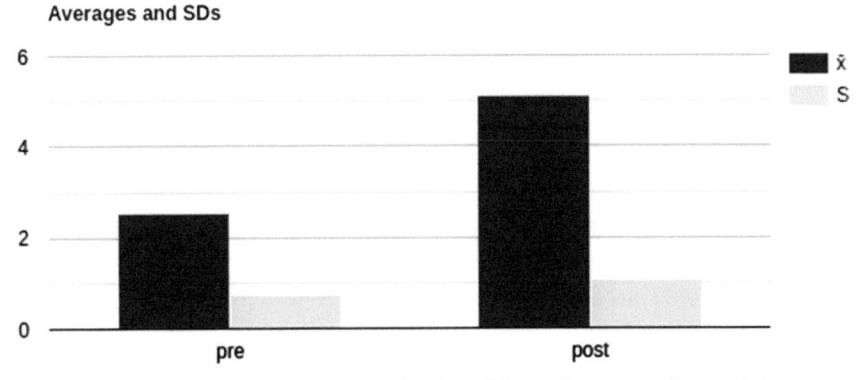

Averages and SDs

FIGURE 9.20 Average and standard derivation of the students according to their wisdom.

9.5 NOVELTIES

- This study is a positive approach in the direction of establishing the ancient Indian Vedic methodologies in a more scientific way.
- In this study, a trial has been made to study mental conditions like anxiety, stress, etc., quantitatively through experimental data.
- This study is focusing on one of the major issues raised due to the coronavirus pandemic, i.e., mental health of adolescents, on which the growth of society depends.

- This study is using various software tools like Tableau, Python, and ML for better analysis and to strengthen the fact that Vedic methodologies also have their scientific correlation.
- This study is also a way of encouraging adolescents towards the benefits of the natural environment to rejuvenate mental as well as physical health in this fast-growing world.

9.6 RECOMMENDATIONS

This study primarily focuses on the issue of post-COVID effects on adolescents and the Vedic ancient methodologies to rejuvenate their mental and physical health after the COVID-19 pandemic. Adolescents nowadays are facing problems like anxiety, stress, depression, PTSD, obesity, diabetes, high blood pressure, etc., which are severely affecting their overall growth. This study aims to provide the world with easy-to-practice methods like Yoga and *Yagya* to improve them from the inside as well as from the outside by creating an herbal environment and providing them with well-established herbal formulations.

The study clearly shows improvements in IQ, mathematical skills, stress levels, etc., by consuming *SARASWATI PANCHAK* and following the protocols of *Yajna* and Yoga. Various mental qualitative properties are studied quantitatively by continuously monitoring the participants through various tests over a course of 3 months. This study is a strong point in establishing Indian Vedic Methodologies as a scientific approach.

9.7 FUTURE RESEARCH DIRECTIONS AND LIMITATIONS

9.7.1 LIMITATIONS

- The sample size used in this study is 25 to 30 individuals, but for more accurate results, the sample size can be increased for better analysis.
- This study must comprise individuals of all age groups, and these various age groups can be observed to get more insights regarding the mental health of adults as well as elders.
- The time duration for the experiment can be increased from 3 months to more months to get a more visible and highlighted effect on the individuals.

- The latest technologies and software tools can be used to get more precise analysis.

9.7.2 FUTURE DIRECTIONS

- This study can be further used in the directions of curing mental diseases using Ayurvedic medicinal herbs.
- This can also be used in the study of the role of daily Vedic protocols in decreasing the tendency of attempting suicide or getting depressed among youngsters.
- Also used as a source of knowledge about herbal dietary supplements which can be used to promote the overall fitness of growing children instead of giving them chemical-based dietary supplements.
- Can be used as a reference for studies establishing Indian ancient Vedic sciences.

9.8 CONCLUSION

The study had compellingly proved the virtue of Vedic science, Ayurveda, and nature in building a sustainable, disease-free, happy world. An orderly lifestyle and a good environment are the essentials for good health. The power of herbs as rasayana and curatives is no longer a question of debate but scientifically proven knowledge, acceptable around the whole world.

Herbs described in ancient texts as brain tonics are successful prevention and cure for the ever-rising mental health problems for all age groups. Adolescence has several ups and downs in life, but every problem has solutions if not around us, maybe in those enriched ancient texts. A good lifestyle, practicing Yajna, intake of a balanced diet, and support of herbs are enough to pave the way for adolescence from the period of dilemma, stress, and transformation to a successful, healthy, and happy life.

The data shows improvement of individuals in all the studied parameters (i.e., their understanding ability, i.e., the power of comprehending, their altruistic behavior, i.e., tendency to help, mathematical ability, memory power, honesty, sense of responsibility, courageousness, intelligence). The scale improved to double the earlier score and even higher in most cases. While this was the norm in scoring of individual parameters, the overall integrated score showed even better results. The increase from 1 to 13, 4 to 17, and 0 to 7 are some of the startling numbers observed from the study.

KEYWORDS

- **adolescents**
- **control group**
- **experimental group**
- **mental trauma**
- **obesity**
- *Saraswati Panchak*
- *yajna*
- **yoga**

REFERENCES

(2023). What is the Data, Information, Knowledge, Wisdom (DIKW) Pyramid? *Ontotext*. https://www.ontotext.com/knowledgehub/fundamentals/dikw-pyramid/ (accessed on 5 July 2024).

(2023). What-is-behavioral-data-science-and-how-to-get-into-it. Medium. https://medium.com/behavior-design-hub/what-is-behavioral-data-science-and-how-to-get-into-it-e389ed20751f (accessed on 5 July 2024).

Ashwin, A., Cherukuri, S. D., & Rammohan, A. (2022). Negative effects of COVID-19 pandemic on adolescent health: Insights, perspectives, and recommendations. *Journal of Global Health, 12*, 03009. https://www.ncbi.nlm.nih.gov/pmc/articles/PMC9123917/#:~:text=Decreased%20physical%20activity%2C%20loss%20of,can%20adversely%20affect%20mental%20health (accessed on 5 July 2024).

Castro, D., Coral, W., Rodriguez, C., Cabra, J., & Colorado, J. (2017). Wearable-based human activity recognition using an IoT approach. *Journal of Sensors and Actuator Networks, 6*(4), 28. https://www.mdpi.com/240424 (accessed on 5 July 2024).

Cikanavicius, D. (2019). The effects of trauma from growing up too fast. *Psych Central*. https://psychcentral.com/blog/psychology-self/2019/12/trauma-growing-up-fast#1 (accessed on 5 July 2024).

Damgaard, P. (2023). The knowledge pyramid. https://cognifirm.com/the-knowledge-pyramid/ (accessed on 5 July 2024).

Gururaja, D., Harano, K., Toyotake, I., & Kobayashi, H. (2011). Effect of yoga on mental health: Comparative study between young and senior subjects in Japan. *International*

Journal of Yoga, 4(1), 7–12. https://pubmed.ncbi.nlm.nih.gov/21654969/#:~:text=Con clusion%3A%20Decrease%20in%20Salivary%20amylase,health%20in%20both%20 the%20groups (accessed on 5 July 2024).

Khedkar, N. P., Singh, S., & Deodas, M. (2018). Role of Ayurveda in adolescent age. *International Ayurvedic Medical Journal, 6*(3), 617–623. http://www.iamj.in/posts/2018/ images/upload/617_623.pdf (accessed on 5 July 2024).

Koach, M. (2004). Homa Therapy the Ancient Science of Healing. https://homatherapy. org/product/homa-therapy-the-ancient-science-of-healing-english/.

Loades, M. E., Chatburn, E., Higson-Sweeney, N., Reynolds, S., Shafran, R., Brigden, A., & Crawley, E. (2020). Rapid systematic review: The impact of social isolation and loneliness on the mental health of children and adolescents in the context of COVID-19. *Journal of the American Academy of Child & Adolescent Psychiatry, 59*(11), 1218–1239. https://doi.org/10.1016/j.jaac.2020.05.009.

Mondal, S. (2013). Science of exercise: Ancient Indian origin. *The Journal of the Association of Physicians of India, 61*. https://pubmed.ncbi.nlm.nih.gov/24818341/.

Pradhan, B., Bhattacharyya, S., & Pal, K. (2021). IoT-based applications in healthcare devices. *Journal of Healthcare Engineering, 2021*, 6632599. https://www.hindawi.com/ journals/jhe/2021/6632599/ (accessed on 5 July 2024).

Rafaj, P., Kiesewetter, G., Gül, T., Schöpp, W., Cofala, J., Klimont, Z., Purohit, P., Heyes, C., Amann, M., Borken-Kleefeld, J., & Cozzi, L. (2018). Outlook for clean air in the context of Sustainable Development Goals. *Global Environmental Change, 53*. https:// reader.elsevier.com/reader/sd/pii/S0959378018304035?token=6DFD7E294B6FEB4E 4F00FEF0A34470E25B4DE7902F83BC521FFE8D59F5D1AFEFCF42094556659D 03F9E0F7590A6F594D&originRegion=eu-west-1&originCreation=20211225112138 (accessed on 5 July 2024).

Rahman, M. M., Saifuzzaman, M., Ahmed, A., Mahin, M. F., & Shetu, S. F. (2021). Impact of COVID-19 on mental health: A quantitative analysis of anxiety and depression based on regular life and internet use. *Current Research in Behavioral Sciences, 2*(2021), 100037. https://doi.org/10.1016/j.crbeha.2021.100037.

Rastogi, R., Saxena, M., Chaturvedi, D. K., Gupta, M., Rastogi, M., Srivatava, P., Jain, M., Kumar, P., Sharma, U., Choudhary, R., & Gupta, N. (2021). Computing analysis of Yajna and mantra chanting as a therapy: A holistic approach for all by Indian continent amidst pandemic threats. In P. Kumar, V. Jain, & V. Ponnusamy (Eds.), *The Smart Cyber Ecosystem for Sustainable Development*. https://doi.org/10.1002/9781119761655.ch16.

Rathi, P. (2019). Effects of Yagya on environment purification and human health: A review. *Research Journal of Chemical and Environmental Sciences, 7*, 9–18. http://aelsindia. com/rjces_oct_dec_2019/8.pdf (accessed on 5 July 2024).

Russ, T. C., Woelbert, E., Davis, K. A. S., et al. (2019). How data science can advance mental health research. *Nature Human Behavior, 3*, 24–32. https://doi.org/10.1038/ s41562-018-0470-9.

Schmidt, J., Marques, M.R.G., Botti, S. et al. (2019) Recent advances and applications of machine learning in solid-state materials science. npj Comput Mater 5, (83). https://doi. org/10.1038/s41524-019-0221-0

Singh, R. (2020). Saraswati Panchak–A novel herbal combination for mental health. *Interdisciplinary Journal of Yagya Research, 3*(2), 9–18. https://www.researchgate.net/

publication/348308824_Saraswati_Panchak_-_A_Novel_Herbal_Combination_for_ Mental_Health (accessed on 5 July 2024).

Tariq, M. U., Babar, M., Poulin, M., Khattak, A. S., Alshehri, M. D., & Kaleem, S. (2023). Human Behavior Analysis. *Frontiers in Psychology, 12.* https://www.frontiersin.org/ articles/10.3389/fpsyg.2021.686610/full.

Trivedi, P. (2020). To study the effect of Yagya therapy on the level of emotional maturity. *Webinar on Public Health Journal, S(2), 5,* Osaka, Japan. Retrieved from: https://www. alliedacademies.org/articles/to-study-the-effect-of-yagya-therapy-on-the-level-of-emotional-maturity.pdf.

Xiang, M., Liu, Y., Yamamoto, S., Mizoue, T., & Kuwahara, K. (2022). Association of changes of lifestyle behaviors before and during the COVID-19 pandemic with mental health: A longitudinal study in children and adolescents. *International Journal of Behavioral Nutrition and Physical Activity, 19,* 92. https://ijbnpa.biomedcentral.com/ articles/10.1186/s12966-022-01327-8 (accessed on 5 July 2024).

ANNEXURE

> **Additional Readings:**

1. Delhi's air quality improves to 'poor' category; AQI drops to 280 (https://www.business-standard.com/article/current-affairs/delhi-s-air-quality-improves-to-poor-category-aqi-drops-to-280-121032000148_1.html).

2. The Impact of Economic Growth and Air Pollution on Public Health in 31 Chinese Cities (https://www.ncbi.nlm.nih.gov/pmc/articles/PMC6388246/).

3. Economic Impacts from PM2.5 Pollution-Related Health Effects in China: A Provincial-Level Analysis (https://pubmed.zncbi.nlm.nih.gov/27063584/).

4. Public health and air pollution in Asia (PAPA): a combined analysis of four studies of air pollution and mortality (https://pubmed.ncbi.nlm.nih.gov/21446215/).

5. Computational Analysis of Air Quality and the Potential of Rich Indian Tradition for Healthcare 4.0 (https://www.researchgate.net/publication/352883834_Computational_Analysis_of_Air_Quality_and_the_Potential_of_Rich_Indian_Tradition_for_Healthcare_40).

6. Construction of an Improved Air Quality Index: A Case Report (https://www.ncbi.nlm.nih.gov/pmc/articles/PMC7145911/).

7. Yajna and Mantra Therapy Applications on Diabetic and Other Disease Subjects: Computational Intelligence Based Experimental Approach (https://papers.ssrn.com/sol3/papers.cfm?abstract_id=3515800).

8. Analytical Study of Large-Scale Household Yagya Effects on Ambient Air Pollution: A Study in NCR, India (https://www.researchgate.net/publication/341200761_Analytical_Study_of_Large-Scale_Household_Yagya_Effects_on_Ambient_Air_Pollution_A_Study_in_NCR_India).

9. Yajna and Mantra Science Bringing Health and Comfort to Indo-Asian Public: A Healthcare 4.0 Approach and Computational Study (https://www.researchgate.net/publication/339809276_Yajna_and_Mantra_Science_Bringing_Health_and_Comfort_to_IndoAsian_Public_A_Healthcare_40_Approach_and_Computational_Study).

10. Happiness Index and Gadget Radiation Analysis on Yajna and Mantra Chanting Therapy in South Asian Continent: COVID-19 vs. Ancient Rich Culture from Vedic Science (https://www.igi-global.com/gateway/article/270952#pnlRecommendationForm).

11. Treatment Case Studies and Emissions Analysis of Wood in Yagya: Integrating Spirituality and Healthcare with Science (https://www.igi-global.com/article/treatment-case-studies-and-emissions-analysis-of-wood-in-yagya/282493).

➤ **Key Terms and Definitions:**
- **Climate Change:** This includes both human-induced global warming and its large-scale impacts on weather patterns. There have been previous periods of climate change, but the current changes are more rapid than any known events in Earth's history.
- **Yajna:** It refers in Hinduism to any ritual done in front of a sacred fire, often with mantras. *Yajna* has been a Vedic tradition, described in a layer of Vedic literature called *Brahmanas*, as well as *Yajurveda*.
- **Mantra:** A mantra is a sacred utterance, a numinous sound, a syllable, word or phonemes, or group of words in Sanskrit, Pali, and other languages believed by practitioners to have religious, magical or spiritual powers.
- **Human Health:** Health, according to the World Health Organization, is "a state of complete physical, mental, and social well-being and not merely the absence of disease and infirmity."
- **Economic Growth:** It can be defined as the increase or improvement in the inflation-adjusted market value of the goods and services produced by an economy over time. Statisticians conventionally measure such growth as the percent rate of increase in the real gross domestic product, or real GDP.
- *Havan Kund:* It is the center place in a *Havan* in which the fire is put, and all the oblations' offerings are made. It could be considered like a sanctum sanctorum for a *Yajna*.
- *Havan Samagri:* It is a mixture of dried herbal roots and leaves that are burned during *Yajna* and *Homa*. Contents of the *Samagri*: Made from Ayurvedic Havan exotic herbs, Black

til, Jau, 32 types of dhoop, Bhimseni Kapoor (camphor), rose petals, sandalwood powder, lobaan, Ghee, Agarbatti, Chandan, and Turmeric.

In physical terms, *Yajna* is a process aimed at refinement of the subtle energy existing in matter with the help of thermal energy of the Mantras. The experiments of Yajna, when performed at a small scale in a day-to-day life are called – Havan or Agnihotra.

- **Knowledge Management:** It is the process when an organization extracts, collects, stores, shares, uses, and dismisses information in a refined way.
- **Knowledge Pyramid:** It is orderly transmission of data to information to further knowledge and finally wisdom is said to be the DIKW hierarchy or the knowledge pyramid.

DATA SETS

TABLE 1 Sample Dataset: The Parameters Studied with Respect to Individual Subject for the Analysis of the Experimental Results (2022)

शिक्षक द्वारा भरना है:–		Date:– 26-5-22	Date:–1-7-22
	गुण	स्केल (पूर्व) (1-10)	(पश्चात्) (1-10)
1	बात को समझने की शक्ति	2	5
2	मदद् करने की प्रवृत्ति	1	3
3	गणित को समझने की शक्ति	1	4
4	याद् करने की क्षमता	2	3.6

TABLE 2 Sample Dataset: The Parameters Studied with Respect to Individual Subject for the Analysis of the Experimental Results (2022)

शिक्षक द्वारा भरना है:–		Date:– 26-5-22	Date:–1-7-22
Name	Raja	5/26/2022	7/1/2022
	गुण	स्केल (पूर्व) (1-10)	(पश्चात्) (1-10)
1	बात को समझने की शक्ति	3	6
2	मदद् करने की प्रवृत्ति	3	5
3	गणित को समझने की शक्ति	3	6
4	याद् करने की क्षमता	2	6.4

TABLE 3 Sample Dataset: Integrated Scores of All Test Parameters Studied Pre- and Post-Experiment

Sl.No	Student	Experiment Goup		Control Goup	
		Exp. Pre	Exp. Post	Control Pre	Control Post
1	khusi	6	5	9	13
2	Khushbu	7	7	7	7
3	krishna	1	7	11	11
4	Pooja	4	18	4	6
5	Prince	8	8	6	5
6	Gobinda	0	7	8	5
7	Raja	9	14	2	2
8	Rajkumar	1	13	9	5

TABLE 4 Sample Dataset: Integrated Scores of All Test Parameters Analyzing Memory Ability Studied Pre- and Post-Experiment

Ion	Havan G	Date:- 26-5-2022	Date:- 01-7-2022
	Details	Memory game	Memory game
Sl.No	Student Name	Ctrl. Gr. Pre.	Ctrl. Gr. Post
1	Neha	9	13
2	Chanchal	7	7
3	Aarti	11	11
4	Chandni	4	6
5	Sani	6	5
6	Varsa	8	5
7	Puspa	2	2
8	Mohit	9	5

CHAPTER 10

Statistical Surveillance on Effect of Ayurvedic Herbs on Improvement in Brain Power of Children

ROHIT RASTOGI,[1] MAMTA SAXENA,[2] CHARU TRIPATHI,[3] YATI VARSHNEY,[4] RAYUSH JAIN,[4] and PRABHINAV MISHRA[4]

[1]*Associate Professor, Department of CSE, ABES Engineering College, Ghaziabad, Uttar Pradesh, India*

[2]*Ex-DG, MoS-PI, GoI, Delhi, India*

[3]*BAMS, MD(Ayu.) CMO, MCD, Delhi, India*

[4]*Student, Department of CSE, ABES Engineering College, Ghaziabad, Uttar Pradesh, India*

ABSTRACT

Ayurveda is one of the ancient established therapies in India, and Yagyopathy or Yagya therapy was one of the main modes of therapy in Ayurveda during ancient times, not only for humans but also for animals, plants, and environmental management. In medieval and modern times, this wonderful science lost its sheen and is now being practiced as a religious ritual in many ceremonies and *Sanskaras*. *Yagya* is known to heal humans in multiple dimensions: (i) physical; (ii) mental; (iii) spiritual; (iv) social; and (v) environmental. This chapter is an effort to re-establish Yagyopathy as a therapeutic science for holistic (complete) healing, complementing Ayurvedic treatment in its present form. As we know, the Western medicinal system has established its supremacy in research characteristics of processes

Yoga and Meditation: Past and Present Evidence. Sachi Nandan Mohanty, Rabindra Kumar Pradhan, & Sugyanta Priyadarshini (Eds.)

where they use validated research and develop advanced techniques. Hence, this study has been conducted to validate the basic principles of Yagyopathy as well as herbs and other inputs used in therapeutic systems with the help of modern research tools and techniques, along with statistical analysis. The study, conducted on 24 children, showed marked improvement in the cognitive function of the brain and also in several behavioral aspects of the children who participated in the study.

➢ **Role of Authors:** Dr. Mamta Saxena is the main experimenter who designed and conducted this study and generated the data. Dr. Rohit Rastogi is the team leader. He coordinated among all the co-authors and also prepared the format of the research paper. Dr. Mamta and Dr. Charu proposed the topic introduction and background contents. Mamta Saxena also contributed to the main methodology of the experiment and assessment of participants in this study. Ms. Yati did the data analysis with statistical t-tests. Mr. Prabhinav and Mr. Rayush prepared the analytical remarks. All the co-authors compiled the literature survey. Ms. Yati and Dr. Mamta contributed to the results and concluding remarks with discussions.

➢ **Deliverables:**
1. The data were measured based on the memory games and quizzes.
2. Results have been presented through proper mathematical models such as graphs, block diagrams, and charts.
3. Statistical analysis has been done through paired t-tests to provide scientific interpretation and conclusions for this study.

➢ **Stakeholders:**
1. Students nowadays are facing several mental issues due to their hectic schedules, ever-increasing competition, and memory weakness. Hence, they can take advantage of this therapy for better performance and a happier lifestyle.
2. Young adolescents can undergo this therapy to strengthen their cognitive capabilities, which will help them get rid of mental pressure and have an edge over others.
3. Parents are the ones who handle all the stress and pressure for their children. This study will help parents make their children more mentally strong, active, and enhance their lifestyle in a harmless way.

4. Society consists of all kinds of people from children to adults, and in today's scenario, people live very hectic lives, suffering from various mental problems such as depression, anger, frustration, and obsessive-compulsive disorder, among others. They simultaneously want to excel in life as well. This therapy will help them achieve that.

➢ **Research Objective:** Objective of this study is to expose children to Yagyopathy with special herb preparation called Saraswati Panchak, known for its effect in improving memory, and assess its impact. As Yagya is known for affecting the inner core of human beings, it is to be seen if it can bring about some change in the human values and behavior of children (Callahan, 2007).

➢ **The Scope of Research:** This study is intended to study the effect of Yagyopathy done with special *Saraswati Panchak Havan Samagri* on children aged 5 to 15 years (listed in Annexure), both male and female. It has been decided to select children from the underprivileged class to avoid the effects of the rich category. Children from the weaker section of society usually do not have access to Yoga, Meditation, *Pranayama*, and *Yagya*. They also do not have a rich and nutritional diet. Therefore, clear visible results were expected within a 30-day period. Since most of the children were attending school, the one-month period was chosen in June, during their summer holidays, so that they could attend the Yagyopathy camp daily.

➢ **Background and Motivation:** *Yagya* therapy has been hereafter referred to as Yagyopathy. It has immense potential for healing not only humans and animals both physically and mentally, but also various components of the environment such as air, water, soil/earth, and vegetation including medicinal plants. There are innumerable references in our ancient Vedic texts that mention the cures for various ailments being done through *Yagya. Atharva Veda* 1/2/3132, 4, 37, 5/23, 29 are a few of the mantra verses that clearly mention how *Yagya* clears the atmosphere and indoor spaces of houses of pathogenic microflora and renders the atmosphere bacteriostatic. A lot of scientific work has been done recently to validate this. It has been seen that indoor atmospheric bacteria and fungi are reduced by more than 78% even after the 7th day of Yagya (Nautiyal et al., 2007; Samanth et al., 2018; Saxena et al., 2018; Verma et al., 2018).

There is, however, a significant difference in the behavior of air microflora in the *Yagya* atmosphere and in the atmosphere of ordinary fumes. Whereas in the *Yagya* atmosphere the bacteria and fungi tended to decrease, those in the ordinary fumes' atmosphere increased by 111% to 257%. This decremented effect was also seen in the outdoor air microflora. As pathogenic microflora are responsible for all types of infectious diseases, it was an established fact in ancient times that all infectious diseases including Tuberculosis could be cured by Yagyopathy using herbs specific for curing that disease (Atharva Veda); (Raghuvanshi et al., 2004, 2009; Saxena et al., 2007, 2008).

In the present times, several studies have been performed on individuals of various age groups, where it has been found that *Yagya* has been effective in controlling lifestyle diseases like blood sugar, asthma, joint pains, thyroid, and more. It was observed that while the patient received therapy for a specific issue, other related and unrelated problems also improved (Rastogi et al., 2020a–c).

Mental health is equally important, if not more, for physical well-being. Currently, there is a high number of people suffering from mental ailments such as forgetfulness, depression, OCD, mental weakness, and emotions like jealousy, anger, hate, and various fears. Even though they may seem normal, they are going through a difficult time and causing distress to their families. Modern medicine has limited capabilities in treating mental health issues. Therefore, it was believed that performing Havan and Agnihotra, along with herbs that have a positive effect on brain function, could yield good results. This study has been conceptualized with this in mind.

This present study is an effort to re-establish Yagyopathy as a therapeutic science for holistic (complete) healing, complementing Ayurvedic treatment in its present form. The Ayurvedic Rishi Charak has said that those seeking a quick and more effective cure should drink the herbal concoctions and also do daily *Yagya* with the same herbs (Jacqui, 2013; Rastogi, 2020).

Considering that there is a perceptible decrease in the memorizing capability of humans today and also degradation of human values resulting in a society lacking in values like coordination, cooperation, honesty, responsibility, bravery, etc., it was felt to conduct a study on a group of young children (below 15 years) and expose them to

Yagyopathy along with a unique combination of medicinal herbs known as Saraswati Panchak and mantras for a month and then see its effect on them in their cognitive functions as well as value-based behavioral functions. Hence, this study has been conducted.

10.1 INTRODUCTION

Yagya therapy is a traditional approach that was only known to very few people due to its stickiness to primitive methods, but now recent research on *Yagya* therapy to use it as a therapeutic measure has helped in the growth of *Yagya* therapy. These studies helped us to understand how *Yagya* therapy helped people in curing various kinds of diseases without any harmful aftereffects.

10.1.1 MENTAL HEALTH AND ITS IMPORTANCE

Human beings are considered the most evolved among all creations of the universe, especially because of their marvelous mental faculties of intelligence, memory, decision-making, and various emotional and behavioral capacities that place them above the rest of the creatures. But these boons yield results only when the person has sound mental health and the person, along with society, continuously makes efforts for improvement using various methods. This will include above-average intelligence and memory, positive emotions, socio-emotional intelligence, and subjective well-being.

10.1.2 YAGYA THERAPY – AN ALTERNATE THERAPY OF FUTURE

Yagya Therapy is totally a scientific process, wherein Hawan Samagri containing herbs for specific purposes along with goghritha are offered in fire of particular herbal woods with medicinal properties in *Hawan Kund* designed in a specific shape for it. The dynamic effects of *Yagna* are produced as a combination of the following procedures:

1. **The Effect of Heat Energy:** The herbal products offered in fire are sublimated in a controlled manner, so as to release medicinal vapors and phytochemicals. It is well proved that medicines have the best and fastest results when taken in the form of vapors.

2. **The Effect of Sound Energy:** The use of specific mantras for specific ailments creates special electromagnetic waves and sonic effects that are very helpful in intensifying and spreading the benefits of yagna widely (Pandya, 2018).

10.1.3   YAGYOPATHY AS A MULTIDIMENSIONAL HEALER

Yagyaopathy has its own identity as the most ancient and Traditional System of healing in India. Though lesser known now for the purpose of healing, it is associated with the whole life of human beings affecting it from the prenatal state to the end of life. *Yagya* in Indian philosophy demonstrates the art of living, and it is a science of life that disciplines human lives and affects them to the inner core, thereby healing the mental as well as physical knots resulting in diseases and leading to a happy and long life. Yagyopathy has been one of the main modes of therapy during ancient times, not only for humans but also for animals, plants, and also for environmental management. In medieval and modern times, this science lost its significance and is now practiced as a religious ritual in many ceremonies and sanskaras. *Yagya* is believed to heal humans in various dimensions: Activity, Feelings, Consciousness, Group Behavior, and Environment.

10.2   LITERATURE REVIEW

The study has been conducted to present Yagyopathy as a multidimensional and scientific method which can be used as an alternative to the mainstream drugs which show immediate results but have several side effects. It is our traditional Indian method present in our ancient Vedic literature and recently several research and studies have been done on this subject of which few are discussed in subsections.

10.2.1   VEDIC LITERATURE

The Vedic literatures, especially Ayurveda, the science of life of human beings, are considered as a tripod of body, mind, and soul. Ayurveda is based on the principles of the total well-being of an individual, i.e., balance of all the three. Soul and mind represent the conscious entity. The body connects with the conscious entity through the brain, the most developed and sensitive organ of the body, and it communicates with the outer world through the sense organs.

As per Vedic literature, the knower is one who feels emotions, has memory, has mood, thought, intellect, and various other abilities and is thus the conscious entity with their corresponding special areas in the brain. The mind, which is an integral part of the conscious entity, is in close contact with the brain. Broadly, the mind has the following three layers:

1. Inner mind consists of a deep core of feeling and emotions;
2. Intermediate mind is our capacity to bring outer impressions to the inside and vice-versa;
3. Outer mind is dominated by senses, gathering impressions and acting in the outer world.

Ayurveda is deeply concerned with the concept of balance between all the above factors. Practicing the right use of mind and following values in life helps one to achieve one's highest potential (Charak Samhita Sutra Sthana 1).

Yagyopathy is one such strong healing methodology to develop the above virtues and bring about balance between the conscious entity and the body. The medicated fumes of the Yagya have a quick positive effect on the brain and nervous system. The sonic effect of the divine mantras used during *Yagya* affects the conscious entity positively.

This therapy has been widely used in Ayurveda for effective control of communicable diseases like *kshaya* (T.B.), psychological disorders, epilepsy, joint pains, various fevers, etc.

10.2.2 REVIEW OF MODERN LITERATURE

Modern science considers understanding and defining the mind and mental health a challenge. There are various views, some of which are being discussed as follows:

1. Plato identified only one soul/psyche consisting of three parts:

   i. **Thymos:** Emotions, located in the chest.
   ii. **Logos:** Reasoning, located in head.
   iii. **Pathos:** Id, located in liver.

2. Identity Theory states that all mind functions are a kind of brain functions. Scientists tried to find the exact location of brain structures representing consciousness but couldn't succeed.

Our mind consists of three parts:

1. **Cognition:** It refers to a person's intelligence, ability to read, write, speak, learn new things, memory, problem solving, etc.
2. **Affective:** It refers to the emotional interpretation of knowledge.
3. **Conative:** It refers to that part of mind that connects knowledge and effects to behavior.

Scientists have found that various brain areas are involved in accomplishing single mental and emotional functions as follows.

The specific regions of the cerebral cortex are associated with various cognitive functions like language, perception, and memory. The hippocampus and thalamus are specially related to the formation of new memories.

The affective and cognitive aspects of the brain work faster than the conative aspects. The amygdala is responsible for activating emotions, the frontal lobes help in regulation, and the hippocampus in appreciating the context of emotional arousal.

Research shows that these areas continuously change as a result of new learning through life experiences at the neural and receptor levels.

10.2.3   *YAGYA THERAPY IN VEDIC AND AYURVEDIC LITERATURE*

Verma et al. (2018) and her team demonstrated that in Vedic and Ayurvedic literature Yagya has been referred to for its various applications namely social development, ecological balance, spiritual development and curing or prevention from different types of diseases. The healing properties of the *Yagya* process have been described and applied in Yagyopathy. During the process, some forest woods with medicinal properties are burned on fire in a *Hawan Kund*, which results in the generation of smoke, or if we term it properly, medicinal smoke. Inhaling the smoke via performing Pranayama helps in curing diseases.

The study began by researching Vedic and Ayurvedic literature (with a special reference to Pt. Shriram Sharma Acharya Vangmay). Through the study, it was discovered that various common diseases such as infections, fever, malaria, goiter, etc., can be easily treated with Yagya therapy. Further research on *Yagya* therapy revealed that Yagyopathy was also used in the prevention and removal of epidemic diseases. The *Rig Veda* describes Yagyopathy in two ways: first, the inhaled medicinal smoke enhances the strength and immunity of the body, and second, the exhaled breath removes poisonous elements from the human or animal body.

Vedic literature extensively describes Yagyopathy treatment for various types of diseases along with detailed procedures. The current study provides a general review of organizing, curing, treatment, and recovery from different diseases through *Yagya* therapy, as well as its procedures and mechanisms (Verma et al., 2018).

10.2.4 *YAGYOPATHY (YAGYA THERAPY) FOR VARIOUS DISEASES*

Shrivastava et al. (2019) and her team demonstrated the idea of a therapy system with the help of *Yagya*. *Yagya* therapy is a popular and effective method for psychosomatic diseases and also helps in improving human psychology. *Yagya* is a method of utilizing the properties of sacrificial matter with the help of heat energy (*oorja*) and sound energy (*mantras*). In the *Yagya* process, plants and herbs are sacrificed in the fire and transformed into vapors. Inhalation therapy is at the core of Yagya therapy.

Yagya therapy is considered the best method of pulmonary drug administration for plant medicines. The *Hawan Samagri* is made up of various dry plant medicines and during the *Yagya* process, it transforms from a solid to a vapor state. Inhaling this medicinal smoke along with continuous chanting of *mantras* (which enhances pulmonary administration) helps in preventing and curing certain diseases. Sitting near the *Yagya* fire allows the patient to experience bright light and thermal energy, providing relief from depression and stress. Research also discusses various diseases specific to *Hawan Samagri,* dietary advice, and *Pranayama.*

Yagya therapy is a modern approach for treating various diseases through pulmonary administration and continuous chanting of Vedic hymns. Positive results have been observed with *Yagya* therapy, indicating its potential for future use and further research (Shrivastava et al., 2019).

10.2.5   IMPACT OF YAGYA ON PARTICULATE MATTER

Saxena et al. (2018) and their team demonstrated that particulate matter (PM) resulting from air pollution is the cause of several lung-related problems and hazardous diseases. The measures taken to reduce these pollutants are important, but there is one method proposed in our ancient Vedic literature called *Yagya*, which can help reduce air pollutants, especially PM and CO_2.

The team conducted an indoor experiment at two locations in which they performed a *Yagya* using proper *Yagya Samagri* and *vidhi*. In both case studies, the level of PM did not significantly reduce on Day 0 but did so on Day 1 and Day 2 of the Yagya. The CO_2 level also showed the same patterns.

The results are significant because the Yagya involves combustion through the burning of woods and herbs, which should increase the levels of CO_2 and PM. The levels increased on Day 1, but on Day 2, the levels of PM and CO_2 decreased. This may be due to the volatilization of the ghee to which the PM stuck or due to the complete combustion of the Samagri (Saxena et al., 2018).

10.2.6   THE CASE STUDY OF THE EFFECT OF YAGYA ON THE LEVEL OF STRESS AND ANXIETY

Nilachal et al. (2019) and his team demonstrated that stress and anxiety are one of the major issues from which a major section of our society is suffering and people suffering from these disorders takes use of mainstream drugs and medicines which provides instant relief but has several devastating effects not only on the body but also on the mental health which may arise later. But instead of using these drugs, we can follow our traditional Indian approach suggested in our ancient Vedic texts known as *Yagya*.

The team conducted the experiment on children between the ages of 8 and 22 years, and they were made to sit in the Yagya performed with proposed methods. Sinha's Comprehensive Anxiety Test (SCAT) for anxiety and Galvanic Skin Response (GSR) for stress were performed, and recordings were taken before and after the Yagya. The study suggested that during the 30-day curing process, there was a significant reduction in pain, stress levels, negative feelings, and anxiety.

Therefore, *Yagya* Therapy is a very effective method with no harmful effects. It can not only reduce stress and anxiety but also help in the treatment of several mental health-related problems (Nilachal et al., 2019).

10.2.7 EXPLORING INDIAN YAJNA AND MANTRA SCIENCES FOR PERSONALIZED HEALTH

Rastogi et al. (2021) and his team researched that the *Yajna* and *Mantra* science can control disease, pollution, cause rain and also give effect on the animals and humans productivity positively and on mental fitness. *Yajna* and *mantra* have been researched by the ancestors, which have an effect on health and well-being. *Yajna* is a combination of heat, light, and sound science in *Hawan Kund* with fire. *Mantras* are represented as the energy of God, like the Lakshmi Mantra as '*Shreem*.' If you repeat the words of the *Mantra*, they imbibe with the brain, heart, and consecutively the blood of the human body. The fumigations emitted in the *Yajna* prevent the clouds from dispersing.

There were some mantra therapies and cures reviewed by researchers, like disease prevention mantras and safety *mantras* such as *apad-rakshardhamahuti*, etc. Some Hindu traditions are scientifically proven by researchers, like no marriage in the same *Gotra*, touching the feet of elders, clapping during *Aarti*, etc.

The team also analyzes the data with data analytic tools like Python, SPSS, and Excel. This is performed through online platforms over a duration of 150 days. Some protocols are included such as *Asanas*, *Mantra* chanting, breathing exercises, and alternate therapies. Some mudras are used like Surya, *Pran*, *Apan*, *gyan mudras* for 5 minutes. According to the data, it is concluded that the smoke of *Yagya* had no effect on the pollution level (Rastogi et al., 2021).

10.2.8 YAJNA AND MANTRA THERAPY APPLICATIONS ON DIABETIC AND OTHER DISEASE SUBJECTS

Rastogi et al. (2020) and his team researched on some patients suffering from diabetes and many others. These diseases can be Diabetes, TTH, stress, Anxiety, Hypertension, and Obesity. The team also explained about machine vision for the analysis of the applications. Machine vision can involve medical images and analysis, machine learning in healthcare, big data, and the Internet of Things. These are the technologies used to analyze medical records. The third field is the science and philosophy of *Yagya*. *Yagya* means sacrificing the selfless for the noble. *Yagya* is deciphered by Rishis. The last field is *Mantras*. In ancient times, it was the most important technological invention. It is basically a form of sound energy. It is a collection of special words which may not have a clear meaning but form bioenergy that combines with a person's will.

Researchers aim to treat Type 2 diabetes conditions and promote Yagyopathy. This study is based on research from the Yagyopathy Research and Development Association (YRDA) and involved the use of *Hawan Samagri*, cow milk, and jaggery. Additionally, a special Hawan Samagri was used in a 2:1 ratio with a common one. The Hawan took place at 8:00 am in the morning for about 60 minutes per day. There were 11 patients in the Hawan, aged between 38 and 70 years, who followed a specific diet plan.

Their symptoms were recorded based on their PP blood sugar levels. The research showed a reduction in physical problems and improvement in health. It was also found to be beneficial in fighting infections. Yagyopathy helps in healing the body and creating a balanced internal environment. It is a beneficial treatment for diabetes patients without any side effects (Rastogi et al., 2020).

10.3 THE METHODOLOGY AND THE PRESENT STUDY

10.3.1 *EXPERIMENT DESIGN*

A group of 24 children, in the age group of 5 to 14 years, were taken from economically weaker sections and categorized into two groups of 12 each. The first group of 12 children was not given any therapy or herbal concoction. They were labeled as Control Group C0. The second group of 12 children, hereafter referred to as group C1, were brought to the center for 30 days and were exposed to Yagyopathy in the morning. Additionally, they were given *Saraswati Panchak Kadha* (concoction) 10 ml both in the morning and evening and were told stories with good moral lessons every day. Moreover, they were provided with sprouted chickpeas, moong Dal, peanuts, and raisins for breakfast daily after the Yagyopathy sessions. They were under the direct observation and mentoring of one teacher who conducted the daily *Yagya*, gave the children of the C1 group daily math lessons, and read stories with good moral lessons to them. He also prepared daily kadha from *Saraswati Panchak Samagri* herbs and gave it to the children of the C1 group twice a day.

As shown in the Figure 10.1, 24 students are selected from weaker sections in which 12 students are taken in the experimental group and the remaining 12 are taken in the control group. The various activities are performed by the experimental group which are as follows:

- Yoga Asanas;
- Yagya;
- Meditation;
- Pranayama;
- Drink saraswatipanchakkadha (twice a day);
- Healthy breakfast;
- Learn math and moral lessons.

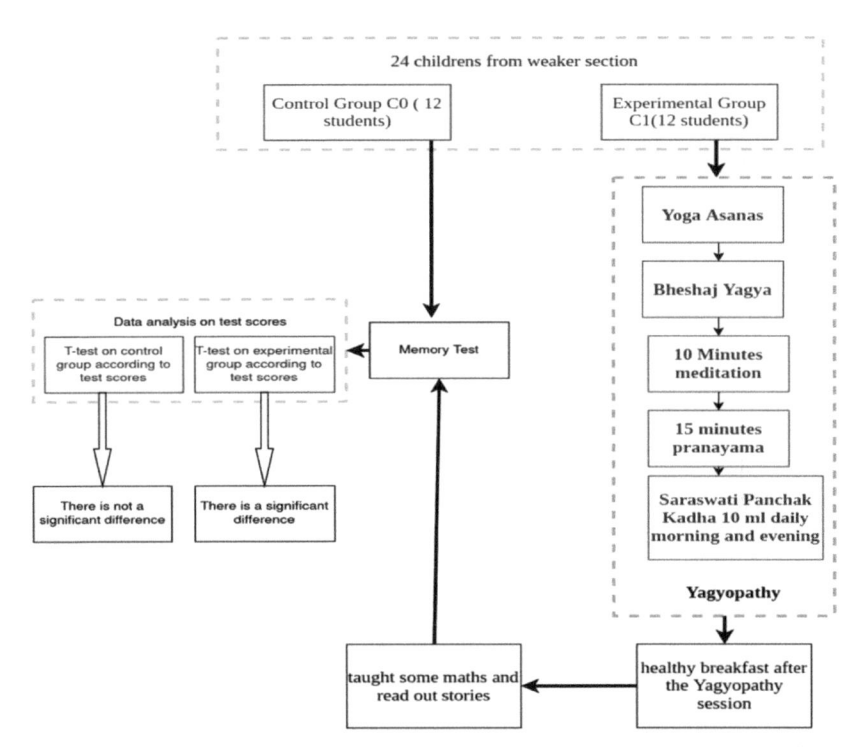

FIGURE 10.1 Block diagram of the experimental design to perform the present study with conclusions.

On the basis of the conclusion, the memory test was conducted to test the performance of the groups after the experiment. The researchers analyzed the test scores achieved by the students in both groups and found that the experimental group showed a significant difference in performance before and after, while there was no significant difference in the performance of the control group.

10.3.2   THE YAGYOPATHY EXPERIMENT PROTOCOL/METHODOLOGY

The Yagyopathy process includes the following sub-processes:

1. Simple Yoga Asanas for children to activate their mind and body.
2. *Bheshaj Yagya*: This consisted of simplified procedures listed in the book "Saral and Sankshipt Gayatri Havan Vidhi" by Pt. Shriram Sharma Acharya. The basic steps followed for this experiment included Shatkarma for the purification of body, mind, and spirit, Devavahan, Fire or *Agni sthapanam*. Then, 24 oblations (aahuties) were given with the *Saraswati Gayatri Mantra* using *Saraswati Panchak Havan Samagri* mixed with Ghee (clarified butter) Gur, followed by 3 oblations of *Mahamritunjay mantra*, 1 with *Swishtikrit Mantra*, and then Poornahuti. This was followed by *Ghritavghranam, bhasmdharanam*, a prayer for the well-being of everybody in this world, and *Shantipath*.
3. 10 Minutes meditation and 15 minutes *Pranayama* to calm the mind and absorb the positive *Pranas* in the atmosphere after *Yagya*.
4. As a part of this experiment, children of group C1 were given *Saraswati Panchakadha* 10 ml daily in the morning and evening.
5. In addition, they were given a healthy breakfast of sprouted moong dal, chickpeas, peanuts, and raisins, soaked a day before and sprouted, after the Yagyopathy session was over.
6. After breakfast, children were taught some math to improve their mental math abilities and were read stories in Hindi based on moral lessons, after which discussions were held with children to help them understand.

10.3.3   SARASWATI PANCHAK

1. *Saraswati Panchak* is a combination of five herbs, invented and developed by Param Pujya Gurudev Pandit Shri Ram Sharma

Acharya ji for the improvement of mental health, namely *Brahmi, Shatavari, Gorakhmundi, Shankhpushpi*, and *Mithi Buti*.

Each of these herbs is an excellent mental tonic and known for their positive impact on the brain and its various cognitive functions. Three of these herbs, namely *Brahmi, Vacha,* and *Shankhapushpi*, are *Medhya Rasayana* or nootropic herbs, known as memory enhancers or cognitive enhancers (Singh, 2020).

10.3.4 ASSESSMENT OF CHILDREN

10.3.4.1 MEMORY TESTS

All the children in groups C0 and C1 were assessed for their memory through online wiki-fun memory test videos both before the experiment and immediately after the experiment. These are online screen tests where children are shown initially 6 cards with some object pictures on one side and card numbers 1–6 behind them, which they had to memorize with the numbers shown at their back. Then one object is shown on the screen, and they have to tell the card number of that object.

There were four difficulty levels where the number of cards increased from 6 to 8 to 10 and 12, respectively, and children were assessed accordingly. For each correct answer, they were given one point for level one to four points for level four.

Figure 10.2 demonstrated methodology was applied for scoring children, and the outcomes were analyzed. The scoring process and various steps of Yagyaopathy have been demonstrated in Figures 10.2–10.4.

Figure 10.3 shows various children performing *Yagya* with *Saraswatipanchakhavan Samagri* and inhaling the medicinal smoke generated when the *Havan Samagri* is burned in the *Havan Kund*. This smoke enhances their mental power to a large extent and also gives immunity and strength to their body. In Figure 10.4, we can see that children are doing Yoga as it is a part of the Yagya therapy process. The Yoga part will help the children in activating their mind and body, which will enhance the therapeutic effect of the medicinal smoke inhaled by the children.

In Figure 10.5, we can see that children are meditating after the *Yagya* process because it is a part of the Yagyopathy process. The children need to meditate to calm their minds and absorb the positive Pranas in the atmosphere after *Yagya* (as per Figure 10.5).

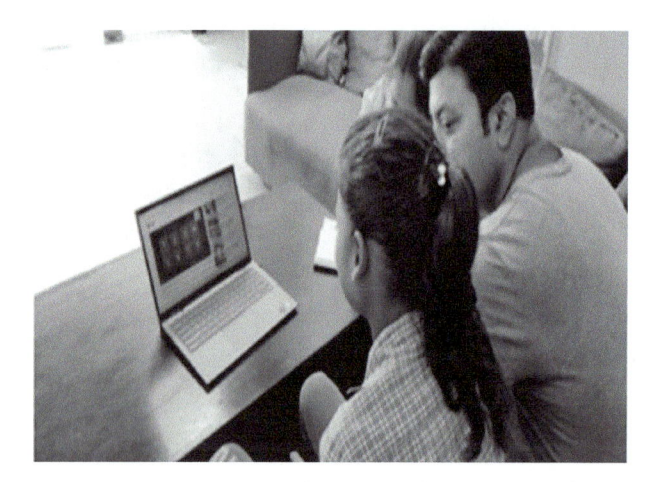

FIGURE 10.2   Children giving online memory tests for assessment after 30 days.

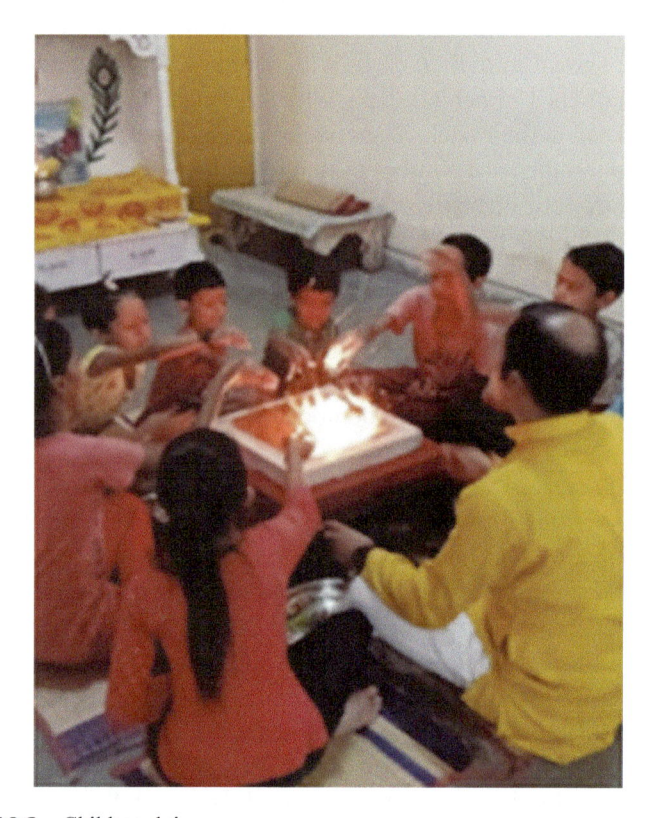

FIGURE 10.3   Children doing *yagya*.

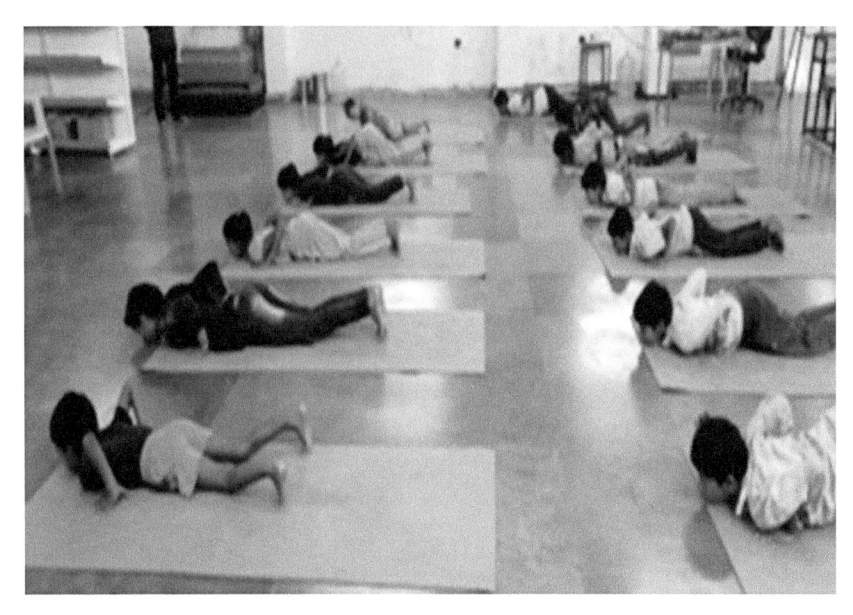

FIGURE 10.4   Children doing yoga as a part of the yagyopathy.

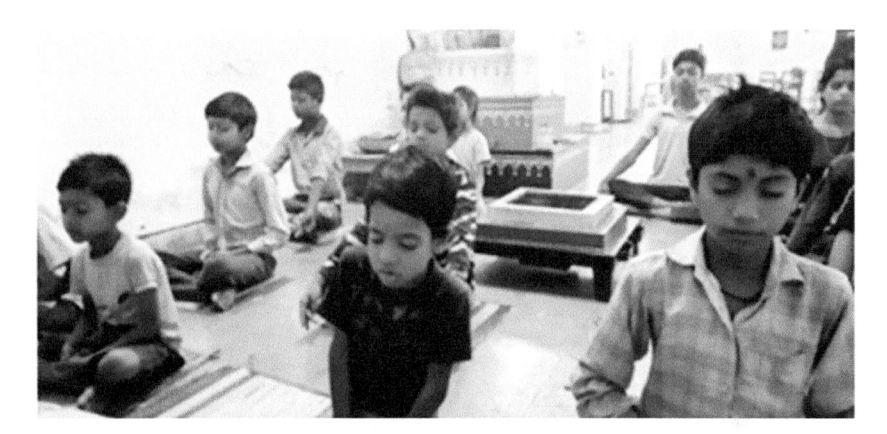

FIGURE 10.5   Children doing meditation as a part of the yagyopathy process.

10.4   RESULTS AND DISCUSSION

After the memory test assessment, the test scores are recorded based on the students' performance. The following is the statistical analysis of the test scores of different groups, including the experimental and control groups.

10.4.1   *MEMORY GAME ASSESSMENT RESULTS OF THE CONTROL GROUP*

According to the results of the statistical analysis from the table provided for the memory game assessment, the students' performance is recorded (*please refer to* Table 10.2).

10.4.1.1   *GRAPHICAL REPRESENTATION OF THE TEST SCORES*

As shown in Figure 10.6, there are 12 students' test score records based on their previous and post-performance. The blue line shows the previous performance, and the green line shows the post-performance (*please refer to* Figure 10.6).

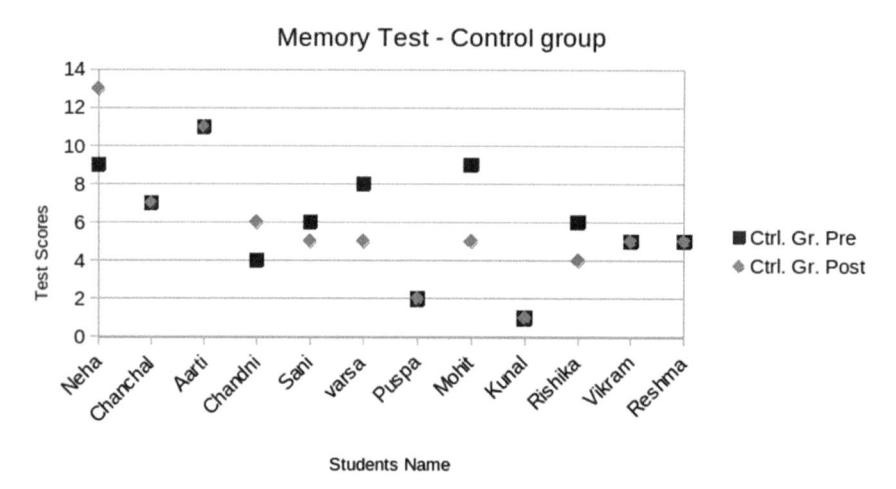

FIGURE 10.6   Graphical representation of the non-Havan group students in the memory game assessment.

As shown in Figure 10.7, there are 12 students' test score records based on their previous and post-performance. The red bar shows the previous performance, and the pink bar shows the post-performance of the students. This graph also displays the respective test score values (*please refer to* Figure 10.7).

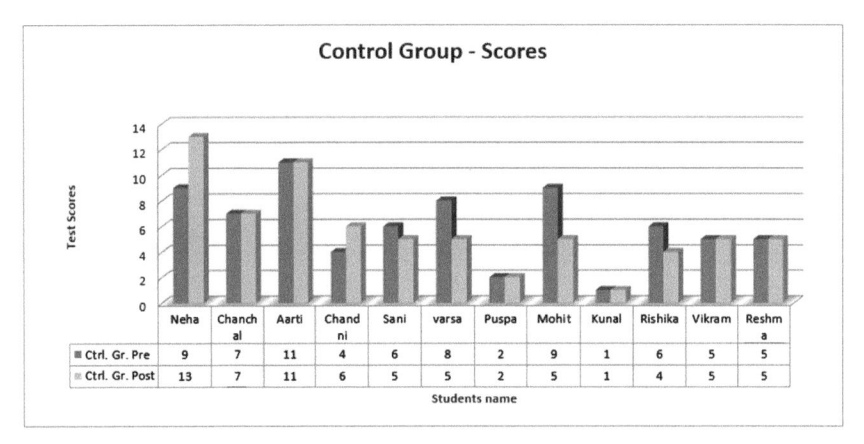

FIGURE 10.7 Representation of the performance of the non-Havan group students through bar graph with their respective test scores.

10.4.1.2 ANALYSIS OF THE STUDENTS' SCORES ACCORDING TO THEIR AGES

In Figure 10.8, the graph represents the students' test scores according to their ages. The bar graph shows the previous test scores and the post-test scores of the non-haven group through a memory game. Additionally, the line graph shows the students' ages accordingly.

10.4.1.3 PAIRED SAMPLE T-TEST RESULTS ANALYSIS

The test statistic T equals 0.4979, which is in the 95% region of acceptance: [–2.201, 2.201]. The 95% confidence interval of post minus previous is: [–2.2805, 3.6138] (*please refer* Figure 10.8).

Here, the team also performed paired t-tests to compare the previous (i.e., ctrl. gr. pre.) and post-test scores (i.e., ctrl. gr. post.) of the students who are not in the haven group. There was not a significant difference in a memory game assessment in the non-haven group between the Control Group previous (M=6.1, SD=2.9) and Control Group post (M=6.8, SD=4.9); t(11) = 0.5489, p = 0.628, where M represents the mean, SD represents the standard deviation, t(df) represents the t-value with respect to the degree of freedom, and p represents the p-value (*please refer to* Table 10.1).

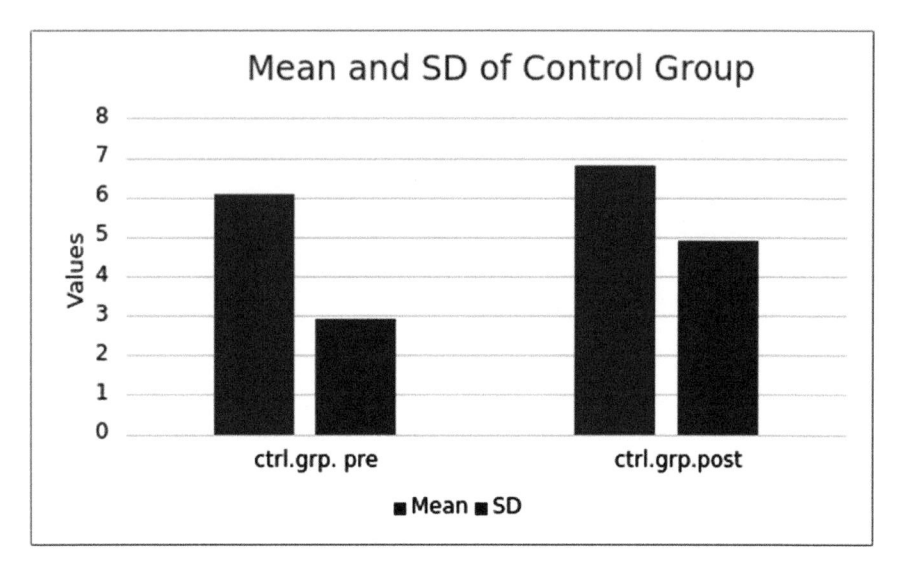

FIGURE 10.8   Mean and standard deviation of the control group using paired t-test.

TABLE 10.1   Resultant Table of the Paired T-Test Performed on the Non-Havan Group

Alpha	0.05	
	Ctrl. Grp. Pre	**Ctrl. Grp. Post**
Mean	6.1	6.8
SD	2.9	4.9
T-value	0.5	–
P-value	0.628	–
Sample size	12	–
Degree of freedom	11	–
Average of difference	0.6667	–
SD of difference	4.6384	–

10.4.2   MEMORY GAME ASSESSMENT RESULTS OF THE EXPERIMENTAL GROUP

According to the results of the statistical analysis based on the given table for the memory game assessment, the performance of the students is recorded (*please refer to* Table 10.1).

10.4.2.1 GRAPHICAL REPRESENTATION OF THE TEST SCORES

As shown in Figure 10.9, there are 12 students' test score records based on their previous and post-performance. The blue line represents the previous performance, and the red line represents the post-performance. This graph visually displays the difference between the previous and post-performance of the experimental students (*please refer to* Figure 10.9).

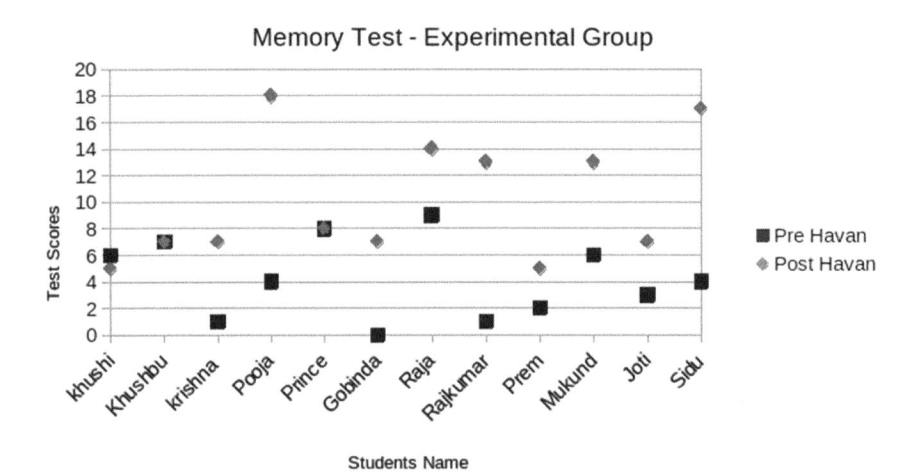

FIGURE 10.9   Graphical representation of the experimental group students in the memory game assessment.

As shown in Figure 10.10, there are 12 students who are involved in Havan. The effects and performance were measured pre and post experiments. There are some test scores on their performance which are in the form of bar graph representation with their respective scores. It clearly shows the difference between the performance of the students through all the activities (*please refer to* Figure 10.10).

10.4.2.2 ANALYSIS OF THE STUDENTS' SCORES ACCORDING TO THEIR AGES

In Figure 10.11, the graph represents the students' test scores according to their ages. The bar graph shows the previous test scores and the post-test score of the experimental group through a memory game. Also, the line graph shows the students' age accordingly. It is concluded that the experiment positively affects the students at any age.

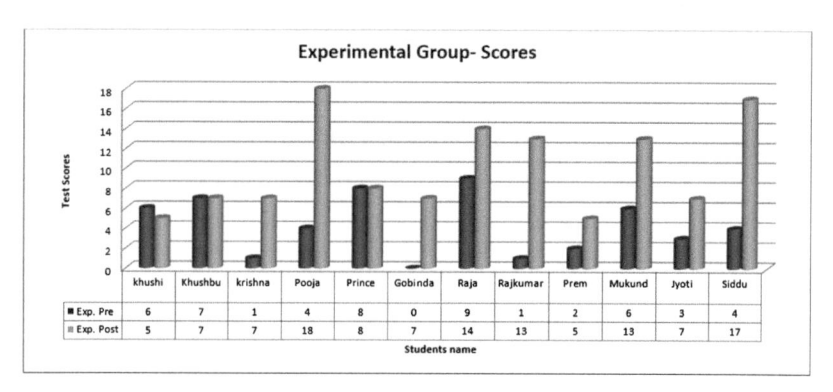

FIGURE 10.10   Representation of the performance of the experimental group students through bar graph with their respective test scores.

10.4.2.3   PAIRED SAMPLE T-TEST RESULTS ANALYSIS

The test statistic T equals 3.9653, which is not in the 95% region of acceptance: [−2.201, 2.201]. The 95% confidence interval of after minus Before is: [2.5955, 9.0712] (as per Figure 10.11).

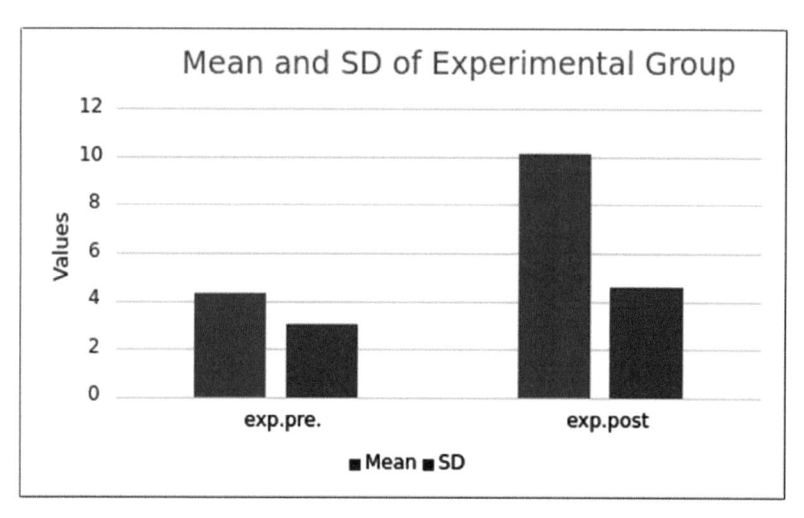

FIGURE 10.11   Mean and standard deviation of the control group.

Here, the team also performed paired t-tests to compare the previous (i.e., exp. pre.) and post-test scores (i.e., exp. post.) of the experimental group students who participated in the *Havan*. There was a significant difference in a memory game assessment in the experimental group between the previous (M=4.25, SD=2.958) and post (M=10.083, SD=4.640) scores of the experimental group; t(11) = 3.965, p = 0.0022, where M represents the mean, SD represents the standard deviation, t(df) represents the t-value with respect to the degrees of freedom, and p represents the p-value (as per Table 10.2).

TABLE 10.2 Resultant Table of the T-Test Performed on the Experimental Group

Alpha	0.05	
	Exp. Pre.	**Exp. Post**
Mean	4.3	10.1
SD	3	4.6
T-value	3.965	–
P-value	0.002	–
Sample size	12	–
Degree of freedom	11	–
Average of difference	5.8333	–
SD of difference	5.096	–

10.5 NOVELTIES

1. In the present system of Ayurvedic therapy, people are given medicinal herbs in tablets, powdered, or liquid form and are cured slowly through a one-to-one process. However, with the Yagya therapy, the smoke generated by herbs is inhaled by a number of people at a time, which is a one-to-many process. If given along with oral medicines, the recovery is much faster.

2. The medicinal smoke generated in the *Yagya* therapy cures not only the diseases in the body but also builds immunity and energizes the person through the Pranic energy that is developed massively after the Yagya.

3. Direct intake of herbs in solid or liquid form has a slower and lesser effect in comparison to the medicinal smoke because it is

directly absorbed by the lungs and is infused with the blood, which helps in enhancing the curing process at a faster rate.

10.6   RECOMMENDATION

Problems related to mental health are one of the major concerns of people nowadays, and a simple and cost-effective process of Yagyopathy, which is a one-to-many type of method, has been presented here. In this process, a large number of people can benefit at a time from the smoke released due to the combustion of Saraswatipanchak herbs. Along with this, the Ayurvedic medicinal kadha prepared from Saraswati Panchak, given to children to increase their memory power, has enhanced the power of therapy. The results of the experiments have been inspiring, as the children performed significantly better in the memory tests and quizzes conducted after the Yagyopathy than the ones who did not participate. Therefore, it is recommended that this therapy should be further tried by individuals in various age groups and strata of society to establish the results.

10.7   FUTURE RESEARCH DIRECTION AND LIMITATIONS

10.7.1   *LIMITATIONS*

1. It is difficult to obtain pure Saraswati Panchak Samagri for the Yagya, especially in big cities.
2. The experiment was conducted on a very small sample size and may show some variation in the results if the sample size were to increase.
3. The instruments used to calculate the memory score of the children were those available online for their age, so scores may vary for different instruments.

10.7.2   *FUTURE DIRECTIONS*

1. The experiment can be conducted on a large sample size and for a longer time period.

2. The concluding parameters may also be increased such as sleep, concentration power, violence, behavioral changes, etc., for better study.
3. The study can be conducted in different demographic regions and also on people of different genders, castes, ages, educational qualifications, etc.
4. The methods can be proposed so that the surrounding atmosphere can also benefit from the Yagya.

10.8 CONCLUSION

This study has shown that after 30 days of *Yagya* therapy with *Saraswati Panchak Havan Samagri*, there has been a significant improvement in the memory of the children who participated in the experiment. Though the sample size was small, these results can be taken as an indication of a trend of improvement in the cognitive power of humans after *Yagya* therapy with *Saraswati Panchak* composition *Havan Samagri*.

So, it can be concluded that the study has proved to be successful and has paved the way for more studies on the subject with different medicinal Hawan Samagri and a larger group.

The data analytics are performed using Python and Excel. The analysis is done in two groups, i.e., the Experimental group and the control group. Control Group and experimental group test score records are recorded according to their performance. After the data analysis, it is found that:

- The control group students do not have a significant difference in a memory game assessment in the non-Havan group between the Control group previous (M=6.1, SD=2.9) and Control Group post (M=6.8, SD=4.9); t(11) = 0.5489, p = 0.628.
- Experimental groups have a significant difference in a memory game assessment in the experimental group between the experimental group previous (M=4.25, SD = 2.958) and experimental Group post (M=10.083, SD=4.640); t(11) = 3.965, p = 0.0022.

It is found that the Saraswati Panchak Samagri plays an important role in the effective performance of the experimental group. This study successfully proved the difference between the performances of the experimental group.

KEYWORDS

- **control group**
- **experimental group**
- **memory game assessment**
- **memory tests**
- **test scores**
- **T-test**
- **yagyopathy**

REFERENCES

Atharva Veda Chapter 19/38/12; 3/10; 3/11/13, Published by Sri Vedmata Gayatri Trust, Shantikunj, Haridwar, India.

Callahan, D. (2007). *The Role of Complementary and Alternative Medicine: Accommodating Pluralism*. Georgetown University Press. Retrieved from: https://www.jstor.org/stable/j.ctt1qd9028 (accessed on 5 July 2024).

Jacqui, W. (2013). Herbal products are often contaminated, study finds. *BMJ Journals, 1*(1), 1–10. https://doi.org/10.1136/bmj.f6138.

Kumar, K. (2011). Yagyopathy: A new dimension of research in therapy system. *ResearchGate, 10*(01), 1–3. Retrieved from: https://www.researchgate.net/publication/215639095_Yagyopathy_A_New_dimension_of_Research_in_Therapy_System (accessed on 5 July 2024).

Mishra, A., Batham, L., & Shrivastava, V. (2019). Yagyopathy (Yagya Therapy) for Various Diseases–An Overview. *Ayurveda Evam Samagra Swasthya Shodhamala, 1*(1), 1–11. Retrieved from: https://www.researchgate.net/publication/339484294_Yagyopathy_Yagya_Therapy_for_Various_Diseases_-_An_Overview (accessed on 5 July 2024).

Nautiyal, C. S., Chauhan, P. S., & Nene, Y. S. (2007). Medicinal smoke reduces airborne bacteria. *Journal of Ethnopharmacology, 114*(3), 446–451. http://dx.doi.org/10.1016/j.jep.2007.08.038.

Nilachal, N., & Trivedi, P. (2019). A case study of the effect of Yagya on the level of stress and anxiety. *Dev Sanskriti Vishwavidyalaya Interdisciplinary Journal of Yagya Research, 2*(2), 7–10. https://doi.org/10.36018/ijyr.v2i2.44.

Pandya, P. (2018). *Applied Science of Yagya for Health & Environment*. Shri Vedmata Gayatri Trust, Shantikunj, 1–160.

Raghuvanshi, M., Pandya, P., & Joshi, R. R. (2004). Yagyopathic Herbal Treatment of Pulmonary Tuberculosis–A Clinical Trial. *Mary Ann Libert, Inc. Publisher, 10*(2), 101–105. https://doi.org/10.1089/107628004773933352.

Raghuvanshi, M., Pandya, P., & Joshi, R. R. (2009). In-vitro testing of an ethnobotanical inhalation therapy against pulmonary tuberculosis phytotherapies. *ResearchGate, 7*(5), 243–249. http://dx.doi.org/10.1007/s10298-009-0413-8.

Rastogi, R., Saxena, M., Gupta, U. S., Sharma, S., Chaturvedi, D. K., Singhal, P., Gupta, M., Garg, P., Gupta, M., & Maheshwari, M. (2020a). Yajna and mantra therapy applications on diabetic subjects: Computational intelligence based experimental approach. *SSRN Journals, 1*(1), 1–14. https://dx.doi.org/10.2139/ssrn.3515800.

Rastogi, R., Saxena, M., Sagar, S., & Tandon, N. (2021). Exploring Indian Yajna and mantra sciences for personalized health: Pandemic threats and possible cures in twenty-first-century healthcare. *De Gruyter Publications, 1*(1), 17–36. https://doi.org/10.1515/9783110708127-002.

Rastogi, R., Saxena, M., Sharma, S. K., Muralidharan, S., Beriwal, V. K., Singhal, P., Rastogi, M., & Shrivastava, R. (2020c). Evaluation of efficacy of yagya therapy on T2–diabetes mellitus patients. *SSRN Journals, 01*(01), 1–13. https://papers.ssrn.com/sol3/papers.cfm?abstract_id=3514326 (accessed on 5 July 2024).

Rastogi, R., Saxena, M., Sharma, S. K., Murlidharan, S., Beriwal V., Jaiswal, D., Sharma, A., & Mishra, A. (2020b). Statistical analysis on efficacy of yagya therapy for type-2 diabetic mellitus patients through various parameters. *Springer Link Journal, 1120*(01), 181–197. http://dx.doi.org/10.1007/978-981-15-2449-3_15.

Samanth, T. U. et al. (2018). Effect of smoke from medicinal herbs on nosocomial infections in the ENT outpatient department. *Indian Journal of Otology, 24*(01), 09–12. Retrieved from: https://www.indianjotol.org/article.asp (accessed on 5 July 2024).

Saxena, M., Sengupta, B., & Pandya, P. (2007). Comparative Study of Yagya vs Non-Yagya Microbial Environments. *Indian Journal of Air Pollution Control, 07*(01), 16–24.

Saxena, M., Sengupta, B., & Pandya, P. (2008). Controlling the Microflora in Outdoor Environment: Effect of Yoga. *Indian Journal of Air Pollution Control, 8*(2), 30–36.

Saxena, M., Sengupta, B., & Pandya, P. (2018). Impact of Yagya on Particulate Matters. *Dev Sanskriti Vishwavidyalaya Interdisciplinary Journal of Yagya Research, 1*(1), 1–8. Retrieved from: http://ijyr.dsvv.ac.in/index.php/ijyr/article/view/5/6 (accessed on 5 July 2024).

Singh, R. (2020). Saraswati Panchak–A Novel Herbal Combination for Mental Health. *Interdisciplinary Journal of Yagya Research, 03*(02), 09–18. http://dx.doi.org/10.36018/ijyr.v3i2.59.

Verma, S., Mishra, A., & Shrivastava, V. (2018). Yagya Therapy in Vedic and Ayurvedic Literature: A Preliminary exploration. *Dev Sanskriti Vishwavidyalaya Interdisciplinary Journal of Yagya Research, 1*(1), 15–20. https://doi.org/10.36018/ijyr.v1i1.7.

ANNEXURE

> ### ➤ Additional Readings:

Acharya S. S. (2001). *The Integrated Science of Yagna*, IIT Bombay.

Ayurvedic texts of Charaksamhita, Sushrutsamhita, Ashtangasamgraha.

Bansal, P., Kaur, R., Gupta, V., Kumar, S., & Kaur, R. P. (31 Dec. 2015). Is There Any Scientific Basis of *Hawan* to be used in Epilepsy-Prevention/Cure?, *5*(2), 33–45, *Doi:* 10.14581/jer.15009.

Buelteman R. (2012). Shocks Flowers With 80,000 Volts of Electricity, *BSIIJ.*

Chhabra G. (2015). Human Aura: a new vedic approach in it, *University of Petroleum and Energy Studies.*

Chig, T. T. (1998). What is Yin Yang? Always Dream Even When Awake, *Taoist Articles.*

Corsini, R. J., *Encyclopedia of Psychology.*

Dudeja J. (2017). Scientific Analysis of Mantra-Based Meditation and its Beneficial Effects: An Overview, *ResearchGate.*

Ferrara, L. A., (Nova Publishers, 2006). *Focus on Body Mass Index and Health Research.*

Gaiam.com/blogs/discover/how-does-meditation-affect-the-body.

Grimnes S., & Martinsen G. (2015), *Bioimpedance, and Bioelectricity Basics,* ResearchGate 3.

Grujin, J. (2016), What is Kirlian Photography? Aura Photography Revealed, *Light Stalking.*

Hershberg, W. A., *Psychology as Cognitive Science.*

http://en.wikipedia.org/wiki/Conation-acessed.

https://blog.sivanaspirit.com/sp-gn-scientific-benefits-chanting/.

https://qz.com/1630159/bioelectricity-may-be-key-to-fighting-cancer/ANDhttps://onlinelibrary.wiley.com/doi/abs/10.1111/jtsb.12101.

https://rationalwiki.org/wiki/Quantum_consciousness.

https://www.chakra-anatomy.com/human-aura.html.

https://www.doyou.com/how-mantras-work-39322/.

https://www.encyclopedia.com/medicine/encyclopedias-almanacs-transcripts-and-maps/bioelectricity.

https://www.worldpranichealing.com/en/energy/what-is-pranic-energy/ AND.

Humberto, N., *Basic Psychoanalytic Concepts on the Theory of Instincts.*

Mills, A. (29 June 2009). Kirlian Photography, *History of Photography, 33*(3).

Prabhat, S., (January 7, 2010). (http://www.differencebetween.net/miscellaneous/difference-between-yin-and-yang/).

Pranav Pandya. *Applied Science of Yagna for Health and Environment.*

Sia, P. D. (2016). Mindfulness: Consciousness and Quantum Physics, *University of Padova.*

Smith, J. A., Suttie, J., Jazaieri, H., & Newman, K. M. (2018). Things We Know About the Science of Meditation, *Mindfulness Research.*

Sui, C. K. (2012), Pranic Energy: Feel Divinity All Around You, *IJITEE.*

Sui, C. K., The Ancient Science and Art of Pranic Healing & Advanced Pranic Healing.

Varman, H. (2014), *Five Important Levels of the Human Consciousness*, BSIII.

Wertheimer, M. *Productive Thinking.*

Wikipedia (https://simple.wikipedia.org/wiki/Chakra).

Williams, M. (McGraw-Hill, 2006). *Nutrition for Health, Fitness, and Sport*, 8th Edn.

Wisneski, Leonard A., (2010). *The Scientific Basis of Integrative Medicine*, IJITEE.

➢ **Key Terms and Definitions:**

- *Yajna*: It literally means "sacrifice, devotion, worship, offering," and refers in Hinduism to any ritual done in front of a sacred fire, often with mantras. *Yajna* has been a Vedic tradition, described in a layer of Vedic literature called *Brahmanas*, as well as *Yajurveda*. The tradition has evolved from offering oblations and libations into sacred fire to symbolic offerings in the presence of sacred fire (Agni).

- *Mantra*: A *mantra* is a sacred utterance, a numinous sound, a syllable, word or phonemes, or group of words in Sanskrit believed by practitioners to have psychological and/or spiritual powers. Some mantras have a syntactic structure and literal meaning, while others do not.

- ***Jap*:** It is the meditative repetition of a *mantra* or a divine name. It is a practice found in Hinduism, Jainism, Sikhism, Buddhism, and Shintoism. The mantra or name may be spoken softly, enough for the practitioner to hear it, or it may be spoken within the reciter's mind. *Jap* may be performed while sitting in a meditation posture, while performing other activities, or as part of formal worship in group settings.
- **Ayurveda:** This system of medicine with historical roots in the Indian subcontinent. Globalized and modernized practices derived from Ayurveda traditions are a type of alternative medicine. In countries beyond India, Ayurvedic therapies and practices have been integrated in general wellness applications and in some cases in medical use. The main classical Ayurveda texts begin with accounts of the transmission of medical knowledge from the Gods to sages, and then to human physicians. In *Sushruta Samhita* (Sushruta's Compendium), Sushruta wrote that Dhanvantari, Hindu god of Ayurveda.
- **Sanskrit:** It is an Indo-Aryan language of the ancient Indian subcontinent with a 3,500-year history. It is the primary liturgical language of Hinduism and the predominant language of most works of Hindu philosophy as well as some of the principal texts of Buddhism and Jainism. Sanskrit, in its variants and numerous dialects, was the lingua franca of ancient and medieval India. In the early 1st millennium AD, along with Buddhism and Hinduism, Sanskrit migrated to Southeast Asia, parts of East Asia and Central Asia, emerging as a language of high culture and of local ruling elites in these regions.
- **Vedic:** The Vedic period or Vedic age (c. 1500–c. 500 BCE), is the period in the history of the northern Indian subcontinent between the end of the urban Indus Valley Civilization and a second urbanization which began in the central Indo-Gangetic Plain c. 600 BCE. It gets its name from the Vedas, which are liturgical texts containing details of life during this period that have been interpreted to be historical and constitute the primary sources for understanding the period. These documents, alongside the corresponding archaeological record, allow for the evolution of the Vedic culture to be traced and inferred.

- **Energy Measurements:** There are various kinds of units used to measure the quantity of energy sources. The Standard unit of Energy is known to be Joule (J). Also, another mostly used energy unit is kilowatt/hour (kWh) which is basically used in electricity bills. Large measurements may also go up to terawatt/hour (TWh) or also said as billion kW/h.

  Other units used for measuring heat include BTU (British Thermal Unit), kilogram calorie (kg-cal) and most commonly Ton of Oil Equivalent. Actually, it represents the quantity of heat which can be obtained from a ton of oil.

  Energy is also measured in some other units such as British Thermal Unit (BTU), calorie, therm, etc., which varies generally according to their area of use.

- **PM Level-Particulates:** This also known as atmospheric aerosol particles, atmospheric particulate matter, particulate matter (PM), or suspended particulate matter (SPM) – are microscopic particles of solid or liquid matter suspended in the air. The term aerosol commonly refers to the particulate/air mixture, as opposed to the particulate matter alone. Sources of particulate matter can be natural or anthropogenic. They have impacts on climate and precipitation that adversely affect human health, in ways additional to direct inhalation. Types of atmospheric particles include suspended particulate matter, thoracic and respirable particles, inhalable coarse particles, designated PM10, which are coarse particles with a diameter of 10 micrometers (μm) or less, fine particles, designated PM2.5, with a diameter of 2.5 μm or less, ultrafine particles, and soot.

- **Emission of Gases:** A greenhouse gas (sometimes abbreviated GHG) is a gas that absorbs and emits radiant energy within the thermal infrared range. Greenhouse gases cause the greenhouse effect on planets. The primary greenhouse gases in Earth's atmosphere are water vapor (H_2O), carbon dioxide (CO_2), methane (CH_4), nitrous oxide (N_2O), and ozone (O_3). Without greenhouse gases, the average temperature of Earth's surface would be about $-18°C$ ($0°F$), rather than the present average of $15°C$ ($59°F$). The atmospheres of Venus, Mars, and Titan also contain greenhouse gases.

- **Machine Learning (ML):** It is the study of computer algorithms that improve automatically through experience. It is seen as a subset of artificial intelligence. Machine learning algorithms build a mathematical model based on sample data, known as "training data," in order to make predictions or decisions without being explicitly programmed to do so. Machine learning algorithms are used in a wide variety of applications, such as email filtering and computer vision, where it is difficult or infeasible to develop conventional algorithms to perform the needed tasks.
- **Sensor and IoT:** The Internet of things (IoT) is a system of interrelated computing devices, mechanical and digital machines provided with unique identifiers (UIDs) and the ability to transfer data over a network without requiring human-to-human or human-to-computer interaction. Sensors are devices that detect and respond to changes in an environment. Inputs can come from a variety of sources such as light, temperature, motion, and pressure. Sensors output valuable information and if they are connected to a network, they can share data with other connected devices and management systems. They are an integral part of the Internet of Things (IoT). There are many types of IoT sensors and an even greater number of applications and use cases.
- **Pollution:** It is the introduction of contaminants into the natural environment that cause adverse change. Pollution can take the form of chemical substances or energy, such as noise, heat or light. Pollutants, the components of pollution, can be either foreign substances/energies or naturally occurring contaminants. Pollution is often classed as point source or nonpoint source pollution. In 2015, pollution killed 9 million people in the world. The major kinds of pollution, usually classified by environment, are air pollution, water pollution, and land pollution. Modern society is also concerned about specific types of pollutants, such as noise pollution, light pollution, and plastic pollution. Pollution of all kinds can have negative effects on the environment and wildlife and often impacts human health and well-being.

DATA SETS

TABLE 1   Sample Dataset for Experiment Group

Details		Experiment Group	
SL. No	**Student Name**	**Pre-Havan**	**Post-Havan**
1.	Khushi	6	5
2.	Khushbu	7	7
3.	Krishna	1	7
4.	Pooja	4	18
5.	Prince	8	8
6.	Gobind	0	7
7.	Raja	9	14
8.	Rajkumar	1	13
9.	Prem	2	5
10.	MuKund	6	13
11.	Joti	3	7
12.	Sidhu	4	17

TABLE 2   Sample Dataset for Control Group

SL. No	**Non-Havan Group**	**Date: 26-5-2022**	**Date: 01-7-2022**
	Details	**Memory Game**	**Memory Game**
	Student Name	**Ctrl. Gr. Pre**	**Ctrl. Gr. Post**
1.	Neha	9	13
2.	Chanchal	7	7
3.	Aarti	11	11
4.	Chandni	4	6
5.	Sani	6	5
6.	Varsha	8	5
7.	Pushpa	2	2
8.	Mohit	9	5
9.	Kunal	1	1
10.	Rishika	6	4
11.	Vikram	5	5
12.	Reshma	5	5

SNAPSHOTS

The practice starts by encouraging the fire god to enter the *Havan Kund* and bless the premises for the success of the *Havan*. Then all the participating members offer their respective *Aahutis* to the *Agni Dev* (as per Figure A).

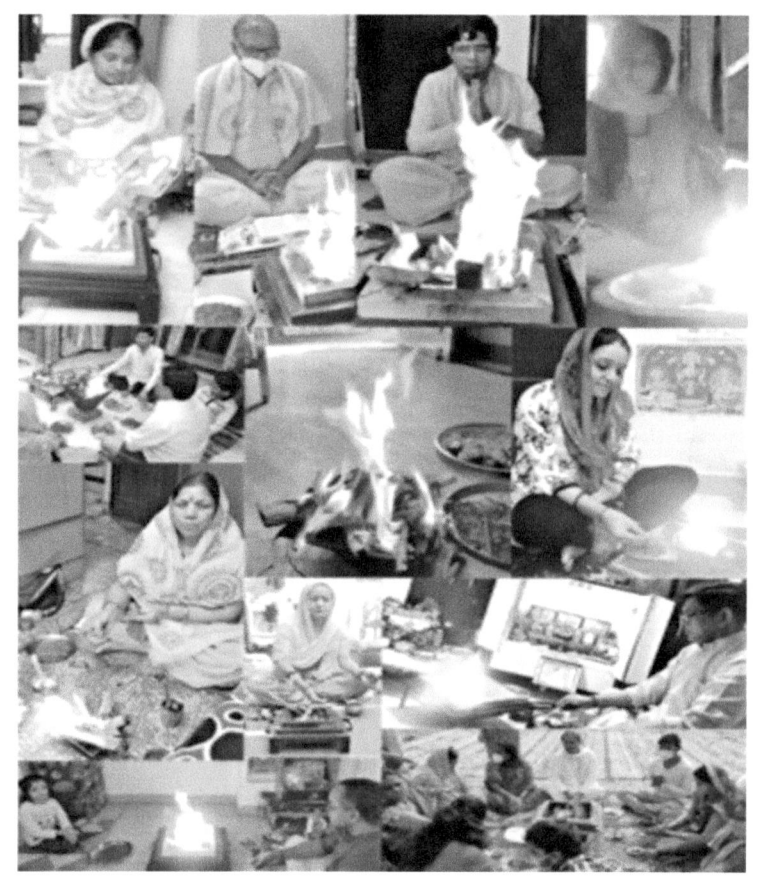

FIGURE A   *Havan* process is done by the persons by giving *Aahuti* to *Agni Dev*.

- **Om:** The Original sound/The primeval sound;
- **Bhur:** The physical body;
- **Bhuvah:** The life force/the mental realm;
- **Suvah:** The soul/spiritual nation;

- **Tat:** That God;
- **Savitur:** The Sun, Creator (source of all life) or that which gives birth;
- **Vareñyam:** Adore or to choose;
- **Bhargo:** Effulgence (divine light); or the self-luminous one;
- **Devasya:** Superior Lord; or the divine Grace;
- **Dhimahi:** Meditate; or who's wisdom and knowledge flow, like waters;
- **Dhiyo:** The intellect (a faculty of the spirit inside the body, life activity);
- **Yo:** May this light;
- **Nah:** Our (of us);
- **Prachodayat:** Illumine/inspire (to move in a specific direction) (as per Figure B).

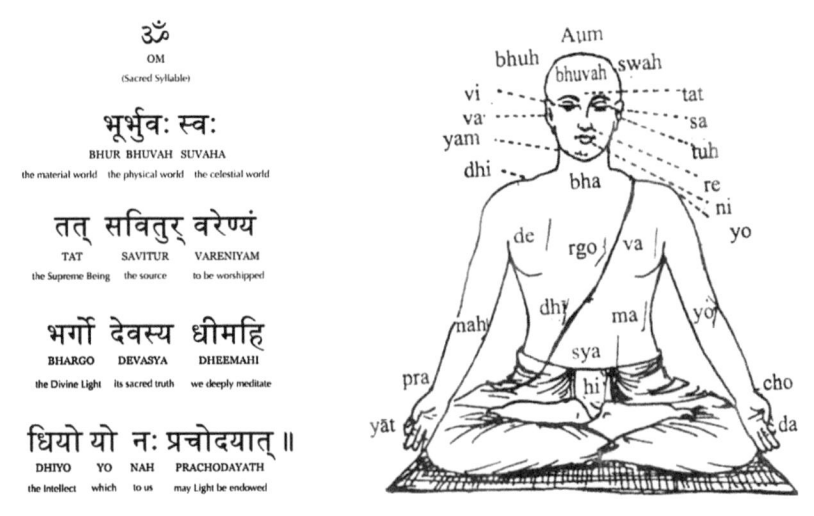

FIGURE B   *Gayatri Mantra* with their meaning and benefits.

Source: Vedicfeed. https://vedicfeed.com/gayatri-mantra-meaning-significance-and-benefits/

Samidha, i.e., *Agni Dhan* (+) *Samvida* or *Samvida*, i.e., *Yajna* Wood. Mango wood starts burning due to the removal of carbon dioxide in small amounts, being highly flammable and even when moist, air from hand fan. As much as possible, mango wood should be used in the sacrificial spirit according to the environment (as per Figure C).

Before, rinse the *Hawan Kund* with water and place 4 pieces of wood in the *Kund*, place them in an overlapping square in the shape of a hash# (as per Figure D).

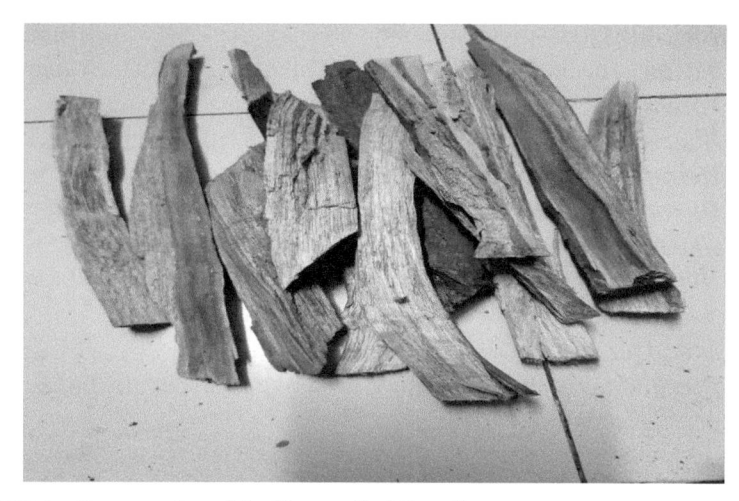

FIGURE C   *Yajna* wood used for *Yagya* called *Samidha*.

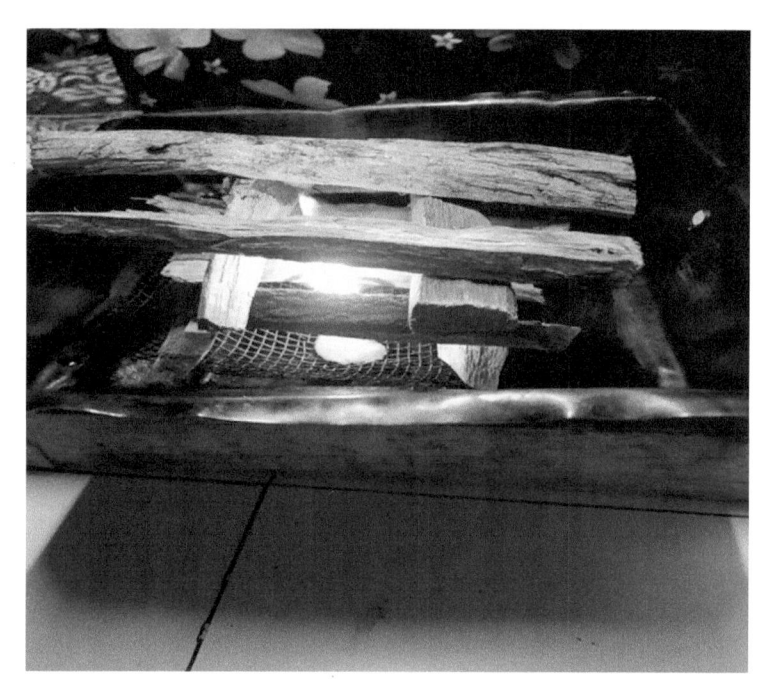

FIGURE D   Way to put the *Samidha* in the *Hawan Kund*.

The fumigation of specific ingredients used in the *Yagya* fire is the scientific method of subtilization of matter into energy that unveils its potential and impacts the environment positively. The electromagnetic waves generated due to the fire ceremony are helpful in transmitting the desired sonic signals "embedded" in the *Yagya*'s mantras which are chanted during the process of sacrificing the natural ingredients and materials in the fire (as per Figure E).

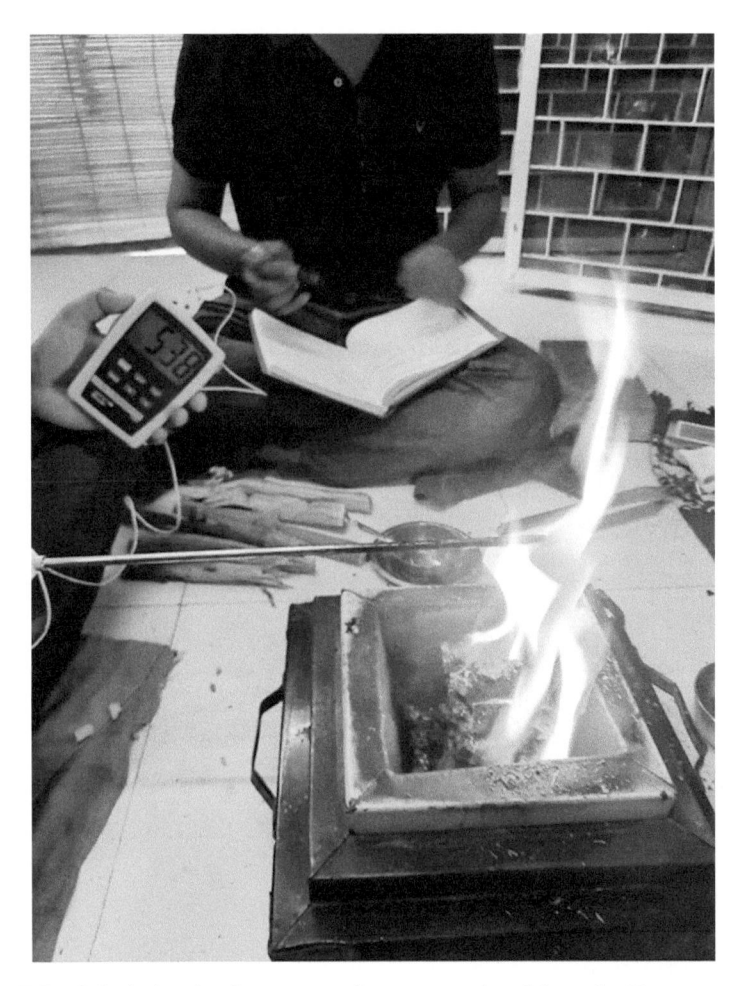

FIGURE E   Calculating the electromagnetic waves produced from the *Havan*.

Using Python, it is showing the previous and post test scores and calculating the difference between them. It is clearly concluded that there is not a major difference between both performances (as per Figure F).

```
In [7]: _,p_value=stats.ttest_rel(a=pre,b=post)
```

```
In [8]: print(p_value)
```

```
0.0022139262950176732
```

```
In [9]: if p_value < 0.05:
            print("Not accepted null hypothesis")
            print("THERE IS A SIGNIFICANT DIFFERENCE BETWEEN TWO SAMPLES")
        else:
            print("Accepted null hypothesis")
            print("THERE IS NOT A SIGNIFICANT DIFFERENCE BETWEEN TWO SAMPLES")

        Not accepted null hypothesis
        THERE IS A SIGNIFICANT DIFFERENCE BETWEEN TWO SAMPLES
```

```
In [10]: #control group
```

```
In [11]: c_pre=[9,7,11,4,6,8,2,9,1,6,5,5]
         c_post=[13,7,11,18,5,5,2,5,1,4,5,5]
         weight_df1=pd.DataFrame({"control_pre":np.array(c_pre),
                                  "control_post":np.array(c_post),
                                  "change":np.array(c_post)-np.array(c_pre)})
```

```
In [12]: weight_df1
```

Out[12]:

	control_pre	control_post	change
0	9	13	4
1	7	7	0
2	11	11	0
3	4	18	14
4	6	5	-1
5	8	5	-3
6	2	2	0
7	9	5	-4

FIGURE F   Calculating the difference between the before and after test scores of control group.

Using Python, it is showing the previous and post test scores and calculating the difference between them. It is clearly concluded that there is a major difference between both performances (as per Figure G).

```
In [1]: #Experimental group
```

```
In [2]: import numpy as np
```

```
In [3]: import numpy as np
        import pandas as pd
        import scipy.stats as stats
        from scipy.stats import ttest_1samp
        import math
```

```
In [4]: print("NULL HYPOTHESIS- THERE IS NOT A SIGNIFICANT DIFFERENCE BETWEEN TWO SAMPLES")

        NULL HYPOTHESIS- THERE IS NOT A SIGNIFICANT DIFFERENCE BETWEEN TWO SAMPLES
```

```
In [5]: pre=[6,7,1,4,8,0,9,1,2,6,3,4]
        post=[5,7,7,18,8,7,14,13,5,13,7,17]
        weight_df=pd.DataFrame({"experimental_pre":np.array(pre),
                                "experimental_post":np.array(post),
                                "change":np.array(post)-np.array(pre)})
```

```
In [6]: weight_df
```

Out[6]:

	experimental_pre	experimental_post	change
0	6	5	-1
1	7	7	0
2	1	7	6
3	4	18	14
4	8	8	0
5	0	7	7
6	9	14	5
7	1	13	12
8	2	5	3
9	6	13	7

FIGURE G   Calculating the difference between the before and after test scores of experimental groups.

CHAPTER 11

Yoga as a Protective Factor for Arresting Cognitive Impairment and Promoting Well-Being Among Institutionalized Seniors

ESHVA SHAH[1] and URMI NANDA BISWAS[2]

[1]*Ahmedabad University, Ahmedabad*

[2]*Department of Psychology, Faculty of Arts, Delhi University*

ABSTRACT

The prevalence of dementia is 7.4% in India for the population above 60 years in 2023. Cognitive impairment is the antecedent of dementia. This research aims to study the effects of Yoga training on cognitive functioning, physical fitness, and subjective well-being of Institutionalized Seniors with Mild Cognitive Impairment (SWMCI) in Ahmedabad, Gujarat. A pre-post experimental design with a waitlist control group was used. It was hypothesized that the experimental group's pre-post difference score would vary significantly from the control group on (a) cognitive impairment; (b) positive affect; (c) negative affect; and (d) physical fitness. Seniors were recruited from elderly care NGOs with permission from the management. Mini-Mental State Examination (MMSE) was used to identify participants with mild cognitive impairment (MCI). Once the willingness to participate and consent was received, the participants were then randomly allocated to the experimental (n=45) and control (n=43) groups. A standardized chair Yoga module was delivered for 12 weeks (2 days a week, one hour a day) based on the recommendation of a Yoga

Yoga and Meditation: Past and Present Evidence. Sachi Nandan Mohanty, Rabindra Kumar Pradhan, & Sugyanta Priyadarshini (Eds.)

doctor and expert. The independent sample t-test statistical test comparing the means of pre-post phases of experimental and control groups reported a significant difference. There was better cognitive functioning, reduced negative affect, and improved physical fitness for the experimental group compared to the control group. These findings imply the development of a low-cost, non-invasive, and sustainable Yoga intervention module to promote well-being and physical fitness, arrest the progression of cognitive impairment, and prevent dementia.

11.1   INTRODUCTION

According to the World Health Organization (WHO, 2023), dementia is considered the seventh leading cause of death. Globally, there are 55 million people diagnosed with dementia. Based on the reports published by the World Alzheimer Report (2022), 60% of the population with dementia is in low-middle-income countries. The number of dementia cases is expected to increase; by 2050, there will be approximately 148 million people with dementia. The cost to treat dementia globally is approximately 1.3 trillion US dollars. Dementia prevalence, treatment costs, and the senior population are all expected to increase annually.

The reports published by the Population Census in 2011 claim that there are approximately 104 million seniors in India. By 2026, there is a prediction of an increase in the senior population to 173 million (National Population Commission, 2011). Based on the reports published by Statista (2016), in 2021 in India, there is a rural population of 909.38 million and an urban population of 498.18 million. However, Swargiary & Roy (2022) claim that the literacy rate for the urban population is higher compared to the rural population in 2022. The senior population in India does participate in activities, but the reports published by Kar (2023) suggest that the majority of seniors do not engage in a variety of activities. Seniors living in institutionalized settings have reported they face difficulty in coping with the feeling of loneliness, financial instability, and emotional disputes with family members (Rajeev & Ajikumar, 2015). In terms of access to resources and medical check-ups, there is an urban-rural gap. The ratio of cost between a private and public hospital is varied and not affordable for many. The institutes also do not have adequate resources and are of poor quality to provide care and service for the seniors (Kar, 2023).

In India, the prevalence of dementia is 7.4% in 2023 (Lee et al., 2023). In 2021, approximately 20 cases of dementia were reported out of 1,000 people in India (Choudhary et al., 2021). Chaudhary et al. (2021) claimed that the prevalence rate of dementia is similar among both sexes. The findings also suggest that there was a higher prevalence rate of dementia in rural areas compared to urban. There are many risk factors for dementia in India: illiteracy, aging, hypertension, diabetes, addiction, poor socioeconomic status, familial or genetic factors, nutrition, stroke, lack of access to resources, and financial constraints.

In the Diagnostic and Statistical Manual 5 (DSM-5), dementia is characterized by the "evidence of significant cognitive decline from a previous level of performance in one or more cognitive domains (complex attention, executive function, learning, memory, language, perceptual-motor, or social cognition)." Dementia in DSM-5 is referred to as Major Neurocognitive Disorder. DSM-5 defines Mild Cognitive Impairment (MCI) as "evidence of modest cognitive decline from a previous level of performance in one or more cognitive domains (complex attention, executive function, learning, memory, language, perceptual-motor, or social cognition)." Kelley & Petersen (2007) claimed that individuals diagnosed with MCI are prone to have dementia. The prevalence of MCI is between 3 and 42% worldwide, and in India, the prevalence is between 15 and 33% (Das et al., 2007; Sosa et al., 2012; Swarnalatha, 2007). This implies that arresting the progression of MCI can benefit seniors from the risk and onset of dementia.

11.2 WELL-BEING AND PHYSICAL ACTIVITY

According to the study conducted by Taspinar et al. (2014), individuals who regularly engage in physical activity experience a feeling of well-being. Recent studies have concluded that physical activity has a profound impact on developing well-being and inner satisfaction for seniors (Barrows & Fleury, 2016; Chen et al., 2010; Hariprasad et al., 2013; Jha, 2003; Youkhana et al., 2016). According to the study conducted by Choudhary et al. (2019), high well-being is associated with a low prevalence of diseases, longevity, and healthy aging (Freedman et al., 2017; Steptoe et al., 2015).

Escuder-Mollon et al. (2014) claimed that there is a correlation between life-long learning and the general well-being of seniors. Cognitive abilities are also affected by environmental factors like lighting (Riemersma-Van Der Lek et al., 2008), spatial layout (Marquardt & Schmieg, 2009), access to outdoor areas (Detweiler et al., 2008), and the design of dining rooms (de

Graaf et al., 2006). This is indicative of the fact that performing daily life activities is complex, involving cognitive as well as physical components. There are many types of research claiming that a deterioration in performing executive functions is associated with poor performance in daily life activities (Arrighi et al., 2013; Clemmensen et al., 2020; Suh et al., 2004; Wajman et al., 2014). A combination of cognitive-physical intervention is beneficial for patients with dementia and MCI (Karssemeijer et al., 2017).

An increase in physical activity leads to a minimal burden on social and health care, enabling healthy aging for an individual (Chodzko-Zajko et al., 2009; Davis & Fox, 2007; Sampaio et al., 2020). Particular components of physical fitness are required to conduct daily life activities. A few of the components include taking a shower, lying or sitting position, walking, and avoiding obstacles when walking (Hesseberg et al., 2016; Rikli & Jones, 2013b). For people with dementia, exercise interventions have resulted in a positive impact and a comparatively better ability to perform daily life activities (Forbes et al., 2015; Sampaio et al., 2020).

11.3   YOGA AND COGNITIVE FUNCTIONING

Yoga is considered a mind-body practice that has ancient Indian roots. The National Centre for Complementary and Integrative Health claims that Yoga is identified as a complementary health approach (Brenes et al., 2019). Yoga aids mental, spiritual, and physical well-being. Yoga can be practiced improving well-being, maintain health, and lessen certain symptoms that are frequently linked to bone discomfort.

Yoga incorporates various postures (asanas), meditation techniques, and breathing exercises (Pranayama) (Hariprasad et al., 2013). Yoga is a Sanskrit term; the root of the term Yoga is '*Yuj*.' The translated meaning of the term *Yuj* is "to bind, attach, and yoke, join, to use, apply, to direct, and concentrate one's attention on" (Bonura, 2007; Iyengar, 1979). Chair Yoga (CY) is when breathing exercises and modified postures are practiced while seated or supported by a chair. CY is a non-invasive and non-pharmacological intervention (Park et al., 2022) and valid for seniors.

Brenes et al. (2019) claimed a lack of available literature on the impact of Yoga on the cognitive functioning of seniors with MCI and dementia. Nulkar et al. (2019) claimed that there is a need for healthcare facilities that are continuous, integrated, and holistic for people with dementia. Yoga-based intervention would be cost-effective for low-middle-income countries. Thus, the present study aims to examine the effect of Yoga training on cognitive functioning, well-being, and physical fitness of insti-tutionalized seniors with mild cognitive impairment aged 65 years and above in Ahmedabad, Gujarat, India.

11.4   METHOD

11.4.1   RESEARCH DESIGN

A Pre-test/Post-test control group design was used for this study, which is a classical controlled experimental design, where the participants were randomly assigned to control and experimental group. This study includes three phases – pre-intervention, intervention, and post intervention phase. Based on the inclusion and exclusion criteria a total of 102 participants were recruited. The participants were recruited from multiple local elderly care institutes in Ahmedabad, Gujarat, India.

11.4.1.1   SAMPLE

- **The Population for the Study:** This comprised seniors living in old age homes without any acute physical or mental problems. Thus, assisted living for seniors and other types of elder care were not part of the study population. After contacting several old age homes within Ahmedabad city and seeking their permission to cooperate with the research, only three institutes were finalized for the selec-tion of samples. Participants who were willing to participate in the research and agreed to complete the intervention were considered for the study. A total of 102 participants completed the questionnaire.
- **Inclusion and Exclusion Criteria:** Only participants aged above 65 years with MCI were included in the study. Participants who were normally healthy, not suffering from any acute physical or mental health conditions, or not suffering from any terminal diseases were included in the study. Seniors staying in elderly care institutes in Ahmedabad, Gujarat, which provided free boarding, lodging, and medical care (when needed) to the seniors were considered for the research. The exclusion criteria included seniors suffering from moderate to severe MCI, seniors diagnosed with

depression, psychopathology, chronic disease, alcohol dependence, Down Syndrome, brain injury, Huntington's disease, Parkinson's disease, and stroke.

- **Sample Characteristics:** Following the exclusion and inclusion criteria and the willingness of the seniors, and their continuous participation in the study, 88 participants were finally retained for the study. These participants were randomly allocated to the experimental group (n=45) and control group (n=43). The sample breakdown according to gender and age was as follows: There were 44 (46.8%) female participants and 50 (53.2%) male participants. The majority of the participants, 44.7%, belonged to the age group 65–70 years, 30.9% of the participants were of age 71–75 years, 6.4% belonged to the age group of 81–85 years, and 3.2% were more than 86 years old. The majority of the participants belonged to a lower socio-economic class and had school education only. According to the self-report of the participants, 7.4% of the participants belonged to the middle to higher socio-economic class and only 3.2% of the participants have completed undergraduate and postgraduate studies.

11.4.1.2 TOOLS/MEASURES

The following tools were included in the questionnaire: Mini Mental State Examination (MMSE), Addenbrooke's Cognitive Examination III (ACE-III), Positive, and Negative Affect Schedule (PANAS), and Physical Fitness tests: 30-Second Chair Stand, 30-Second Arm Curl, 2-Minute Step Test, Back Scratch, 8-Foot Up and Go, Chair Sit and Reach.

Folstein et al. (1983) created the Mini-Mental State Examination. The Mini-Mental State Examination is a valid tool to diagnose cognitive impairment (Molloy & Standish, 1997). The MMSE is regarded as a global measure of cognitive abilities. The test is widely accepted because it covers a wide range of cognitive domains such as long-term memory, short-term memory, orientation to time and space, constructional ability, registration, recall, language, and the ability to follow commands and understand instructions (Molloy & Standish, 1997). The tool is used to determine whether or not a person has Mild Cognitive Impairment (MCI). The MMSE consists of 11 questions that take about 10 minutes to complete, making it a practical and straightforward instrument. MMSE excludes the categories of mood, aberrant experiences, and thinking. It focuses on the cognitive element of mental functions in particular (Folstein et al., 1983). The MMSE has many advantages for the participant, including the ability to complete the exam quickly and easily without the use of any additional devices or equipment. However, there are a few drawbacks: the tool does not examine long delay recall, which may result in erroneous findings (Velakoulis et al., 2007); and because it is an MMSE, the short form of the test may also result in many inconsistencies. According to Bernard & Goldman (2010), the MMSE has a moderate-high level of dependability. Because it is connected with other dementia screening exams, it has been reported to have moderate construct validity.

Addenbrooke Cognitive Examination III (ACE) was developed by Mathuranath et al. (2000). The objective of the test was to detect dementia and differentiate it from Alzheimer's dementia and frontotemporal dementia. It is considered an extension of the cognitive screening technique. The Addenbrooke Cognitive Examination was also developed to address the limitations of the Mini-Mental State Examination (MMSE). The aim of the ACE is to be used as a screening technique to evaluate cognitive functions. Administration typically takes 1–15 minutes and is also useful in detecting dementia syndromes (Bruno & Schurmann Vignaga, 2019). ACE focuses on the following cognitive domains: memory, orientation, language, visual perception, visuospatial skills, and attention. One major advantage of ACE is that it detects dementia syndromes without the use of other equipment (Mathuranath et al., 2000).

ACE III is composed of five major cognitive domains: attention, language, memory, verbal fluency, and visuospatial abilities. The total score one could obtain in ACE III is 100, and the higher score is indicative of better cognitive functioning. In the attention section, the maximum score obtained is 18 points, 26 points in the memory section, 14 points in the fluency section, 26 points in the language section, and 16 points in the visuospatial section (Bruno & Schurmann Vignaga, 2019). The internal reliability of ACE III is measured by calculating Cronbach's alpha coefficient, which is 0.88 (Noone, 2015). ACE III also has construct validity.

The Positive and Negative Affect Scale is developed by Watson et al. (1988). It is also considered one of the most widely used self-report scales that measure subjective well-being (Gellman, 2020). PANAS is developed to measure and assess different emotional states (subjective well-being)

(Watson & Clark, 1994). The expanded version of PANAS consists of 60 items, and the shorter version of PANAS consists of 20 items. This study will use the 20-item version of PANAS. Positive affect refers to the extent to which an individual feels alert, energetic, and active. It is considered a state of increased concentration, high energy, and pleasurable engagement. Whereas negative affect refers to the extent to which a person feels distressed, unpleasant, feeling aversive moods like anger, disgust, guilt, and fear (Watson et al., 1988).

The 20-item version of PANAS consists of 10 items of positive affect and 10 items of negative affect. Each of the items is to be rated on a 5-point Likert scale (Gellman, 2020). The major advantage of this tool is that it is brief and easy to administer (Watson & Clark, 1994). To score a teste, the score of positive affect needs to be summed up and the score of negative affect needs to be scored. The total score can range from 10–50. A higher total score represents high levels of positive affect, and a lower total score represents a lower level of negative affect (Watson & Clark, 1994; Watson et al., 1988). PANAS also demonstrates test-retest reliability, internal consistency reliability, and convergent and divergent validity (Merz et al., 2013; Watson & Clark, 1994; Watson et al., 1988).

The physical fitness tests proposed by Jones & Rikli (2002) have good interrater and intrarater reliability and good validity as well. As part of standardization, the criterion-referenced points are provided for both men and women. The age range for both women and men is 60–94 plus (as part of standardization). The criterion-referenced points help identify if the participant is at risk of functional mobility loss (Jones & Rikli, 2002). Physical fitness exams help seniors improve functional mobility and delay physical frailty (Jones & Rikli, 2002). The parameters tested are muscle endurance/strength, flexibility, aerobic endurance, motor ability, and body composition. Jones & Rikli (2002) offered the following tests: 30-second chair stand, 30-second arm curl, 2-minute step test, back scratch, 8-foot up and go, chair sit and reach. The proposed tests assess participants' capacity to execute everyday tasks such as walking, standing up, and stair climbing.

11.4.1.3 PROCEDURE

Various institutions were approached in Ahmedabad, Gujarat, India for this research study. The pre-test phase was initiated once the management team of the institute was debriefed. The participants were also debriefed about the research, and their consent was also obtained. This study included a total of 88 participants. Once the informed consent was received, the motivated participants were further instructed on what they as participants were supposed to do for this research. As part of the pre-phase, MMSE (MCI), Addenbrooke (ACE), PANAS, 30 Second Chair Stand, Arm Curl, 2 Minute Step Test, Chair Sit and Stand, Back Scratch, 8 Foot Up and Go (physical fitness) were conducted. The tests were conducted only when the participants were clear with what they were supposed to do, and if they had any questions or doubts those were also cleared before conducting the tests. The tests were conducted in a language comfortable and convenient to the participants.

Based on the results obtained from the recruited participants for MMSE (MCI), participants were randomly allocated to the experimental and control groups. Microsoft Excel was used to randomly allocate the participants. Only participants with low MCI were selected. Because to explore the impact of the intervention, participants with low MCI were suitable for this study as low MCI is an indication of the stage between normal aging and expected decline in cognitive functions and serious decline of dementia. Thus, participants aged 65 years and above with low MCI were selected and randomly divided into two respective groups. The experimental group went through Yoga training, and the control group continued their daily activities.

The intervention phase began once the randomized groups were formed. Methodologically, this phase is very crucial; high maintenance and safety precautions were required to be followed. The experimental group went through the Yoga training module for 6 weeks and 2 days for one hour. The Yoga intervention module was validated by a Yoga expert and doctor. The influence of specific postures/exercises was taken from available valid literature. During the training, Yoga cameras were recording the participants (for this permission and consent were taken during the consent form itself). The video was taken for the module conducted on two respective days for the institute. Emergency contact for doctors was available with the management team of the institute. They were called in case of any emergency during and after the sessions. The nearby hospitals were also available. Attendance was also taken for all the participants present during the sessions. Once the 6 weeks of training for the experimental group is completed, the post-test phase was initiated.

After the completion of the 6 weeks of training for an experimental group–Yoga training, the two groups–the experimental group and the control group went through the post-test phase. In this phase, the above-mentioned tests were conducted, and the results were obtained. The data remained confidential throughout the research.

11.4.1.4   THE INTERVENTION MODULE

Table 11.1 represents the Yoga exercises and training modules. Om chanting, prayer, Sukshma kriya, Pranayama, flexibility exercises (chair Yoga postures), deep breathing exercises, mindfulness, and relaxation activities are all part of the Yoga intervention module. The Yoga exercises presented to the experimental group members are shown in Tables 11.1 and 11.2. The exercises were divided equally among the aforementioned groups. Every week, the module was taught for an hour on both days. Yoga practitioners and professionals from Sir Sayajirao Institute of Research in Yoga, Ayurveda, Naturopathy, Music, and Allied Sciences from Vadodara have validated the modules. A compilation of YouTube videos for different kriyas and asanas was used to teach the module. On each day, a feedback session was also arranged following the end of the lesson. The feedback session was held to ensure that any potential injuries were reported and addressed.

11.5   RESULTS

Table 11.3 shows the findings after performing an independent sample t–test between the difference scores of pre and post intervention. Using an independent sample t–test, researchers compared the d score means of the experimental and control groups before and after the tests. The results of the t test are presented in Table 11.3. Refer to Table 11.3 to see the mean difference between the experimental and control groups pre and post the test.

As the results presented in Table 11.3, there is a significant difference between the pre-post difference score of the experimental and control groups. Comparison of the mean values on the d score of both groups indicates that post the intervention, the experimental group's cognitive functioning has improved significantly compared to their counterparts.

TABLE 11.1   The Yoga Training Module for the First Day

Sr no.	Yoga	Details	Set	Time
1	Om chanting	–	More than 10 times	10 mins
2	Prayer	–	5–7 times and hold	7 mins
3	Head stretching	Up and down	5–7 times and hold	5–7 mins
4	Head stretching	Left and right	5–7 times and hold	5–7 mins
5	Head stretching	Side	5–7 times and hold	5–7 mins
6	Neck stretching	Side	5–7 times and hold	5–7 mins
7	Neck stretching	Circular and reverse	5–7 times and hold	5–7 mins
8	Shoulder stretching	Up and down	5–7 times and hold	5–7 mins
9	Shoulder stretching	Circular and reverse	5–7 times and hold	5–7 mins
10	Hand stretching	Side	5–7 times and hold	5–7 mins
11	Hand stretching	Up and down	5–7 times and hold	5–7 mins
12	Hand stretching	Circular and reverse	5–7 times and hold	5–7 mins
13	Wrist stretching	Up and down	5–7 times and hold	5–7 mins
14	Wrist stretching	Circular and reverse	5–7 times and hold	5–7 mins
15	Loosening fingers	Open and close	5–7 times and hold	5–7 mins
16	Ankle stretching	Up and down	5–7 times and hold	5–7 mins
17	Ankle stretching	Circular and reverse	5–7 times and hold	5–7 mins
18	Ankle stretching	Finger open and close	5–7 times and hold	5–7 mins
19	Tadasana	–	5–7 times and hold	5–7 mins
20	Deep breathing	–	5–7 times and hold	7–9 mins

TABLE 11.1 *(Continued)*

Sr no.	Yoga	Details	Set	Time
21	Anuloma Viloma	–	5–7 times and hold	7–9 mins
22	Bhastika Pranayama	–	5–7 times and hold	7–9 mins
23	Bhramari Pranayama	–	5–7 times and hold	7–9 mins
24	Om chanting	–	More than 10 times	10 mins
25	Prayer	–	2–3	7 mins

TABLE 11.2 Represents the Yoga Training Module for the Second Day

Sr no.	Yoga	Details	Set	Time
1	Om chanting	–	More than 10 times	10 mins
2	Prayer	–	2–3	7 mins
3	All stretching	Up and down	5–7 times and hold	10–12 mins
4	Remind about exercises	–	–	5–7 mins
5	Forward bending	–	5–7 times and hold	5–7 mins
6	Backward bending	Side	5–7 times and hold	5–7 mins
7	Side bending	–	5–7 times and hold	5–7 mins
8	Twisting	Standing and sitting	5–7 times and hold	5–7 mins
9	Instant relaxation exercises	Deep breathing	5–7 times and hold	5–7 mins
10	Heel stretching	Up and down	5–7 times and hold	5–7 mins
11	Ardh– kati chakrasana	–	5–7 times and hold	5–7 mins
12	Marijari Asana	Seated	5–7 times and hold	5–7 mins
13	Standing relaxation pose	Deep breathing	5–7 times and hold	5–7 mins
14	Mindfulness	Walk around	5 rounds of walk and hold	5–7 mins
15	Mindfulness – sense activity	All senses	Once and hold	5–7 mins
16	Deep breathing	–	5–7 times	7–9 mins
17	Anuloma viloma	–	5–7 times	7–9 mins
18	Kapalbhati	Abdominal breathing	5–7 times	7–9 mins
19	Vibhagiya Pranayama	3 stages	5–7 times	7–9 mins
20	Om chanting	–	More than 10 times	10 mins
21	Prayer	–	2–3	7 mins

TABLE 11.3 The Mean Differences between the Difference Score from Pre–Post Stage for the Experimental and Control Group

Group	Experimental group			Control group			
Variable	Pre (Std. dev)	Post (Std. dev)	d mean (Std. dev)	Pre (Std. dev)	Post (Std. dev)	d mean (Std. dev)	t
MMSE	22.06 (1.21)	25.31 (1.83)	3.23	22.07 (1.21)	23 (1.83)	0.93	4.37**
PANAS Positive	35.84 (11.55)	25.71 (4.65)	−6.07	36.72 (11.55)	32.83 (4.65)	4.19	−4.87**
PANAS Negative	31.78 (8.01)	22.97 (5.37)	−8.80	28.65 (8.01)	30.37 (5.37)	1.72	−6.41**
ACE III	75.8 (5.82)	78.8 (4.75)	3.00	75.95 (5.82)	76.65 (4.47)	0.70	2.41
Chair stand	10.64 (4.18)	13.71 (3.71)	3.07	11.16 (4.18)	11.39 (3.88)	0.23	4.15**
Arm curl	13.08 (3.28)	16.06 (3.57)	2.98	13.53 (3.28)	12 (3.33)	−1.53	7.16**
2 min step	64.91 (11.54)	70.57 (14.22)	5.67	70 (11.54)	64.44 (11.50)	−5.56	6.17**
Chair sit and reach	3.37 (3.62)	1.62 (1.63)	−1.76	2.46 (3.62)	2.97 (1.34)	0.51	−4.40**
Back stretch	9.63 (3.64)	7.37 (3.87)	−2.26	7.97 (3.64)	9.23 (2.99)	1.26	−6.07**
8 foot up and go	2.02 (1.42)	1.31 (1.52)	−0.71	1.72 (1.42)	3.20 (1.02)	1.49	−7.42**

Based on the results indicated in Table 11.3, there is a significant difference between the pre-post difference score of the experimental and control groups. The findings suggest a reduction in the negative affect mean value on the d score and an increase in the positive affect mean value on the d score. This suggests that the intervention has benefited the participants of the experimental group in terms of reducing negative affect. However, post the intervention, the reduction in positive affect is one of the limitations of this study.

The scores for the tests of physical fitness are presented in Table 11.3. There is a significant difference in the mean values on the d scores of chair stand, arm curl, 2 min step, chair sit and reach, back scratch, and 8-foot up and go. Post the intervention, compared to the control group, the findings suggest that the intervention has significantly benefited physical fitness performance. In particular, relating to body strength, upper body strength, aerobic endurance, lower body flexibility, shoulder flexibility strength, agility, and dynamic balance, the findings suggest an improvement post the intervention.

11.6   PROFILE GRAPHS

There is a significant difference in the post and pre-test scores for the experimental group. After the intervention, the MCI and ACE III scores have increased, indicating an improvement in cognitive functioning. Positive and negative affect scores have decreased. The yoga training module has benefited the experimental group in reducing negative affect. Scores for chair stand, arm curl, and 2-minute step have increased post-intervention, indicating improved performance. After the intervention, the scores for chair sit and reach, back scratch, and 8-foot up and go have decreased, indicating improvement in physical fitness performance (Figures 11.1 and 11.2).

The mean for pre-test MMSE score is 22 and the mean for post-test score is 25. The range for pre-test MMSE score is 5, whereas the range of post MMSE score is 8. The majority of the participants have received a score closer to 30 post the intervention, which indicates that the overall score of cognitive functioning has increased. The graph suggests that for the experimental group post the intervention, there is an improvement in the MCI score. A higher score is indicative of better cognitive functioning.

In this case, the graph suggests that for the majority of the participants, the MCI score has significantly increased (Figure 11.3).

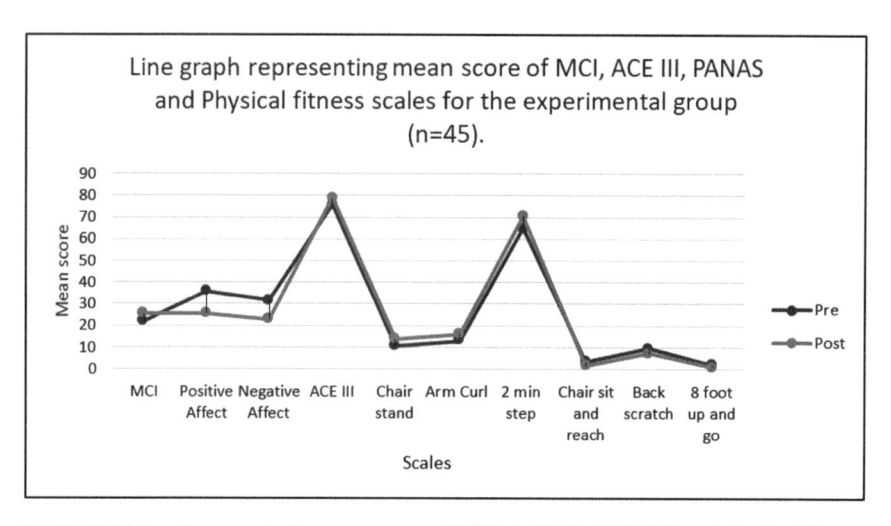

FIGURE 11.1   Represents the mean score of MCI, ACE III, PANAS, and physical fitness scales for the experimental group.

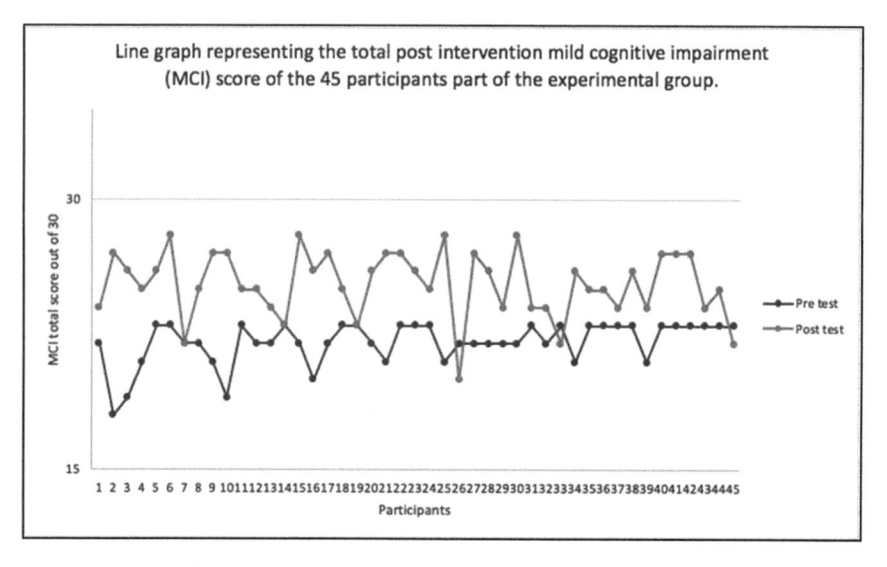

FIGURE 11.2   Line graph representing the pre- and post-intervention score on MCI for the experimental group.

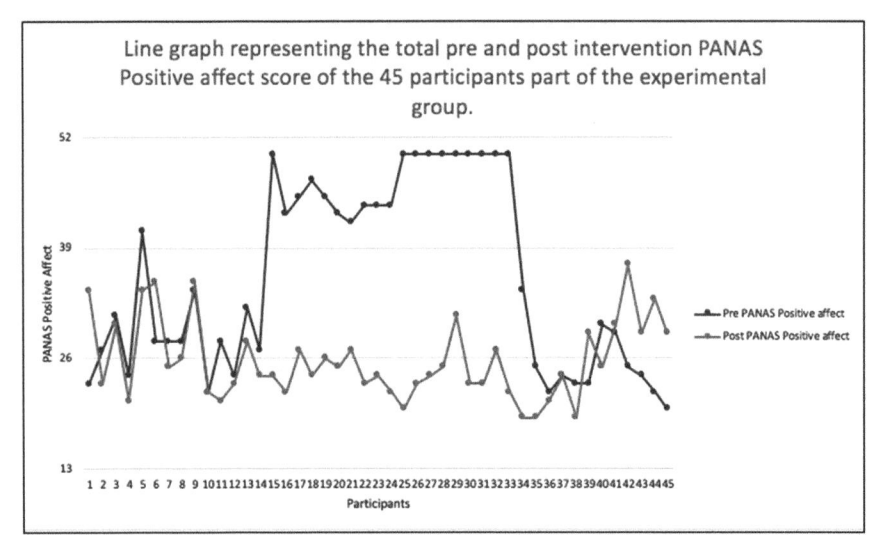

FIGURE 11.3 Line graph representing the pre- and post-intervention scores of experimental groups on positive affect.

The mean for pre-test PANAS Positive Affect score is 35.44 and the mean for post-test score is 25.71. The range for pre-test PANAS Positive Affect score is 30, whereas the range of post PANAS Positive Affect score is 18. The graph shows that pre-test PANAS Positive Affect score is higher for participants than the post-test scores for the experimental group. Thus, for the experimental group post the intervention, the positive affect has not increased. This is one of the limitations of the study. A possible interpretation for a reduction in positive affect is in the choice of the scale (Figure 11.4).

The mean for pre-test PANAS Negative affect score is 31.78 and the mean for post-test score is 22.97. The range for pre-test PANAS Negative affect score is 39, whereas the range of post PANAS Negative affect score is 24. The graph shows that pre-test PANAS Negative affect score is higher for participants than the post-test scores. Thus, this indicates that post-intervention the PANAS negative affect score has reduced. Post the intervention, the graph indicates a reduction in the scores of negative effects. It suggests that the participants of the experimental group have benefited from the reduction of negative affect scores.

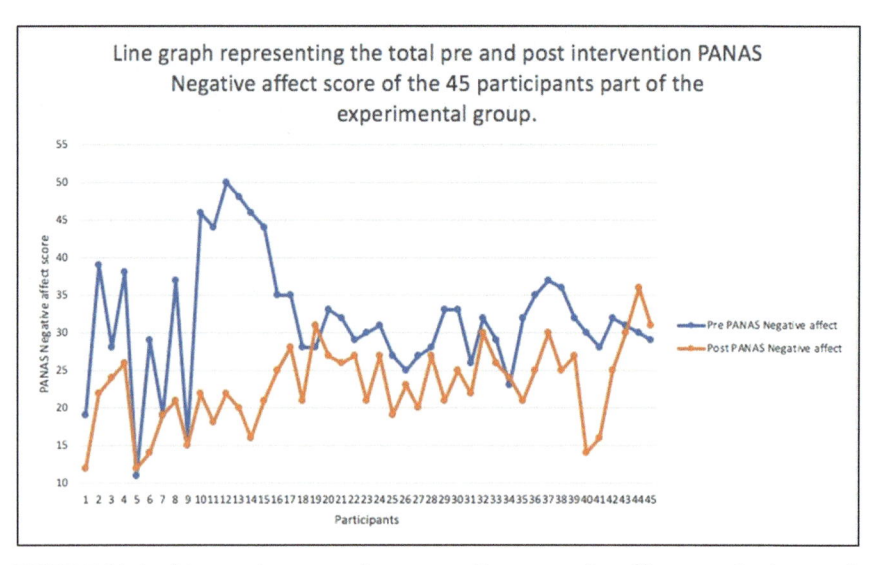

FIGURE 11.4   Line graph representing pre-post Panas negative affect score for the experimental group.

11.7   DISCUSSION

The first hypothesis suggests that there will be a significant difference between the experimental and control groups' pre-post difference scores on a. MCI, b. Addenbrooke ACE III, c. Positive affect, d. Negative affect, and e. Physical fitness (Chair stand, arm curl, 2-minute step, chair sit and reach, back scratch, and 8-foot up and go). There is a significant difference between the experimental and control groups' pre-post test scores. This means that the intervention has a significant impact on the previously indicated psychological elements. However, the PANAS positive affect scores obtained imply that the positive affect on the experimental group individuals has decreased following the intervention. However, the post-test results for the remaining components indicate a beneficial impact. The post-test scores for the control group differ slightly from those of the experimental group.

According to the findings of this study, the post-test scores for the experimental group, MMSE, have increased, indicating that cognitive processes have improved. This is also corroborated by a study by Chatterjee et al. (2021), which concluded that Yoga training improves the cognitive functioning of middle-aged adults. The findings of this study demonstrate that the outcome, in this case, the intervention, affected the participants (improvement in attention and alertness). After Yoga training, the middle-aged group improved in terms of serial learning (short-term memory). Physical fitness, nutrition, cognitive training, and social interventions are factors that improve the cognitive abilities of patients with dementia (Ballesteros et al., 2015; Bangalore & Varambally, 2012).

Choudhary et al. (2019) found that high well-being is linked to lower disease rates, longer life, and healthy aging (Freedman et al., 2017; Steptoe et al., 2015). The study conducted by Choudhary et al. (2019) aims to analyze Yoga's effect on well-being and multiple health outcomes in elders. The researchers hypothesized that Yoga intervention groups would show moderate improvement in self-reported subjective well-being and secondary outcomes like pain, sleep, mobility, mood, cognition, and stress. The study concluded that Yoga could provide a wide range of physical and mental health advantages to the elderly. Based on the obtained results, PANAS positive affect score has reduced. However, PANAS negative affect has been reduced. This is also well supported by the study conducted by Taspinar et al. (2014) claiming individuals who regularly engage in physical activity experience a feeling of well-being. Studies have also concluded that physical activity has a profound impact on developing well-being and inner satisfaction for seniors (Barrows & Fleury, 2016; Chen et al., 2010; Hariprasad et al., 2013; Jha, 2003; Youkhana et al., 2016).

The participants' chair stand, arm curl, and 2-minute step of the physical fitness scale have also improved. The scores for chair sit, reach, and back scratch have decreased, showing an increase in performance. The range of 8-foot up and go has been reduced, yet it is not suitable for the range stated in the physical fitness manual. Regular physical fitness participation provides significant health benefits to persons of all ages (Sampaio et al., 2020). Exercise therapies have shown a positive influence on patients with dementia, resulting in a comparatively greater ability to undertake daily living tasks (Sampaio et al., 2020). Physical activity is essential for seniors since it aids in disease prevention, increased quality of life or subjective well-being, and sustains independence (Sampaio et al., 2020). Engaging in regular physical fitness offers important health advantages for individuals of all ages (Sampaio et al., 2020).

The 12-week (12-hour) intervention benefited the participants by demonstrating a substantial difference in the aforementioned dependent variables.

11.7.1   *LIMITATIONS*

One of the significant limitations of this study is the selection of the scale to assess subjective well-being. PANAS was chosen because it provides an attribute checklist that must be completed within a week. However, the acquired skewed results, particularly for PANAS positive affect, show that the elders may have some difficulties in communicating their answers. The challenge may be in establishing a relationship/connection with the presented traits or states on the scale. One of the significant drawbacks of this study is the necessity for a follow-up test. Due to time constraints, the follow-up test phase was not carried out; therefore, in future studies for this research, a follow-up test phase would be desirable to test the validity of the data. It would also reveal whether or not seniors are practicing, as well as the influence on the dependent variables. Another significant limitation of this study is the Yoga training intervention. Even though the intervention module was approved by a yoga practitioner, the description and impact of their work would be different if taught by a yoga teacher. The videos for each module were taken specifically for each day for this research study. They were not shared with the participants because they did not have access to electronics. As a result, the ability to monitor the continuity of the intervention module is hindered. It is challenging to determine if the participants understood the importance of engaging in physical activity of any kind following the intervention test phase. Furthermore, the target population of this study is older adults over the age of 65 who live in institutionalized settings. The study was able to obtain demographic information on each participant; however, more information on the educational and economic backgrounds of these participants is needed.

11.7.2   *IMPLICATIONS*

The findings of this study have special relevance for policymakers, health care professionals, primary caregivers to seniors with mild cognitive impairment, management teams of senior living organizations, and volunteers. Caregivers at senior living organizations and at home could be taught to provide the intervention module to the elderly. The management team of the old age homes/senior homes might be trained to make the seniors practice Yoga for better cognitive functioning and physical fitness. The top management should be sensitized about the value and utility of Yoga practices for seniors to protect them from cognitive impairment, improve their physical and mental health. The findings have implications for the non-profit organizations which partner with institutionalized settings for seniors in teaching, practicing, and entertaining seniors. Institutions which shelter abandoned seniors, or lonely seniors could also promote their physical and emotional wellness, and thus; healthy aging with these low-cost non-invasive interventions. A low-middle-income country like India, with very little financial support for these institutionalized seniors, can protect them from a deadly neurodegenerative disease like Dementia by incorporating this Yoga module into their daily schedule of activities, preventing and arresting cognitive impairment. This, in turn, will promote their right to live healthily and happily.

11.8 CONCLUSION

The participants benefited from the Yoga training intervention. The results indicate an improvement in cognitive performance and physical fitness, and a decrease in negative affect. The findings indicate that Yoga as an intervention helps slow the progression of cognitive impairment and has a good influence in preventing seniors from developing dementia. This Yoga intervention study is both safe and beneficial for future research.

KEYWORDS

- **dementia**
- **emotional wellness**
- **institutionalized seniors**
- **mild cognitive impairment**
- **negative affect**
- **physical fitness**
- **positive affect**
- **subjective well-being**
- **yoga training**

REFERENCES

Arrighi, H. M., Gélinas, I., McLaughlin, T. P., Buchanan, J., & Gauthier, S. (2013). Longitudinal changes in functional disability in Alzheimer's disease patients. *International Psychogeriatrics, 25*(6), 929–937.

Ballesteros, S., Kraft, E., Santana, S., & Tziraki, C. (2015). Maintaining older brain functionality: A targeted review. *Neuroscience & Biobehavioral Reviews, 55*, 453–477.

Bangalore, N. G., & Varambally, S. (2012). Yoga therapy for schizophrenia. *International Journal of Yoga, 5*(2), 85.

Barrows, J. L., & Fleury, J. (2016). Systematic review of yoga interventions to promote cardiovascular health in older adults. *Western Journal of Nursing Research, 38*(6), 753–781.

Bernard, B., & Goldman, J. G. (2010). MMSE-mini-mental state examination. In *Encyclopedia of Movement Disorders* (pp. 187–189). Elsevier Inc.

Bonura, K. B., & Tenenbaum, G. (2014). Effects of yoga on psychological health in older adults. *Journal of Physical Activity and Health, 11*(7), 1334–1341.

Bowman, L. J. (2002). Statista. *Journal of Business & Finance Librarianship, 27*(4), 304–309.

Brenes, G. A., Sohl, S., Wells, R. E., Befus, D., Campos, C. L., & Danhauer, S. C. (2019). The effects of yoga on patients with mild cognitive impairment and dementia: A scoping review. *The American Journal of Geriatric Psychiatry, 27*(2), 188–197.

Bruno, D., & Schurmann Vignaga, S. (2019). Addenbrooke's cognitive examination III in the diagnosis of dementia: A critical review. *Neuropsychiatric Disease and Treatment, 15*, 441–447.

Chatterjee, S., Mondal, S., & Singh, D. (2021). Effect of 12 weeks of yogic training on neurocognitive variables: A quasi-experimental study. *Indian Journal of Community Medicine: Official Publication of Indian Association of Preventive & Social Medicine, 46*(1), 112.

Chen, K.-M., Chen, M.-H., Lin, M.-H., Fan, J.-T., Lin, H.-S., & Li, C.-H. (2010). Effects of yoga on sleep quality and depression in elders in assisted living facilities. *Journal of Nursing Research, 18*(1), 53–61.

Chodzko-Zajko, W. J., Proctor, D. N., Singh, M. A. F., Minson, C. T., Nigg, C. R., Salem, G. J., & Skinner, J. S. (2009). Exercise and physical activity for older adults. *Medicine & Science in Sports & Exercise, 41*(7), 1510–1530.

Choudhary, A., Pathak, A., Manickam, P., Purohit, M., Rajasekhar, T. D., Dhoble, P., Sharma, A., Suliya, J., Apsingekar, D., Patil, V., et al. (2019). Effect of yoga versus light exercise to improve well-being and promote healthy aging among older adults in central India: A study protocol for a randomized controlled trial. *Geriatrics, 4*(4), 64.

Choudhary, A., Ranjan, J. K., Asthana, H. S., et al. (2021). Prevalence of dementia in India: A systematic review and meta-analysis. *Indian Journal of Public Health, 65*(2), 152.

Clemmensen, F. K., Hoffmann, K., Siersma, V., Sobol, N., Beyer, N., Andersen, B. B., Vogel, A., Lolk, A., Gottrup, H., Høgh, P., et al. (2020). The role of physical and cognitive function in performance of activities of daily living in patients with mild-to-moderate Alzheimer's disease–A cross-sectional study. *BMC Geriatrics, 20*, 1–9.

Das, S., Bose, P., Biswas, A., Dutt, A., Banerjee, T., Hazra, A., Raut, D., Chaudhuri, A., & Roy, T. (2007). An epidemiologic study of mild cognitive impairment in Kolkata, India. *Neurology, 68*(23), 2019–2026.

Davis, M. G., & Fox, K. R. (2007). Physical activity patterns assessed by accelerometry in older people. *European Journal of Applied Physiology, 100*, 581–589.

de Graaf, C., Kok, F. J., van Staveren, W. A., et al. (2006). Effect of family style mealtimes on quality of life, physical performance, and body weight of nursing home residents: Cluster randomized controlled trial. *BMJ, 332*(7551), 1180–1184.

Escuder-Mollon, P., Esteller-Curto, R., Ochoa, L., & Bardus, M. (2014). Impact on senior learners' quality of life through lifelong learning. *Procedia-Social and Behavioral Sciences, 131*, 510–516.

Folstein, M. F., Robins, L. N., & Helzer, J. E. (1983). The mini-mental state examination. *Archives of General Psychiatry, 40*(7), 812–812.

Forbes, D., Forbes, S. C., Blake, C. M., Thiessen, E. J., & Forbes, S. (2015). Exercise programs for people with dementia. *Cochrane Database of Systematic Reviews, 2015*(4), CD006489.

Freedman, V. A., Carr, D., Cornman, J. C., & Lucas, R. E. (2017). Aging, mobility impairments and subjective wellbeing. *Disability and Health Journal, 10*(4), 525–531.

Gellman, M. D. (2020). *Encyclopedia of Behavioral Medicine.* Springer.

Hariprasad, V., Varambally, S., Varambally, P., Thirthalli, J., Basavaraddi, I., & Gangadhar, B. (2013). Designing, validation and feasibility of a yoga-based intervention for elderly. *Indian Journal of Psychiatry, 55*(Suppl 3), S344–S349.

Hesseberg, K., Bentzen, H., Ranhoff, A. H., Engedal, K., & Bergland, A. (2016). Physical fitness in older people with mild cognitive impairment and dementia. *Journal of Aging and Physical Activity, 24*(1), 92–100.

Iyengar, B. K. S. (1979). *Light on Yoga: Yoga Dipika.*

Jha, P. (2003). Health and social benefits from improving community hygiene and sanitation: An Indian experience. *International Journal of Environmental Health Research, 13*(sup1), S133–S140.

Jones, C. J., & Rikli, R. E. (2002). Measuring functional. *The Journal on Active Aging, 1,* 24–30.

Kar, N. (2023). Ageing and care related issues: A focus on India. *Journal of Geriatric Care and Research, 10*(1), 1–2.

Karssemeijer, E. E., Aaronson, J. J., Bossers, W. W., Smits, T. T., Kessels, R. P., et al. (2017). Positive effects of combined cognitive and physical exercise training on cognitive function in older adults with mild cognitive impairment or dementia: A meta-analysis. *Ageing Research Reviews, 40*, 75–83.

Kelley, B. J., & Petersen, R. C. (2007). Alzheimer's disease and mild cognitive impairment. *Neurologic Clinics, 25*(3), 577–590.

Marquardt, G., & Schmieg, P. (2009). Dementia-friendly architecture: Environments that facilitate wayfinding in nursing homes. *American Journal of Alzheimer's Disease & Other Dementias®, 24*(4), 333–340.

Mathuranath, P. S., Nestor, P. J., Berrios, G., Rakowicz, W., & Hodges, J. (2000). A brief cognitive test battery to differentiate Alzheimer's disease and frontotemporal dementia. *Neurology, 55*(11), 1613–1620.

Merz, E. L., Malcarne, V. L., Roesch, S. C., Ko, C. M., Emerson, M., Roma, V. G., & Sadler, G. R. (2013). Psychometric properties of positive and negative affect schedule (PANAS) original and short forms in an African American community sample. *Journal of Affective Disorders, 151*(3), 942–949.

Molloy, D. W., & Standish, T. I. (1997). A guide to the standardized mini-mental state examination. *International Psychogeriatrics, 9*(S1), 87–94.

National Population Commission. (2011). Report of the technical group on population projections constituted by the national commission on population, May 2006. Population projections for India and States, 2026.

Noone, P. (2015). Addenbrooke's Cognitive Examination-III. *Occupational Medicine, 65*(5), 418–420.

Nulkar, A., Paralikar, V., & Juvekar, S. (2019). Dementia in India–A call for action. *Journal of Global Health Reports, 3*, e2019078.

Park, J., Heilman, K. J., Sullivan, M., Surage, J., Levine, H., Hung, L., Ortega, M., Wiese, L. A. K., & Ahn, H. (2022). Remotely supervised home-based online chair yoga intervention for older adults with dementia: Feasibility study. *Complementary Therapies in Clinical Practice, 48*, 101617.

Rajeev, M., & Ajikumar, V. (2015). Elderly in India: A quality of life of elderly persons in institutional settings. *International Journal of Development Research, 5*(1), 2845–2851.

Regier, D. A., Narrow, W. E., Kuhl, E. A., & Kupfer, D. J. (2009). The conceptual development of DSM-V. *American Journal of Psychiatry, 166*(6), 645–650.

Riemersma-Van Der Lek, R. F., Swaab, D. F., Twisk, J., Hol, E. M., Hoogendijk, W. J., & Van Someren, E. J. (2008). Effect of bright light and melatonin on cognitive and noncognitive function in elderly residents of group care facilities: A randomized controlled trial. *JAMA, 299*(22), 2642–2655.

Sampaio, A., Marques-Aleixo, I., Seabra, A., Mota, J., Marques, E., & Carvalho, J. (2020). Physical fitness in institutionalized older adults with dementia: Association with cognition, functional capacity and quality of life. *Aging Clinical and Experimental Research, 32*, 2329–2338.

Sosa, A. L., Albanese, E., Stephan, B. C., Dewey, M., Acosta, D., Ferri, C. P., Guerra, M., Huang, Y., Jacob, K., Jimenez-Velazquez, I. Z., et al. (2012). Prevalence, distribution, and impact of mild cognitive impairment in Latin America, China, and India: A 10/66 population-based study. *PLoS Medicine, 9*(2), e1001170.

Steptoe, A., Deaton, A., & Stone, A. A. (2015). Subjective wellbeing, health, and ageing. *The Lancet, 385*(9968), 640–648.

Suh, G.-H., Ju, Y.-S., Yeon, B. K., & Shah, A. (2004). A longitudinal study of Alzheimer's disease: Rates of cognitive and functional decline. *International Journal of Geriatric Psychiatry, 19*(9), 817–824.

Swargiary, K., & Roy, K. (2022). Literacy rate in India in 2022. *Academicia: An International Multidisciplinary Research Journal, 12*(8), 87–93.

Swarnalatha, N. (2007). Cognitive status among rural elderly women. *Journal of the Indian Academy of Geriatrics, 3*(1), 15–19.

Taspinar, B., Aslan, U. B., Agbuga, B., & Taspinar, F. (2014). A comparison of the effects of Hatha yoga and resistance exercise on mental health and well-being in sedentary adults: A pilot study. *Complementary Therapies in Medicine, 22*(3), 433–440.

Velakoulis, D., Walterfang, M., Schapira, A., & Byrne, E. (2007). Clinical assessment of mental status. *Neurology and Clinical Neuroscience*, 2–21.

Wajman, J. R., Oliveira, F. F., Marin, S., Schultz, R. R., & Bertolucci, P. H. (2014). Is there correlation between cognition and functionality in severe dementia? The value of a performance-based ecological assessment for Alzheimer's disease. *Arquivos de Neuro-Psiquiatria, 72,* 845–850.

Watson, D., & Clark, L. A. (1994). The PANAS-X: Manual for the positive and negative affect schedule-expanded form. *Unpublished manuscript, University of Iowa. 47,* 17–23.

Watson, D., Clark, L. A., & Tellegen, A. (1988). Development and validation of brief measures of positive and negative affect: The PANAS scales. *Journal of Personality and Social Psychology, 54*(6), 1063.

World Health Organization. (2013). WHO traditional medicine strategy: 2014–2023. World Health Organization.

Yao, C.-T., Lee, B.-O., Hong, H., & Su, Y.-C. (2023). Effect of chair yoga therapy on functional fitness and daily life activities among older female adults with knee osteoarthritis in Taiwan: A quasi-experimental study. *Healthcare, 11*(7), 1024.

Youkhana, S., Dean, C. M., Wolff, M., Sherrington, C., & Tiedemann, A. (2016). Yoga-based exercise improves balance and mobility in people aged 60 and over: A systematic review and meta-analysis. *Age and Ageing, 45*(1), 21–29.

CHAPTER 12

Yoga and Mindfulness: A Positive Health Framework

KAILASH JANDU[1] and RABINDRA KUMAR PRADHAN[2]

[1]Scientist-B, DRDO, 14 Services Selection Board, Selection Centre East, Prayagraj, Uttar Pradesh, India

[2]Department of Humanities and Social Sciences, Indian Institute of Technology, Kharagpur, West Medinipur, West Bengal, India

ABSTRACT

In recent times, we have seen a paradigm shift in the way health is being conceptualized. Instead of viewing health as a single-dimensional entity, today it is seen as a phenomenon consisting of two separate dimensions representing the health continuum and the illness continuum, respectively. The emergence of the discipline of positive psychology with an emphasis on "what makes life worth living" and the emphatic dominance of biopsychosociospiritual framework in health psychology have made it possible to conceive the notion of health in its totality. The idea of positive health rests on the key assumption of the quintessential presence of biological, subjective, and functional domains, thus making health a multidimensional concept. While positive psychology views health as the presence of what works in life, i.e., well-being; the field of health psychology delineates the role of biological, psychological, social, and spiritual factors in comprehending what does not work in life. In this chapter, we describe how Yoga and mindfulness can contribute to positive health while converging the complementary positions of positive and health psychology traditions such that the optimal functioning of the individuals can be ensured.

Yoga and Meditation: Past and Present Evidence. Sachi Nandan Mohanty, Rabindra Kumar Pradhan, & Sugyanta Priyadarshini (Eds.)

12.1   INTRODUCTION

Health and well-being have always been at the core of human existence. Every civilization has strived to achieve excellence in human productivity while maintaining an optimal state of well-being. The notion of positive health, a new concept in the field of positive psychology, can help us realize human flourishing, a key goal of human survival, as it considers the entirety of human experience. To make progress towards achieving positive health for all, the ancient wisdom embedded in two Eastern health practices, namely Yoga and mindfulness, can serve as valuable tools. In recent times, there has been a significant interest in the revival of these practices within both the scientific community and the general population. This chapter draws on the knowledge of health psychology and positive psychology to present a framework for positive health, illustrating how yogic and mindfulness practices can facilitate positive change in the realm of health and well-being, ultimately working towards the goal of 'health for all.'

12.1.1   HEALTH: THE CONTEMPORARY CONCEPTUALIZATION

The World Health Organization (WHO) has defined health in terms of "a state of complete physical, mental, and social well-being and not merely the absence of disease and infirmity" (WHO, 2006). Though this definition is broad, optimistic, and ostensibly all-encompassing, there is much more to understand with respect to the concept of health. Inasmuch as this definition provides us with a comprehensive theoretical and intellectual understanding, the measurement of health based on this definition remains an ordeal. At a global level, in the United Nations (UN) Sustainable Development Goals (SDGs), the issue of health is covered under the rubric of SDG 3 to ensure and promote health and well-being for all age groups (WHO, 2023). However, there are anticipated challenges in achieving the targets set by the UN, partly owing to the lack of consensus on what health is. While it may be possible to cater to the physical health needs of citizens satisfactorily, as there are well-defined objective systems of measurement, diagnosis, and treatment in place, the same cannot be said to be true when it comes to mental and social well-being. Thus, the notion of health and well-being remains an elusive one.

To begin with history, the traditional notion of health, i.e., the biomedical model, puts forth a clear dichotomy between health and illness wherein you can either be healthy or ill at a particular occasion. This notion, however, has been challenged and attempts have been made to comprehend the concept of health more holistically. To do so, the systemic perspective views individual organisms as open systems relentlessly interacting with their surroundings and other individuals (Ahmadi & Sadeghi, 2017). This dynamic systemic interaction, in turn, affects their health. Further, based on the general system theory, the notion of "health as a continuum" has been forwarded by Neuman (1990) and expressed as "the degree of client wellness that exists at any point in time, ranging from an optimal wellness condition, with available energy at its maximum, to death, which represents total energy depletion" (Neuman, 1990). Thus, the health continuum reflects an illness-wellness continuum with the state of illness representing one end of the continuum whereas wellness exists on the other end of the continuum. In the year 1972, John Travis first proposed that the entire spectrum of the health continuum captured various stages namely "premature death, disability, symptoms, signs, neutral point, awareness, education, growth," and a high level of wellness, from the illness pole to the wellness pole, sequentially (Travis & Ryan, 1988).

Turning to mental health, the WHO states that mental health forms an essential element of overall health and defines it in terms of "a state of well-being in which an individual realizes his or her own abilities, can cope with the normal stresses of life, can work productively, and is able to make a contribution to his or her community" (WHO, 2023). The continuum of mental health is characterized by two opposite ends, namely mental illness and mental health, and spans over five zones, namely crisis, struggling, surviving, thriving, and excelling, in a sequential manner (Delphis, 2020).

The understanding of health as a concept and its nuances has undergone tremendous intellectual scrutiny in the recent past. Today, in lieu of a single continuum for health, dual continuums for both physical and mental health, separately, are in place. To say so, there are two dual continuum models that have been proposed for physical health and mental health, respectively. These dual continuum models advocate that physical health and physical illness can co-exist; and, similarly, mental health and mental illness can co-exist. In other words, a person may suffer from some chronic physical health condition (e.g., diabetes) or may have a physical disability in terms of impaired motor functions, yet she or he may consider herself or himself as physically healthy. The underlying connotation here is that the element of subjectivity of the concerned individual as well as the co-existence of dual states of health and illness prevail in the modern approach to understanding health. Similarly, a person may have some phobic disorder and yet may perceive him/herself as mentally healthy.

In sum, there are a total of four continuums, two for physical health and two for mental health. In the case of physical health, these continuums are the health continuum (with the absence of health at one end and the presence of health at the other end) and the illness continuum (with the absence of illness at one end and the presence of illness at the other end). Thus, the absence of illness is not equal to the presence of health and vice versa. Similarly, for mental health, the two continuums include the mental health continuum (with the absence of mental health at one end (i.e., languishing) and the presence of mental health (i.e., flourishing) at the other end) and the mental illness continuum (with the absence of mental illness at one end and the presence of mental illness (i.e., psychopathology) at the other end) (Keyes, 2002). Therefore, the absence of mental illness is not equal to the presence of mental health and vice versa.

12.2   POSITIVE PSYCHOLOGY: BALANCING THE TRADITIONAL PSYCHOLOGICAL SCIENCE

The field of psychology describes itself as a discipline that tries to understand, diagnose, and treat mental disorders, bring about positive changes in the lives of the people, and cultivate talents in society (Seligman, 2002). However, the field has not made sufficient progress in catering to the needs of the people pertaining to positive changes and nurturing talents. Rather, as Seligman (2002) calls it, psychology became "victimology," looking at human beings as just passive entities at the mercy of environmental stimuli or unconscious determinism without any conspicuous intervention of cognitive rational faculties. Thus, the limitations of the two major schools of thought, namely psychoanalysis and behaviorism, soon became evident in fully accounting for human behavior.

The emergence of the third force in psychology, i.e., the humanistic paradigm, in the mid-20th century paved the way for reconsidering consciousness, rationality, and the goodness of human behavior. Before the dawn of humanism, psychology had predominantly limited itself to a treatment model or deficiency model in order to examine human behavior. The focus of the deficiency model has been on what lacks in a person and how he or she can be helped to fulfill that state of inadequacy. Thus, it was broadly a healing paradigm that exclusively targeted the treatment of sufferings. Nonetheless, humanistic psychology builds on the efficiency model in order to emphasize sufficiently on what is present in a person and how new strengths and resources can be built upon to fully actualize human potential. Two major figures in the field of humanistic psychology, Abraham Maslow and Carl Rogers, highlighted the importance of "self-actualization" and "fully functioning person," respectively (Ciccarelli & White, 2017). Maslow coined the term "positive psychology" in the year 1954 in his book "*Motivation and Personality*" (Maslow, 1954) to describe his work and emphasize the need to shift the focus of psychology from mere pathology to vast human potential. It is against this backdrop that the field of positive psychology started to make its appearance.

Towards the last phase of the 20th century, with the efforts of Martin Seligman who was the then President of the American Psychological Association, the positive psychology movement started to gain momentum. The idea behind the initiation of this movement was, as mentioned partly earlier, that there was a need being felt relentlessly in the intellectual sphere to bring the focus of psychology back to its original mission of positive change and to foster genius talent along with the traditional realm of healing the trauma and getting the person to the so-called *normalcy* state from a state of deviancy. In Seligman's words,

> "The aim of positive psychology is to catalyze a change in psychology from a preoccupation only with repairing the worst things in life to also building the best qualities in life. To redress the previous imbalance, we must bring the building of strength to the forefront in the treatment and prevention of mental illness" (Seligman, 2002).

Thus, positive psychology made an attempt to regain the balance in the field of psychology which, somehow, had been lost owing to certain influential events in the history of mankind such as World War II (Seligman, 2002). As a branch of psychology, positive psychology studies conditions, processes, and traits that facilitate optimal functioning of individuals and societies (Gable & Haidt, 2005). Sheldon & King (2001) describe positive psychology as "the scientific study of ordinary human strengths and virtues." Moving from the *thesis* of traditional psychology preoccupied with distress, disorders, deviance, and dysfunction to the *antithesis* of emphasizing strengths, virtues, happiness, well-being, and optimal functioning, the field of positive psychology has traveled across the path of intellectual evolution and stands today at the juncture of *synthesis* that aspires to study human experience in its totality ranging from loss and trauma to health and well-being (Alex Linley, Joseph, Harrington, & Wood, 2006).

12.2.1 HEALTH PSYCHOLOGY: A BIOPSYCHOSOCIOSPIRITUAL PARADIGM

The end of the 20th century witnessed the emergence of a new sub-field in the discipline of psychology under the broader rubric of behavioral medicine that later became popularized as health psychology, with its primary emphasis on highlighting the role behavioral factors play in determining the health and illness of individuals. Matarazzo (1982) defined health psychology as "the aggregate of the specific educational, scientific, and professional contributions of the discipline of psychology to the promotion and maintenance of health, the prevention and treatment of illness, the identification of etiologic and diagnostic correlates of health, illness, and related dysfunction, and to the analysis and improvement of the health care system and health policy formation." This definition was accepted by the American Psychological Association, and the branch of health psychology became the 38th division of this association (Tran, 2013). Thus, the goal of health psychology is to promote health, prevent illness, diagnose causal factors of health and illness, and inform health care policy formulation.

The field of health psychology, in order to achieve its goals, relies on a holistic framework known as the "biopsychosocial model of health and illness" (Engel, 1977). Under this framework, health psychologists attempt to examine the role of biological factors such as genetic abnormalities, hormonal dysfunction, neurological issues, and biochemical imbalance, psychological factors such as personality traits, mood states, health habits, emotional regulation, cognitive appraisal, etc., and sociocultural factors such as socio-economic status, cultural practices, norms regarding expected health behaviors, etc., in influencing the health status of an individual. In fact, the framework in question has actually served as a philosophical undercurrent for the health psychology discipline along with its practical utility value for acknowledging the multifaceted and multi-layered impact of myriad factors in influencing the health and illness status of the individual. As described by Borrell-Carrió and colleagues (2004), the biopsychosocial framework… is both a philosophy of clinical care and a practical clinical guide. Philosophically, it is a way of understanding how suffering, disease, and illness are affected by multiple levels of organization, from the societal to the molecular. At the practical level, it is a way of understanding the patient's subjective experience as an essential contributor to accurate diagnosis, health outcomes, and humane care. Thus, the framework allows for taking into account the subjective, idiosyncratic experiences of the individual along with the macro-level factors emanating from the surroundings. More recently, we have witnessed the event of the COVID-19 pandemic, a typical case of "bio-psycho-socioeconomic crisis" (Pradhan et al., 2022, 2023), showing how various factors are at play in determining the health status of an individual.

Lately, a new dimension called the spiritual aspect has been added to the biopsychosocial framework in order to account for the individual differences in health and well-being status and to capture the nuances of the concept of health that may vary across societies globally. Thus, the biopsychosociospiritual framework considers the role of relational and existential experience of an individual with others and the universe in understanding the notion of holistic well-being (Sulmasy, 2002). Despite the fact that there are multiple interpretations of the term "spiritual," there is an increasing agreement over the health benefits that spirituality could serve to the human race. For practical purposes, spirituality could be understood as "the search for ultimate meaning, purpose, and significance, in relation to oneself, family, others, community, nature, and the sacred, expressed through beliefs, values, traditions, and practices" (Puchalski, Vitillo, Hull, & Reller, 2014). Some of the key benefits of adding the spiritual dimension to the existing model may pertain to spiritual coping, positive impact of spiritual practice by the doctor, spiritual support for end-of-life care patients, and spiritual therapies (Saad, De Medeiros, & Mosini, 2017). In sum, health psychology has made an attempt to adopt a holistic approach to health and wellness by considering biological, psychological, socio-cultural, and spiritual aspects so that the wholeness of the human experience can be comprehended and a new psychological science of health can be established.

Notwithstanding, the focus of health psychology has largely been on treating chronic health diseases and lifestyle-related disorders such as diabetes mellitus, chronic respiratory diseases, cancer, hypertension, arthritis, irritable bowel syndrome, etc., thus essentially reflecting a healing approach, in line with the traditional psychological endeavor, focused solely on alleviating suffering while running the risk of being oblivious towards the possibility of potential capitalization of human strengths.

12.3   YOGA: AN AGE-OLD TRADITION IN ITS NEW AVATAR IN THE 21ST CENTURY

Yoga, with its more than 30 centuries old origin in the East, has received considerable recognition in the West in this 21st century in the form of a therapeutic and spiritual practice aimed at sustaining and promoting health and well-being. Since the year 2015, International Day of Yoga is being celebrated on June 21 every year across the globe after its due recognition by the UN General Assembly. This itself provides a testimony about the importance and the promising benefits that Yoga can yield for the human race. The precise meaning of the word 'Yoga' is to join or union, and concentrate one's attention (Raub, 2002). At a philosophical level, Yoga means a connection or union of the self with the Universe by being aware of the incessant tremendous energy flow operating between the individual (person) and the cosmos (environment). At a more practical level, it means a harmonious connection between the mind (mental processes) and the body (physical/physiological processes). Thus, in essence, Yoga is a robust mind-body interactional process that involves physical and motor activity as well as mindful self-awareness with sustained attention on one's breathing pattern, energy flow, and the subjective experience of union with the cosmic energy.

The very first description of Yoga is traced back to the classic text, *Yoga Sutras*, written by Patanjali wherein he has described it as a road to enlightenment and conscious awareness (Desikachar, Bragdon, & Bossart, 2005). While a dominant understanding of Yoga may simply focus on *asana*, i.e., the physical aspect of Yoga, the original meaning of it goes much beyond by incorporating diverse aspects such as mindful breathing, meditation, *satvik ahara*, and *anasakti* for materialism. The comprehensive healing system of Yoga is built on the foundation of four basic principles

(Desikachar et al., 2005). The first among them considers the human body as an all-inclusive entity made up of various interconnected aspects that operate in a reciprocal manner; thus, any damage to a particular bodily system will have an inevitable influence on the rest of the systems. The second principle mandates that the requirements of any individual are unique, idiosyncratic to him/her, thus entailing a tailor-made approach in order to suitably and sufficiently address them through the yogic practice. The third principle advocates for the active and autonomous involvement of the individual who practices Yoga. In other words, the person is required to play an active role, free from any external dominance, in influencing his/her health status while undergoing the yogic healing system. The last principle emphasizes the need to possess a positive, balanced, and optimistic mental state to benefit from the fruits of the yogic practice of healing (Desikachar et al., 2005).

As a form of complementary and alternative medicine, Yoga is now widely recognized for its therapeutic effects. It is argued that the integration of physical, spiritual, and psychological components in the yogic practice leads to numerous health-related benefits pertaining to physiological, emotional, and spiritual well-being (Collins, 1998). Research shows that the regular practice of yogic exercises results in physical health benefits such as bodily flexibility, muscular soundness, improved cardiovascular and respiratory functions, de-addiction, sound sleep, and recovery from chronic pain as well as mental health benefits namely decreased stress and anxiety levels, improved psychological adjustment, and enhanced quality of life and overall well-being status (Bharshankar et al., 2003; Cohen et al., 2004; Collins, 1998; Desikachar et al., 2005; Kissen & Kissen-Kohn, 2009; Kolasinski et al., 2005; Marlatt, 2002; Oken et al., 2006). Thus, inferring from the empirical evidence described above, it can reasonably be argued that the yogic healing system contributes to physical, mental, and spiritual health, thereby becoming a promising potential facilitator of positive health.

12.4 MINDFULNESS: BEING IN THE PRESENT

Mindfulness, the art of being present, is a central concept in Buddhist psychology. It is defined as "a moment-by-moment awareness of thoughts, feelings, bodily sensations, and the surrounding environment" (Zhang et al., 2021) without being judgmental about the awareness experience. As an inherently personal journey, the aim of practicing mindfulness is "to eliminate needless suffering by cultivating insight into the workings of the mind and the nature of the material world" (Siegel, Germer, & Olendzki, 2009). The significance of mindfulness in a therapeutic environment lies in the fact that instead of fixing the problems of the patient/client without due consideration for his/her self-understanding, the mindfulness approach advocates for awareness and acceptance to be at the forefront followed by the necessary changes to be brought about in the behavior of the person (Siegel et al., 2009). This shift in the way the client with psychological issues is looked at makes all the difference by addressing the subjectivity and the acceptance in such a manner that the emotional turmoil and cataclysmic psychological experiences can be dealt with successfully.

In an influential paper, Bishop & colleagues (2004) discuss the operationalization of mindfulness for the ease of measurement and systematic inquiry on this elusive and intriguing concept. While there are multiple viewpoints about the notion of mindfulness, a general understanding of this concept asserts that the mindfulness state involves observing thoughts and feelings in the form of mental events without any over-identification or reflexive response to them. The two-component model of mindfulness proposed by Bishop & colleagues (2004) views it essentially as a meta-cognitive process that monitors ongoing attentional activity and describes it as comprising "self-regulation of attention" and "orientation to experience" (Bishop et al., 2004). The comprehensive description of mindfulness delineated by the two-component model states that mindfulness is "a process of regulating attention in order to bring a quality of non-elaborative awareness to current experience and a quality of relating to one's experience within an orientation of curiosity, experiential openness, and acceptance" (Bishop et al., 2004). Thus, the model emphasizes reaching an insight about the mental processes at work by embracing a *de-centered perspective* to acknowledge the subjectiveness and ephemeral, non-permanent nature of cognitive and affective processes (Safran & Segal, 1990).

A major impetus for the use of mindfulness techniques in clinical settings was the mindfulness-based stress reduction program aimed at treating chronic pain, chronic diseases, and emotional-behavioral psychological disorders (Kabat-Zinn, 1998). Empirical evidence suggests the utility of mindfulness in treating psychological morbidity, stress reduction, and enhancement of well-being (Carlson et al., 2001; Salmoirago-Blotcher et al., 2013; Williams et al., 2001). More recent evidence substantiates the importance of mindfulness-based intervention programs in reducing detrimental health behaviors such as substance abuse, and promoting adaptive health behaviors and mental health outcomes (Carlson, 2012; Gawande et al., 2019; Goldberg et al., 2018; Li et al., 2017). Attempts have been made to integrate mindfulness into psychological therapeutic framework in order to understand how mindfulness interventions bring about desired behavioral change through the mechanisms of emotional regulation, attentional control, self-regulation, and motivational and learning strategies (Schuman-Olivier et al., 2020). A recent meta-analytic review on the usefulness of mindfulness-based intervention programs highlights that such programs are effective in improving general health, mental health, well-being, and quality of life indicators with high magnitude effect sizes ranging from 0.89 to 1.87 (Aghaie et al., 2018). More promising evidence comes from a recent overall review of mindfulness-based interventions, performed on existing systematic reviews, meta-analytic reviews, and studies using randomized controlled trial design (Zhang et al., 2021). This overall review yields evidence for a positive influence of mindfulness in dealing with a range of mental health issues (such as stress, anxiety, depression, insomnia, substance use, psychosis, etc.), improving physical health conditions (such as pain, weight control, hypertension, cardiovascular diseases, asthma, and diabetes), maintaining social health (in terms of reducing anger and violence), and promoting prosocial behavior by enhancing ecological sustainability and harmonious connection with fellow human beings and nature, across multiple settings including school, workplace, and the healthcare setup (Zhang et al., 2021). Thus, it becomes evident that mindfulness is not only relevant to physical health per se but its benefits are being realized in the domains of mental and social health as well.

12.5 POSITIVE HEALTH FRAMEWORK

Seeman (1989) proposed a model of positive health based on a comprehensive human-system framework that accounted for the involvement of various sub-systems, namely physiological, psychological (cognitive-perceptual), and social (interpersonal), in influencing health status, thus going beyond the traditional, merely biomedical understanding of health. Mezzich

(2005) views positive health as a broader concept of health aligning with the WHO's spirit of well-being and rooted in the 'wholeness' or totality of human experience. Such an understanding of health specifies resilience, supportive resources, and quality of life as integral elements of positive health (Mezzich, 2005). The more recent development in the field of positive health comes from the work of Martin Seligman, the founding father of positive psychology, who attempted to view health in terms of a state that goes beyond mere absence of disease (Seligman, 2008). The key assumption underlying positive health is that shifting the focus from illness to well-being will not only enhance flourishing status in life but also serve as a great shield to protect against the development of mental disorders (Seligman, Rashid, & Parks, 2006).

The notion of positive health investigates how well a person is doing on biological, subjective, and functional measures of health. To elaborate further, Seligman (2008) argues that the biological measure reflects higher status on physiological functioning as determined by specific medical tests for particular physical diseases; the subjective measure indicates a variety of higher psychological states such as a greater sense of positive physical well-being, absence of somatic symptoms, increased level of hardiness, internal health locus of control, life satisfaction, optimism, and positive emotions; and the functional measure denotes positive physical capacity and adaptation in the form of person-environment fit (Seligman, 2008). The utility of the positive health construct lies in the fact that, on a global scale, when health is conceptualized in terms of a combination of biological, psychological, and functional indicators, it can potentially help lower health expenditure, enhance mental health, improve quality of life, and better predict illness development (Seligman, 2008).

Having discussed the importance of adopting a positive health framework, it is evident that it can serve as a better guide to inform the understanding of health in its totality; thus incorporating both physical and mental health aspects along with their respective illness and health continua. Further, as discussed in the respective sections on Yoga and mindfulness in this chapter, it is incontestable that both yogic and mindfulness practices contribute immensely to physical and mental health in terms of improving physical illness symptoms and coping with psychological ailments on their respective illness continua besides bolstering physical health and mental well-being on corresponding health continua. Thus, while the world is struggling with a number of chronic diseases and psychological disorders in today's times, yoga and mindfulness, nested in the positive health framework, can emerge as possible remedies to these burning health issues.

12.6   THE ROAD AHEAD

While health psychology aims to understand how biological, psychological, social, and spiritual factors contribute to the development of illness and maintenance of health, the field of positive psychology calls for de-monopolizing the illness-biased treatment system and moving towards resource-building and strength development in order to achieve human flourishing. The area of positive health provides a unique opportunity to converge these complementary positions wherein both physical health and mental health are looked at with their respective illness and health continuum, making it possible to conceptualize health in its entirety. Such an approach would help in realizing flourishing or optimal functioning, which is an important aim of psychology (Pradhan & Jandu, 2023).

From the lens of positive psychology, both Yoga and mindfulness can be conceived as positive activities having conspicuous beneficial psychological effects for individuals in terms of optimum engagement, positive emotions, and well-being (Pradhan, Jandu, Hati, & Panda, 2022; Pradhan, Jandu, Samal, & Patnaik, 2022). The major theoretical frameworks in positive psychology such as the broaden and build theory of positive emotions (Fredrickson, 2001), sustainable happiness model (Lyubomirsky, Sheldon, & Schkade, 2005), positive activity model (Lyubomirsky & Layous, 2013), to name a few, can be used to empirically test the role of Yoga and mindfulness in building personal resources in the form of psychological strengths and optimal functioning. Similarly, health psychology views Yoga and mindfulness as desirable health behaviors having a bearing on illness prevention and health promotion. The health psychology theories viz. health belief model (Rosenstock, 2000), transtheoretical model of change (Prochaska & DiClemente, 1982), and the theory of planned behavior (Ajzen, 1991), etc., can be used to understand health behavior change occurring on account of following Yoga and mindfulness practices. Keeping in mind the benefits of Yoga and mindfulness, the targeted interventions based on the positive health model can be accelerated to ensure a happy, healthy, productive, and flourishing society.

KEYWORDS

- **health psychology**
- **illness development**
- **mindfulness**
- **positive health**
- **positive psychology**
- **somatic symptoms**
- **yoga**

REFERENCES

Aghaie, E., Roshan, R., Mohamadkhani, P., Shaeeri, M., & Gholami-Fesharaki, M. (2018). Well-being, mental health, general health and quality of life improvement through mindfulness-based interventions: A systematic review and meta-analysis. *Iranian Red Crescent Medical Journal, 20*(2), 1–7.

Ahmadi, Z., & Sadeghi, T. (2017). Application of the Betty Neuman systems model in the nursing care of patients/clients with multiple sclerosis. *Multiple Sclerosis Journal–Experimental, Translational and Clinical, 3*(3), 1–8. doi: 10.1177/2055217317726798.

Ajzen, I. (1991). The theory of planned behavior. *Organizational Behavior and Human Decision Processes, 50*(2), 179–211.

Alex Linley, P., Joseph, S., Harrington, S., & Wood, A. M. (2006). Positive psychology: Past, present, and (possible) future. *The Journal of Positive Psychology, 1*(1), 3–16.

Bharshankar, J. R., Bharshankar, R. N., Deshpande, V. N., Kaore, S. B., & Gosavi, G. B. (2003). Effect of yoga on cardiovascular system in subjects above 40 years. *Indian Journal of Physiology and Pharmacology, 47*(2), 202–206.

Bishop, S. R., Lau, M., Shapiro, S., Carlson, L., Anderson, N. D., Carmody, J., Segal, Z. V., Abbey, S., Speca, M., Velting, D., & Devins, G. (2004). Mindfulness: A proposed operational definition. *Clinical Psychology: Science and Practice, 11*(3), 230–241.

Borrell-Carrió, F., Suchman, A. L., & Epstein, R. M. (2004). The biopsychosocial model 25 years later: Principles, practice, and scientific inquiry. *The Annals of Family Medicine, 2*(6), 576–582.

Carlson, L. E. (2012). Mindfulness-based interventions for physical conditions: A narrative review evaluating levels of evidence. *International Scholarly Research Notices, 2012*, 651583, 1–12.

Carlson, L. E., Ursuliak, Z., Goodey, E., Angen, M., & Speca, M. (2001). The effects of a mindfulness meditation-based stress reduction program on mood and symptoms of stress in cancer outpatients: 6-month follow-up. *Supportive Care in Cancer, 9*, 112–123.

Ciccarelli, S. K., & White, J. N. (2017). *Psychology* (4th ed.). London: Pearson.

Cohen, L., Warneke, C., Fouladi, R. T., Rodriguez, M. A., & Chaoul-Reich, A. (2004). Psychological adjustment and sleep quality in a randomized trial of the effects of a Tibetan yoga intervention in patients with lymphoma. *Cancer: Interdisciplinary International Journal of the American Cancer Society, 100*(10), 2253–2260.

Collins, C. (1998). Yoga: Intuition, preventive medicine, and treatment. *Journal of Obstetric, Gynecologic, & Neonatal Nursing, 27*(5), 563–568.

Delphis Learning. (2020). The mental health continuum is a better model for mental health. Retrieved from: https://delphis.org.uk/mental-health/continuum-mental-health/ (accessed on 5 July 2024).

Desikachar, K., Bragdon, L., & Bossart, C. (2005). The yoga of healing: Exploring yoga's holistic model for health and well-being. *International Journal of Yoga Therapy, 15*(1), 17–39.

Engel, G. L. (1977). The need for a new medical model: A challenge for biomedicine. *Science, 196*, 129–136. doi: 10.1126/science.847460.

Fredrickson, B. L. (2001). The role of positive emotions in positive psychology: The broaden-and-build theory of positive emotions. *American Psychologist, 56*(3), 218–226.

Gable, S. L., & Haidt, J. (2005). What (and why) is positive psychology? *Review of General Psychology, 9*, 103–110.

Gawande, R., To, M. N., Pine, E., Griswold, T., Creedon, T. B., Brunel, A., Lozada, A., Loucks, E. B., & Schuman-Olivier, Z. (2019). Mindfulness training enhances self-regulation and facilitates health behavior change for primary care patients: A randomized controlled trial. *Journal of General Internal Medicine, 34*, 293–302.

Goldberg, S. B., Tucker, R. P., Greene, P. A., Davidson, R. J., Wampold, B. E., Kearney, D. J., & Simpson, T. L. (2018). Mindfulness-based interventions for psychiatric disorders: A systematic review and meta-analysis. *Clinical Psychology Review, 59*, 52–60.

Kabat-Zinn, J. (1998). Meditation. In J. C. Holland (Ed.), *Psycho-oncology* (pp. 767–779). New York: Oxford University Press.

Keyes, C. L. M. (2002). The mental health continuum: From languishing to flourishing in life. *Journal of Health and Social Behavior, 43*(2), 207–222.

Kissen, M., & Kissen-Kohn, D. A. (2009). Reducing addictions via the self-soothing effects of yoga. *Bulletin of the Menninger Clinic, 73*(1), 34–43.

Kolasinski, S. L., Garfinkel, M., Tsai, A. G., Matz, W., Dyke, A. V., & Schumacher Jr, H. R. (2005). Iyengar yoga for treating symptoms of osteoarthritis of the knees: A pilot study. *Journal of Alternative & Complementary Medicine, 11*(4), 689–693.

Li, W., Howard, M. O., Garland, E. L., McGovern, P., & Lazar, M. (2017). Mindfulness treatment for substance misuse: A systematic review and meta-analysis. *Journal of Substance Abuse Treatment, 75*, 62–96.

Lyubomirsky, S., & Layous, K. (2013). How do simple positive activities increase well-being? *Current Directions in Psychological Science, 22*(1), 57–62.

Lyubomirsky, S., Sheldon, K. M., & Schkade, D. (2005). Pursuing happiness: The architecture of sustainable change. *Review of General Psychology, 9*, 111–131.

Marlatt, G. A. (2002). Buddhist philosophy and the treatment of addictive behavior. *Cognitive and Behavioral Practice, 9*(1), 44–50.

Maslow, A. (1954). *Motivation and Personality*. Harper and Row.

Matarazzo, J. D. (1982). Behavioral health's challenge to academic, scientific, and professional psychology. *American Psychologist, 37*, 1–14.

Mezzich, J. E. (2005). Positive health: Conceptual place, dimensions and implications. *Psychopathology, 38*(4), 177–179.

Neuman, B. M. (1990). Health as a continuum based on the Neuman systems model. *Nursing Science Quarterly, 3*(3), 129–135. doi:10.1177/089431849000300308.

Oken, B. S., Zajdel, D., Kishiyama, S., Flegal, K., Dehen, C., Haas, M., Kraemer, D. F., Lawrence, J., & Leyva, J. (2006). Randomized, controlled, six-month trial of yoga in healthy seniors: Effects on cognition and quality of life. *Alternative Therapies in Health and Medicine, 12*(1), 40–47.

Pradhan, R. K., & Jandu, K. (2023). Evaluating the impact of conscientiousness on flourishing in Indian higher education context: Mediating role of emotional intelligence. *Psychological Studies, 68*(2), 223–235.

Pradhan, R. K., Jandu, K., Hati, L., & Panda, M. (2022). Being nice goes long way: Manifesting compassion for others enacts in experiencing positive emotions and workplace happiness for the employees. *Business Perspectives and Research, 12*(2). doi: 10.1177/22785337221113157.

Pradhan, R. K., Jandu, K., Panda, M., Hati, L., & Mallick, M. (2022). In pursuit of happiness at work: Exploring the role of psychological capital and coping in managing COVID-19 stress among Indian employees. *Journal of Asia Business Studies, 16*(6), 850–867.

Pradhan, R. K., Jandu, K., Samal, J., & Patnaik, J. B. (2022). Does practicing spirituality at workplace make teachers more engaged? Examining the role of emotional intelligence. *International Journal of Ethics and Systems39*(4), 1–16. https://doi.org/10.1108/IJOES-05-2022-0105.

Pradhan, R. K., Panda, M., Hati, L., Jandu, K., & Mallick, M. (2023). Impact of COVID-19 stress on employee performance and well-being: Role of trust in management and psycho-logical capital. *Journal of Asia Business Studies18*(1), 1–18. https://doi.org/10.1108/JABS-01-2023-0023.

Prochaska, J. O., & DiClemente, C. C. (1982). Transtheoretical therapy: Toward a more integrative model of change. *Psychotherapy: Theory, Research & Practice, 19*(3), 276–288

Puchalski, C. M., Vitillo, R., Hull, S. K., & Reller, N. (2014). Improving the spiritual dimension of whole person care: Reaching national and international consensus. *Journal of Palliative Medicine, 17*(6), 642–656.

Raub, J. A. (2002). Psychophysiologic effects of Hatha Yoga on musculoskeletal and cardiopulmonary function: A literature review. *The Journal of Alternative & Comple-mentary Medicine, 8*(6), 797–812.

Rosenstock, I. M. (2000). Health Belief Model. In A. E. Kazdin (Ed.), *Encyclopedia of Psychology* (Vol. 4, pp. 78–80). Oxford University Press.

Saad, M., De Medeiros, R., & Mosini, A. C. (2017). Are we ready for a true biopsychosocial–spiritual model? The many meanings of "spiritual." *Medicines, 4*(4), 79.

Safran, J. D., & Segal, Z. V. (1990). *Interpersonal Process in Cognitive Therapy.* New York: Basic Books.

Salmoirago-Blotcher, E., Hunsinger, M., Morgan, L., Fischer, D., & Carmody, J. (2013). Mindfulness-based stress reduction and change in health-related behaviors. *Journal of Evidence-Based Complementary & Alternative Medicine, 18*(4), 243–247.

Schuman-Olivier, Z., Trombka, M., Lovas, D. A., Brewer, J. A., Vago, D. R., Gawande, R., Dunne, J. P., Lazar, S. W., Loucks, E. B., & Fulwiler, C. (2020). Mindfulness and behavior change. *Harvard Review of Psychiatry, 28*(6), 371–394.

Seeman, J. (1989). Toward a model of positive health. *American Psychologist, 44*(8), 1099–1109.

Seligman, M. E. (2008). Positive health. *Applied Psychology: An International Review, 57,* 3–18.

Seligman, M. E. P. (2002). Positive psychology, positive prevention, and positive therapy. In C. R., Snyder, & S. J. Lopez (Eds.), *Handbook of Positive Psychology*, (pp. 3–12). Oxford University Press.

Seligman, M. E. P., Rashid, T., & Parks, A. C. (2006). Positive psychotherapy. *American Psychologist, 61,* 774–788.

Sheldon, K. M., & King, L. (2001). Why positive psychology is necessary. *American Psychologist, 56,* 216–217.

Siegel, R. D., Germer, C. K., & Olendzki, A. (2009). Mindfulness: What is it? Where did it come from? *Clinical Handbook of Mindfulness*, 17–35.

Sulmasy, D. P. (2002). A biopsychosocial-spiritual model for the care of patients at the end of life. *The Gerontologist, 42*(suppl_3), 24–33.

Tran, V. (2013). Health psychology. In M. D. Gellman & J. R. Turner (Eds.), *Encyclopedia of Behavioral Medicine* (pp. 927–929). Springer, New York, NY. https://doi.org/10.1007/978-1-4419-1005-9_959 (accessed on 5 July 2024).

Travis, J. W., & Ryan, R. S. (1988). *The Wellness Workbook*. Ten Speed Press.

Williams, K. A., Kolar, M. M., Reger, B. E., & Pearson, J. C. (2001). Evaluation of a wellness-based mindfulness stress reduction intervention: A controlled trial. *American Journal of Health Promotion, 15*(6), 422–432.

World Health Organization. (2006). *Constitution of the World Health Organization–Basic Documents, Forty-fifth edition, Supplement, October 2006.*

World Health Organization. (2023). Mental health fact sheet. Retrieved from: https://www.who.int/data/gho/data/major-themes/health-and-well-being (accessed on 5 July 2024).

World Health Organization. (2023). The global health observatory: Explore a world of health data. Retrieved from: https://www.who.int/data/gho/data/themes/world-health-statistics (accessed on 5 July 2024).

Zhang, D., Lee, E. K., Mak, E. C., Ho, C. Y., & Wong, S. Y. (2021). Mindfulness-based interventions: An overall review. *British Medical Bulletin, 138*(1), 41–57.

CHAPTER 13

Yoga for the Management of Diabetes

RAVI SHANKER DATTI

*Assistant Professor, Department of Applied Psychology,
GITAM School of Gandhian Studies, GITAM (Deemed to be University),
Visakhapatnam, Andhra Pradesh, India*

ABSTRACT

Background: The burden of Type II Diabetes Mellitus is growing exponentially globally, with an estimated 134 million affected by 2045. It also accounts for premature morbidity and mortality. One can see the importance of cost-effective interventions in mitigating chronic health conditions like diabetes. Among the available complementary healthcare interventions that can reduce the burden of diabetes is Yoga, which is an ancient mind-body technique with multiple collateral lifestyle benefits. *Method:* The study examined the impact of Yoga on clinical and psychological outcomes in diabetic patients. A stepped care protocol was followed, involving the identification of specific asanas and educating participants on their frequency and practice. Using a pre-post design, all subjects practiced Yoga for 40 days, and changes were measured from baseline to post-intervention. The study included data from 35 participants, with an average age of 50.34 (±8.38), who completed the full 40-day Yoga intervention. Clinical outcome measures included Fasting Plasma Glucose (FPG), Total Cholesterol, and Body Mass Index (BMI), while psychological measures encompassed well-being and self-reported sleep quality. *Results:* The major findings of the study indicate that 40 days of Yoga had brought about positive changes in parameters like BMI,

Yoga and Meditation: Past and Present Evidence. Sachi Nandan Mohanty, Rabindra Kumar Pradhan, & Sugyanta Priyadarshini (Eds.)

absolute FPG, and Cholesterol. More specifically, the BMI has reduced along with a decrease in fasting plasma sugar levels. The findings indicate that Yoga practice has more beneficial effects on psychological states. Participants reported lesser depression and anxiety and more positive well-being and energy. Similar positive changes are observed in reduced sleep disturbances and sleep initiation. *Discussion:* The aforementioned findings suggest that Yoga has a beneficial impact on various outcomes related to diabetes. However, it is crucial to prioritize studying both the immediate and long-lasting effects of Yoga therapy on managing diabetes. Additional research is required to ascertain the full extent of this influence concerning Yoga.

13.1 INTRODUCTION

Diabetes mellitus (DM), a chronic disease, is brought on by insufficient insulin production by the pancreas or inefficient insulin absorption by the body. Type 1 and type 2 diabetes are the two main types. The onset of type 1 diabetes (T1DM), which requires daily insulin injections for life, often occurs throughout childhood and adolescence. On the other hand, type 2 diabetes (T2DM), which accounts for 90% of diabetes cases worldwide, often develops in adulthood (WHO, 2023).

In the 21st century, diabetes mellitus has become a significant public health concern, contributing to a high number of deaths, illnesses, and healthcare costs worldwide (Global Burden of Metabolic Risk Factors for Chronic Diseases Collaboration, 2014). More than 425 million people worldwide had diabetes in 2017, according to recent estimates by the International Diabetic Federation (IDF).

Clearly, it is crucial to identify cost-effective strategies for preventing and managing type 2 diabetes (DM2) that address the various interconnected factors associated with this complex, devastating, and increasingly prevalent condition. Yoga, a traditional mind-body practice that is popular in India for controlling diabetes and high blood pressure, is an intriguing strategy in this regard.

Yoga offers several advantages as a physical activity option for individuals with diabetes: (a) it embraces a holistic philosophy that integrates physical exercises with a comprehensive lifestyle package encompassing diet, relaxation, and stress management, as recognized by Western practitioners; (b) it involves lower cardiovascular demands compared to other forms of exercise; and (c) it is low-impact, making it suitable for individuals who are obese or face difficulties with strenuous physical activity (Skoro-Kondza et al., 2009). Recent systematic reviews have indicated that while the existing evidence does not establish causation, it suggests that Yoga may be effective in managing type 2 diabetes (Innes & Vincent, 2007; Badr et al., 2008).

A brief overview of Asanas:

1. ***Tadasana*–The Mountain Pose:** If practiced daily, aids in improving posture and correcting postural issues. It strengthens the knees, ankles, and thighs while toning the leg muscles.

2. ***Pavana-Mukta-Asana*–The Wind-Releasing Pose:** This asana helps the stomach, and intestines release digestive gas that has been trapped there.

3. ***Utthan Pada Asana*–The Raised Feet Posture:** This asana strengthens the spinal cord and treats back conditions. It reduces a chubby appearance and gets rid of gas, indigestion, and constipation.

4. ***Surya-Namaskar*–Sun Salutation:** It consists of several soft, flowing motions timed to the breath. This is a great warm-up exercise that involves a series of poses that rotate the spine in different directions and increase limb flexibility. Since it aids in the body's increased flexibility, it is especially advantageous to beginners, stiff individuals, and the elderly. Additionally, it controls breathing and sharpens thinking.

5. ***Ardha-Matsyendra-Asana*–The Half Spinal Twist Pose:** It eases stiff necks and upper back stiffness brought on by stress, poor posture, or extended periods of sitting still. The internal organs are massaged, and the abdomen area is flushed with blood as a result of the alternating compression and release. Repeated repetition of the Half Spinal Twist also tones the muscles in the hips and stomach.

6. ***Bhujangasana*–The Cobra Pose:** This posture is the first in a series of backbends. It increases flexibility, revitalizes spinal nerves, and provides the spinal region with a strong blood supply. It stimulates appetite and treats a variety of issues, including indigestion.

7. ***Vajrasana*–Diamond Pose:** This is a great posture for meditation and digestion.

8. *Sasankasana*–**The Hare Pose:** This asana stimulates digestion and tones the organs and muscles of the abdomen.

9. *Janu Sirsasana*–**The Head-to-Knee Pose:** This asana is advantageous for the sciatic nerve. It makes the back muscles and vertebrae flexible and facilitates the digestion process.

10. *Paschimottanasana*–**The Posterior Stretch:** This asana corrects small postural irregularities and deformities in the curvature of the spine. It stretches the spine to its greatest length, making it supple and flexible.

11. *Dhanurasana*–**The Bow Pose:** This pose is a useful exercise for strengthening the back muscles and enhancing posture.

12. *Jathara Parivartanasana*–**Stomach Churning Pose:** This asana gives the spine flexibility and suppleness while relieving lower back and hip strain. It promotes improved circulation, enhances digestion, and lessens hip stiffness and weariness.

13. *Mayurasana*–**Peacock Pose/***Hamsa Asana* **or Swan Pose:** This pose tones the abdominal muscles and directs blood to the abdominal organs. It also aids in digestion, assimilation, and excretion.

14. *Sarvangasana*–**The All-Parts Pose:** This pose helps to treat bronchitis, asthma, difficulty breathing, and shortness of breath.

15. *Halasana*–**The Plough Pose:** This asana stimulates the thyroid and stomach organs. It eases weariness and tension while calming the mind.

16. *Matsyasana*–**The Fish Pose:** The belly and throat muscles are stretched and stimulated by this pose. Additionally, it tones the intestines, kidneys, stomach, and nervous system.

17. *Kati Chakrasana*–**Waist Rotation Posture:** The flexibility of the back will benefit from this pose. Additionally, it strengthens the thighs, tummy, and shoulders and aids in the treatment of digestive issues.

18. *Agnisar Kriya*–**Cleansing Technique:** This purifying method, *Agnisara*, is advised for digestive issues in Yoga treatment.

Pranayama is the fourth stage in Patanjali's eight-stage Yoga. The lungs, heart, diaphragm, abdomen, intestines, kidneys, and pancreas are all exercised by controlling the breath and taking deep breaths. It complements the poses or workout.

13.2 OBJECTIVES

- To examine the effect of Yoga on clinical parameters among Type II Diabetics; and
- To examine the effect of Yoga on psychological states among Type II Diabetics.

13.3 HYPOTHESIS

It is hypothesized that the practice of Yoga would bring about significant improvements in clinical parameters and psychological states in Diabetics.

13.4 METHODOLOGY

13.4.1 RESEARCH DESIGN

All subjects engaged in Yoga practice for a predetermined amount of time, and the difference between baseline and post-intervention was assessed using a pre-post design. The goal of this study is to investigate and put into practice a stepped care protocol for future designs, beginning with the identification of a set of asanas and their effectiveness in the management of diabetes. The set of *asanas* selected for the study have been identified from earlier studies (Malhotra et al., 2002, 2005; Manjunatha et al., 2005) and from the list of *asanas* provided in classical Yoga texts (Shankardevananda, 2002). The *asana* practice period has been set at 40 days because the *Upanishads*, ancient literature, recommend this length of time in order to reap the benefits of the practice.

13.4.2 PARTICIPANTS

The study used a convenience sampling method to select and recruit participants for a 40-day Yoga camp to be held exclusively for patients with Type 2 diabetes in Visakhapatnam. The inclusion criteria include being on oral medication for the management of diabetes and being willing to participate in the Yoga Camp for 40 days. At baseline, 53 eligible participants enrolled for the camp. The participants were screened for any complications (self-reported), provided with all the necessary information, and their consent to participate in the study was taken. The participants were instructed to continue their diabetes medication as advised by their physician. The actual number of persons who successfully completed the 40-day camp was 35, which included 24 men and 11 women.

13.4.3 PROCEDURES

Trained Yoga instructors and doctors held a brief but comprehensive talk on Yoga and diabetes for all the participants. The participants provided demographic details, a list of current medications, and their height and weight were recorded to estimate their Body Mass Index (BMI). The base-line measures included the estimation of clinical parameters, and assess-ment of psychological states were taken. A trained technician did all blood tests initially, and they were repeated after the 40-day Yoga intervention. Data regarding certain dimensions of the quality of sleep experienced by the patients (average sleep duration, average sleep initiation time, and number of sleep interruptions) were also obtained. These measures were also repeated at the end of the 40-day Yoga intervention.

13.4.4 INTERVENTION

For 40 days, the participants took hour-long Yoga courses each day. Depending on their convenience, participants chose morning or evening lessons. A lecture or discussion on the health issues related to better diabetes control took place one day every week.

Following are the Yoga *asanas* included in the study.

Tadasana–The Mountain Pose, *Pavana-mukta-asana*–The Wind-releasing Pose, *Utthan pada asana*–the raised feet posture, *Surya-namaskar*–Sun Salutation, *Ardha-Matsyendra-asana*, *Bhujanga Asana*, *Vajra-asana*–Diamond Pose, *Sasankasana*–The Hare Pose, *Janusirasana*–The Head-to-Knee Pose, *Sarvangasana*–The All-Parts Pose, *Paschimotanasana*–The Posterior Stretch, *Dhanurasana*–The Bow Pose, *Jatara Parivartanasana*–Stomach churning pose, *Mayurasana* peacock pose/*Hamsa asana* or swan pose, *Halasana*–The Plough Pose,

Kati Chakrasana–Waist rotation posture, *Matsyasana*–The Fish Pose, *Agnisar kriya*–This cleansing technique, and *Pranayam*.

It can be noted that the ananas help improve the functioning of the digestive system, increase the flexibility of muscles and enhance the benefits of breathing. The above *asanas* were done under the careful supervision of a Yoga master with regard to frequency, duration, intensity, and content for all participants.

13.4.5 MEASURES

13.4.5.1 PSYCHOLOGICAL MEASURES

13.4.5.1.1 WHO (Bradley) Well-Being Questionnaire (1990)

The Well-being questionnaire was developed by Bradley & Lewis (1990) to provide measures of depression, anxiety, energy, and positive well-being of people with diabetes. The Well-Being Scales were created with the intention of measuring undesirable mood states as well as tracking any changes in them. The Well-being scales were developed from a questionnaire that was initially intended for use with individuals with diabetes treated with insulin, but they have been developed with a population of people who have diabetes treated with tablets and are as appropriate for persons with diabetes treated only by diet. Increasingly, the scales are being used for the purpose of auditing psychological outcomes in diabetes care.

The initial questionnaire consisted of 28 items relating to depression, anxiety, and potential well-being. The scales were administered to samples of 239 outpatients from a hospital and from a multi-center European study. The psychometric analysis of the responses of these samples resulted in the identification of four subscales from 22 items. The four subscales are the following: *Depression, Anxiety, Energy,* and *Positive Well-being*.

13.4.5.1.2 Diabetes Integration (ATT19)

ATT19 was developed by Welch et al. (1994) by augmenting the original ATT39 as a single 19-item scale that is applicable for both insulin-dependent diabetes mellitus and non-insulin-dependent diabetes mellitus patients. On face inspection, the ATT19 looks to assess how much a patient's diabetes has affected both their personality and lifestyle. Anderson (1986), in discussing the importance of the personal meaning of diabetes, drew attention to the fact that "how well diabetes and self-concept are integrated into the self-concept and how much it will become a psychological problem." Anderson's concept of integration comes closest to the characteristic measured by the ATT19.

13.4.5.2   *CLINICAL MEASURES*

13.4.5.2.1   *Biochemical Measures*

The blood was drawn early in the morning, and within an hour of collection, the serum was separated. On the day of the blood draw, individuals were instructed to fast and refrain from physical activity. The determined biochemical tests included lipid profile – total cholesterol (normal values: 140 mg/dL to 200 mg/dL), high-density lipoprotein (HDL normal values: 30 mg/dL to 60 mg/dL), and low-density lipoprotein (LDL normal values: up to 170 mg/dL). Trained lab technicians carried out all laboratory determinations. A semi-automatic biochemistry analyzer was used to determine the fasting blood glucose levels for each group. Each subject had fasting blood drawn from them at the beginning, at the end of 40 days, and at the end of 80 days. Span Diagnostics Ltd. in India provided the reagents for the enzymatic measurements of total cholesterol, triglycerides, LDL, and HDL, which were then analyzed by a semi-automatic biochemistry analyzer (RMS Daksh, India). The Friedewald formula was used to determine the LDL fraction.

13.4.5.2.2   *Fasting Plasma Glucose*

Blood sugar tests assess how efficiently the body metabolizes glucose, or sugar. On an empty stomach, a fasting plasma glucose test is conducted. The subject must fast (consume only water) for eight hours before the test. A lab technician has collected blood from the subject's vein. Blood is drawn and placed in a tube that already has an anticoagulant in it. Anticoagulants prevent blood clots from forming. A person's plasma is mixed with other substances to detect glucose. The amount of glucose in the plasma is calculated from the resulting reaction. Normal results for fasting plasma glucose tests are between 80 mg/dL and 120 mg/dL. Readings were taken using reagents from Span Diagnostics kits (India) and analyzed by a semi-automatic biochemistry analyzer (RMS Daksh, India).

13.4.5.2.3 Body Composition

Body composition was determined with Body Mass Index (BMI), which was measured using the following formula: BMI = body weight (kg)/[height(m)]^2. Body weight and height were measured using a weighing machine and centimeter tape, respectively. Each measurement was obtained twice, and the average was used in the analysis.

13.4.5.3 OTHER MEASURES

Demographic variables like age, gender, disease history, occupation, etc., were obtained from the participants. The study also considered certain sleep variables like average duration of sleep, average sleep initiation time, and total sleep interruptions.

The study considered data collected from 35 participants who had successfully completed the 40 days Yoga intervention. Data were also collected from 10 participants who practiced Yoga for an additional 40 days.

13.5 FINDINGS

The major findings of the study are the following:

> **Changes in BMI and Clinical Parameters After 40 Days of Yoga:**
>
>   1. **Body Mass Index:** A decrease in BMI following 40 days of Yoga is noticed in 94% of the sample, with an average 2.5 kilos reduction. Five participants moved from the above-normal range to the normal range of BMI, i.e., less than 25 kg/m^2.
>   2. **Fasting Plasma Glucose (FPG):** A fall in absolute FPG values is noticed for 57.1% of the sample; there is no change across the ranges.

3. **Total Cholesterol:** 29 participants (82%) had enhanced total cholesterol values after practicing Yoga for 40 days.
4. **HDL:** More than 91% of the sample showed an increase in HDL (good cholesterol) values. Further, 9 participants who were in the below-normal range at baseline moved up to within the normal range.
5. **LDL:** The LDL (bad cholesterol) has increased for 80% of the sample, but they are still within the normal range.

➢ **Changes in Psychological States After 40 Days of Yoga:**
   • Participants reported lesser depression and anxiety, and more positive well-being and energy, though these findings are not statistically significant.

➢ **Gender Differences After 40 Days of Yoga:**
   • Males reported significantly reduced BMI but increased total cholesterol, HDL, and LDL.
   • Females reported significantly reduced BMI but increased HDL
   • There is a significant decrease in Anxiety levels among males.

➢ **Changes After 80 Days of Yoga Practice:**
   • Significant reduction in FPG, Total Cholesterol and LDL levels;
   • Significant improvement of HDL (good cholesterol) levels from baseline;
   • Significantly lowered depression and anxiety levels;
   • Significantly enhanced positive well-being and total general wellbeing;
   • Significantly lesser sleep initiation time and sleep interruptions.

13.6   YOGA AND MANAGEMENT OF DIABETES

Type 2 diabetes has to be managed by the patients by strictly adhering to a treatment regimen that includes exercise, diet, and medication. The usual exercise suggested by endocrinologists is a brisk walk for 40 minutes to 1 hour, which helps to burn the excess calories and facilitate proper usage of insulin. The patients are also required to adhere to a diet that aims to reduce intake of cholesterol and sugar. Finally, the treatment regimen requires the appropriate intake of insulin if required.

It is noted that this treatment regimen is psychologically and behaviorally demanding, and the patient is required to adopt a new lifestyle that should incorporate regular exercise and diet modification. In other words, the regimen necessitates a lifestyle change. Patients who have adopted and adjusted to these changes would be able to manage their diabetes quite satisfactorily. They are likely to feel that they are in control of the disease.

Living with diabetes can cause stress and disrupt the quality of life and well-being of the patients. Earlier studies have shown that women diabetics experience more difficulty living with the disease and that social support facilitates more effective living (Sridhar et al., 2007). It has also been argued that it is necessary to develop an intervention program that facilitates the adoption of an internal locus of control so that the patients would feel capable of managing the disease. Yoga is one such intervention that might help to this extent.

Management of diabetes requires enhancing the positives and reducing the negatives. Proper exercise leads to enhancing the positives in terms of burning excess calories and adequately utilizing insulin. Reducing the negatives involves cutting down on calories and sugar levels. A proper diet can ensure this. Yoga is presumed to facilitate both these changes.

The findings of the present study indicate that Yoga facilitates the management of diabetes in a two-stage process. The first stage, which is the practice of Yoga for a specified period of time (40 days in the present study), helps to enhance the positives. It is noted that BMI levels fall, and the patients report lesser anxiety and depression. In the second stage, Yoga facilitates the reduction of the negatives in the form of reduced cholesterol, LDL, and FPG. Yoga has also been found to improve the quality of sleep in terms of reduced latency and interruptions. In this stage, Yoga further enhances the positives by increasing positive well-being and total general well-being.

The current study outcomes also indicate that Yoga has immense benefits since it brings about changes in the clinical parameters as well as the psychological states. Yoga might very well fit into the biopsychosocial model of disease management, which asserts that psychological and social consequences of coping with diabetes are as important as maintaining normal FPG values (Madhu & Sridhar, 2001; Sridhar et al., 2007).

The results of this study suggest that Yoga is beneficial for several diabetes-related outcomes. Short-term or sustained Yoga can bring about changes in the management of diabetes. Yoga holds promise for a cost-effective and mass-based intervention program for the management of diabetes since it does not require costly equipment, has very few side effects, and can be practiced by anybody under the guidance of a teacher. Yoga can be easily practiced by people from any country because of these advantages. The context of the social environment, including interpersonal relationships and community characteristics, influences the adoption and maintenance of health behaviors (Alexander et al., 2008). Yoga can be adopted for the management of diabetes in specific or chronic diseases in general, as well as maintaining healthy behavior.

13.7 LIMITATIONS OF THE STUDY

The present study was conducted without changing the diet or lifestyles of the participants. Monitoring the diet of the participants (with the help of a diet log) would have given some insights into the fluctuations observed in clinical parameters. Recruitment of participants and retaining the sample size for longer periods in these studies was hard due to participants' practical and motivational barriers to adhering to the program.

13.8 SUGGESTIONS FOR FUTURE RESEARCH

There should be more extensive randomized controlled trials investigating the effectiveness of Yoga for enhancing metabolic markers where the selected asanas can be grouped and tested on different samples. It would be meaningful to examine the influence of the duration for which each of these asanas is practiced in order to evaluate their relative influence. A pruning of these asanas and evaluating their effectiveness would also shed more light on the influence of Yoga in the management of diabetes. Studies on the effect of Yoga on other chronic diseases could also be carried out to scientifically attest to the benefits of Yoga.

It is currently unknown precisely how certain positions and controlled breathing affect both biological and psychological results. Along with nutrition and medical care, Yoga instruction offers crucial metabolic control for the management of diabetes. Small sample numbers, selection bias, a lack of suitable control groups, lifestyle factors, methodological restrictions, exposure to numerous therapies, and other potential confounders limit the interpretation of existing studies. Future studies should conduct rigorous testing to address the significant heterogeneity in the design, length, intensity, and delivery methods of Yoga-based therapies.

KEYWORDS

- **diabetes**
- **heterogeneity**
- **intensity**
- **lifestyle factors**
- **medical care**
- **sleep quality**
- **yoga**

REFERENCES

Alexander, G. K., Taylor, A. G., Innes, K. E., Kulbok, P., & Selfe, T. K. (2008). Contextualizing the effects of yoga therapy on diabetes management: A review of the social determinants of physical activity. *Family & Community Health, 31*(3), 228. doi: 10.1097/01.FCH.0000324487.39481.8c.

Aljasir, B., Bryson, M., & Al-Shehri, B. (2010). Yoga practice for the management of type II diabetes mellitus in adults: A systematic review. *Evidence-Based Complementary and Alternative Medicine, 7*, 399–408. doi: 10.1093/ecam/nen023.

Anderson, R. M. (1986). The personal meaning of having diabetes: Implications for patient behavior and education or kicking the bucket theory. *Diabetic Medicine, 3*(1), 85–89.

Bradley, C., & Lewis, K. S. (1990). Measures of psychological well-being and treatment satisfaction developed from the responses of people with tablet-treated diabetes. *Diabetic Medicine, 7*(5), 445–451.

Global Burden of Metabolic Risk Factors for Chronic Diseases Collaboration. (2014). Cardiovascular disease, chronic kidney disease, and diabetes mortality burden of cardiometabolic risk factors from 1980 to 2010: A comparative risk assessment. *The Lancet. Diabetes & Endocrinology, 2*(8), 634–647. https://doi.org/10.1016/S2213-8587 (14)70102-0.

Innes, K. E., & Vincent, H. K. (2007). The influence of yoga-based programs on risk profiles in adults with type 2 diabetes mellitus: A systematic review. *Evidence-based Complementary and Alternative Medicine, 4*(4), 469–486. doi:10.1093/ecam/nel103.

Madhu, K., & Sridhar, G. R. (2001). Coping with diabetes: A paradigm for coping with chronic illness. *International Journal of Diabetes in Developing Countries, 21*(2), 103–111.

Malhotra, V., Singh, S., Singh, K. P., Gupta, P., Sharma, S. B., Madhu, S. V., & Tandon, O. P. (2002). Study of yoga asanas in assessment of pulmonary function in NIDDM patients. *Indian Journal of Physiology and Pharmacology, 46*(3), 313–320.

Malhotra, V., Singh, S., Tandon, O. P., & Sharma, S. B. (2005). The beneficial effect of yoga in diabetes. *Nepal Medical College Journal: NMCJ, 7*(2), 145–147.

Malhotra, V., Singh, S., Tandon, O. P., Madhu, S. V., Prasad, A., & Sharma, S. B. (2002). Effect of Yoga asanas on nerve conduction in Type 2 diabetes. *Indian Journal of Physiology and Pharmacology, 46*(3), 298–306.

Manjunatha, S., Vempati, R. P., Ghosh, D., & Bijlani, R. L. (2005). An investigation into the acute and long-term effects of selected yogic postures on fasting and postprandial glycemia and insulinemia in healthy young subjects. *Indian Journal of Physiology and Pharmacology, 49*(3), 319–324.

Shankardevananda Saraswati. (2002). *Practices In Yogic Management of Asthma and Diabetes* (3rd ed., pp. 89–198). Yoga Publications Trust.

Skoro-Kondza, L., Tai, S. S., Gadelrab, R., Drincevic, D., & Greenhalgh, T. (2009). Community based yoga classes for type 2 diabetes: An exploratory randomized controlled trial. *BMC Health Services Research, 9*(1), 1–8. doi:10.1186/1472-6963-9-33.

Sridhar, G. R., Madhu, K., Veena, S., Madhavi, R., Sangeetha, B. S., & Rani, A. (2007). Living with diabetes: Indian experience. *Diabetes & Metabolic Syndrome: Clinical Research & Reviews, 1*(3), 181–187.

Welch, G., Dunn, S. M., & Beeney, L. J. (1994). The ATT39: A measure of psychological adjustment to diabetes. In C. Bradley & C. Gamsu (Eds.), *Handbook of Psychology and Diabetes: A Guide to Psychological Measurement in Diabetes Research and Practice* (pp. 223–245).

World Health Organization. (2023). Diabetes. World Health Organization. Retrieved from: https://www.who.int/news-room/fact-sheets/detail/diabetes (accessed on 5 July 2024).

Index

A

Abdominal area, 13, 160
Abhiniveśa, 44
Academic
  deliberations, 2
  disciplines, 33
Acorus calamus, 195
Acquaint, 2
Addenbrooke Cognitive Examination III
  (ACE), 276, 277, 279, 285, 286, 288
Ādhija vyādhi, 46
Adolescents, 113, 114, 124, 126, 127, 175,
  176, 178, 188, 190, 192, 223, 224, 226,
  234
Aerobic endurance, 278, 285
Agility, 285
Agni, 7, 148, 149, 187, 246, 261, 266, 267
Ahaṅkāra, 42
Air quality index (AQI), 84, 188, 229
Aishwarya, 15
Alleviate migraines, 9
Alternate systems, 1
Altruistic behavior, 195, 225
Amenorrhea, 9
Analysis of variance (ANOVA), 119–121
Aṇamaya kosha, 5, 6
Ānanda, 32, 47, 55
Antaḥkaraṇa, 42
Anti-human behavior, 20
Antiquity, 2
Anti-social youth, 20
Anxiety, 13, 21, 27–29, 33, 39, 43, 57,
  69, 82, 83, 114–116, 153, 159, 161,
  163–169, 171, 176, 178, 186, 188–193,
  223, 224, 242, 243, 305, 307, 316, 321,
  324, 325
Anxiousness, 9
Archival veracity, 2
Artery, 9, 164

Artificial intelligence (AI), 82, 87, 103,
  177, 181, 182, 191, 264
Asana, 4, 9, 12–14, 24, 25, 29, 62, 64,
  65, 70, 84, 144, 151, 153, 161, 162,
  165, 168, 179, 243, 274, 280, 304, 315,
  317–321, 326
Asmitā, 44
Asparagus racemosus, 195
Aṣṭanga yoga, 2, 57
Atharva veda, 23, 190, 235, 236
Ātma jñāna, 46
Ātman, 32
Auspicious
  attainments, 15
  posture, 151
Autonomic nervous system (ANS), 162,
  166, 167
Avidyā, 44, 50
Ayurveda, 5, 14, 19, 21, 148, 177, 187,
  225, 233, 238, 239, 262, 280
Ayurvedic
  books, 20
  herbs, 233
  medicinal
    herbs, 225
    kadha, 256
  therapy, 255

B

Bhagavadgītā, 23, 32, 43
Bhakti yoga, 23, 28, 62, 63
Bharatiya parampara, 1
Bhargo, 267
Bhur, 266
Bhuvah, 266
Binding force, 7
Bioelectricity, 260
Bioimpedance, 260
Biopsychosocial model, 302, 325

Blood
  pressure (BP), 69, 144, 150, 166, 169,
    178, 185, 188, 224, 316
  vessels, 5
Body
  chemistry, 6, 9
  conjunction, 5
  mass index (BMI), 164, 167, 260, 315,
    316, 320, 323–325
Brahman, 32, 46, 47, 63
Brahmarandhaṛā, 9
Brahmi, 195
British Thermal Unit (BTU), 263
Brittle nails, 9
Buddhi, 3, 7, 14, 15, 42

C

Cardiovascular
  efficiency, 164
  functions, 27, 169
Causative body, 5
Cell division, 4
Cessation, 3, 5, 20, 47, 50
Chair yoga (CY), 274
Chakra, 16, 152, 260, 261
Chanting, 24, 64, 83, 137, 139, 140, 146,
  230, 241, 243, 260
Character formation, 20
Chronic
  pain, 27, 69, 305, 306
  physical diseases, 6
Chronological narratives, 2
Citta, 2, 3, 7, 14, 42, 48, 51, 62
Cock posture, 151
Cognitive
  concepts, 1
  decline, 273
  function, 186, 234, 237, 240, 247, 271,
    272, 274, 275, 277, 279, 280, 285,
    289, 290
  impairment, 271–273, 275, 276, 290, 291
  performance, 291
  power, 257
  skills, 190
  training, 289
Colleagues, 21, 164, 167, 303, 306
Community members, 21, 66

Comprehensive index, 36
Conditional happiness, 57
Confidence interval, 72–74, 251, 254
Consciousness, 3, 4, 7, 11, 13, 14, 32, 41,
  48, 50, 51, 63, 83, 145–147, 238, 240,
  260, 261, 300
Constipation, 9, 142, 317
Contentment, 14, 38, 48, 56, 67, 68
Control group, 28, 166, 168, 176,
  193–197, 226, 244–246, 249, 251, 252,
  254, 257, 258, 265, 270–272, 275, 276,
  279, 280, 284, 285, 288, 326
Convalescent homes, 27
Convolvulus pluricaulis, 195
Cosmic
  arrangement, 5
  phenomenon, 7
Courageousness, 195, 225
Criminal activities, 22
Criticism, 28
Culture, 21, 35, 39, 48, 66, 71, 86, 107,
  185, 262

D

Darshanas, 23
Data
  Information, Knowledge, Wisdom
    (DIKW), 185, 231
  sciences, 81, 104
  sets, 103, 108
Decision
  difficulty (DD), 124
    scale (DDS), 114, 118–120, 122, 124,
     127
  making, 120, 127
Deep breathing, 148, 280
Defecation, 9, 149
Dementia, 186, 271–274, 277, 279, 289, 291
Democracy, 20
Denser combinations, 5
Depression, 13, 19, 21, 27, 28, 33, 68,
  82–85, 87, 114, 115, 161, 163, 164,
  167–169, 178, 186, 188, 190–193, 224,
  235, 236, 241, 276, 307, 316, 321, 324
Detention homes, 27
Devasya, 267
Dharma, 15, 53, 57

Dhidhrutismrutivibrashtta, 14
Dhimahi, 267
Dhiyo, 267
Dhṛiti, 14
Dhyana, 4, 65, 137, 153, 154
Diabetes, 25, 70, 80, 144, 160, 164, 166, 169, 178, 184, 188, 224, 243, 244, 273, 299, 304, 307, 315–317, 319–322, 324–327
  integration, 321
  mellitus (DM), 25, 304, 315, 316, 321
Diagnostic and statistical manual 5 (DSM-5), 273
Diarrhea, 9
Digital quality of life index (DQLI), 37
Dimensions, 33, 39, 41, 52, 79, 80, 87, 163, 197, 233, 238, 297, 320
Direct
  indicators, 36
  supervision, 23
Domains, 26, 35, 66, 67, 83, 86, 273, 276, 277, 297, 307
Doshas, 1
Dravyas, 4
Drug addiction, 19
Dveṣa, 44
Dysmenorrhea, 9
Dysuria, 9

E

Economic
  growth, 33
  planning, 20
Economically weak class, 27
E-government, 37
Ejaculation, 9
Ekāgra, 44
Electromagnetic waves, 238, 269
Electronic infrastructure, 37
Elementary school quality of life (ESQoL), 87
Elucidation, 50
Emotional
  and spiritual restoration, 153
  health, 96, 97, 166, 194
  intelligence, 237

maturity, 193, 194
  outbursts, 9
  regulation, 124, 125, 302, 307
  stability, 66
  trauma, 15
  well-being, 80, 87, 98, 194
  wellness, 291
Energetic function, 9
Energy
  levels, 25, 149
  measurements, 263
Environmental, 27, 37, 57, 61, 65–67, 71, 74–76, 86, 189, 233, 238, 273, 300
  health, 71, 76
Ephemeral, 48, 306
Erroneous decisions, 6
E-security, 37
Evolutionary process, 6
Executive functions, 274
Exhalation, 51, 149
Experimental
  design, 245, 271
  group, 168, 169, 176, 195, 196, 226, 245, 246, 253–255, 257, 258, 270–272, 275, 276, 279, 280, 285–288
Extrapolates, 1

F

Fasting plasma glucose (FPG), 315, 316, 322–325
Fatigue, 13, 182
Fatty component, 5
Fear of missing out (FOMO), 178
Fellowship program, 28
Fetal development, 5
Fetus blocks, 5
Fibroids, 9
Financial
  insecurity, 19
  status, 31
Five great oaths, 23
Fleshy mass, 5
Flexibility, 27, 69, 144, 164, 166, 278, 280, 285, 305, 317, 318, 321
  exercises, 280

Framing policies, 36
Functional mobility, 278
Fundamental
  nature, 3
  reformation, 1

G

Galvanic skin response (GSR), 242
Garbha pind asana, 13
Garudasana, 13
Gayatri mantra, 139, 140, 142, 246, 267
Gender-sensitive application, 126, 127
Generosity, 34
Global insistence, 33, 37
Glucose metabolism, 164, 170
Gorakhmundi, 195
Government policies, 33
Gross national happiness, 38
Gunas, 3, 11
Gupta gorakshasana, 151
Guptasana, 151
Guru, 23
Gyan yoga, 23, 24

H

Hair loss, 9, 160
Halasana, 9, 318, 320
Hallucinations, 7
Happy planet index (HPI), 37
Harappan civilization, 23
Harmony, 19, 33, 38
Harvesting, 20
Hatha yoga, 24, 25, 32, 40, 42, 43, 49–53,
  62, 63
Havan
  kund, 230, 247, 266
  samagri, 190, 194, 230, 235, 246, 247, 257
Health
  belief model, 309
  benefits, 1, 9, 289, 303, 305
  continuum, 297, 299, 300, 309
  psychology, 65, 68, 297, 298, 302–304,
    309, 310
  related
    problems, 29, 243
    quality of life (HRQOL), 87, 107

Healthy
  aging, 273, 274, 289, 291
  body, 25
  life, 27, 34, 83, 104
  mind, 21
  volunteers, 26
Hedonic treadmill, 47
Hedonism, 35, 48
Herbal
  and spiritual environment, 175, 176, 180
  formulation, 187, 196, 224
Heterogeneity, 327
Hierarchical
  arrangement, 36
  need, 36
High-density lipoprotein (HDL), 322, 324
Higher economic resources, 33
Hirsutism, 159, 160, 165, 169
Holistic health, 32, 104
Homa therapy, 186, 187
Homeostasis, 20
Hormonal, 14, 25, 159–161, 163, 165–167,
  170, 176, 302
  balance, 167
  disorders, 165
  imbalance, 25, 159–161, 163, 165, 170
Housing density, 37
Human
  awareness, 14
  behavior, 5, 15, 20, 181, 182, 300, 301
  development index (HDI), 37
  history, 5
  insight, 23
  needs, 36
  perception, 32
Humanitarian, 33
Hygiene, 46, 66
Hymn, 24
Hypertension, 25, 243

I

Idealist, 35
Illness
  continuum, 297, 300
  development, 308, 310
Illustration, 12, 23, 139

Immortal essence, 41
Immunity, 137, 153, 241, 247, 255
Improper diet, 22
Improved physical fitness, 272
Impulsivity, 29
Income disparities, 37
Indian
  healing systems, 16
  philosophy, 20, 39, 56, 62, 63, 238
Individual
  aspirations, 35
  living, 21
  muscles, 5
Industrial expansion, 33
Inertia, 3, 12, 178
Inexplicable body aches, 6
Infant mortality rate, 36
Infertility, 25, 160, 163
Inhabit status, 21
Injury, 9
Insomnia, 25, 28, 137, 191–193, 307
Instincts, 9
Institutionalized seniors, 271, 275, 291
Insulin
  dependent diabetes, 321
  resistance, 70, 160, 167, 169, 170
  sensitivity, 70, 163, 170
Intellectual
  comprehension, 2
  development, 21
  levels, 20
  pre-eminence, 2
Intelligence, 3, 14, 83, 87, 153, 177, 181,
  185, 191, 195, 225, 229, 237, 240, 264
Intensity, 150, 167, 321, 327
Interlinkages, 48, 57
Internal environment, 20, 244
International
  diabetic federation (IDF), 316
  journals, 26
Internet
  affordability, 37
  of things (IoT), 182–184, 264
  quality, 37
Intricate foray, 2
Inverted posture, 151

J

Jain civilizations, 23
Jap, 262
Jnana yoga, 28, 62, 63, 76
Jnanendriyas, 12
Job insecurity, 19
Journey, 2–4, 9, 41, 47, 144, 306
Joy, 38, 43, 47, 108, 148, 168
Jubilance, 33
Judgment, 15, 146

K

Kāma, 47
Karma, 4
  yoga, 23, 24, 28, 62
Kilowatt/hour (kWh), 263
Kirlian photography, 260, 261
Kleśas, 32, 44, 47, 49, 55
Knowledge, 2, 3, 12, 14, 15, 23, 24, 28,
  39, 42, 46, 48, 54, 56, 63, 66, 67, 83,
  184–186, 225, 231, 240, 262, 267, 298
Kriya yoga, 48
Kṣipta, 44
Kukkutasna, 151
Kundalini yoga, 25
Kurmasana, 13

L

Laghu Yōga Vasiṣṭha, 46
Laya yoga, 25, 62, 64
Legacy, 2, 16, 23
Liberation, 1–3, 7, 9, 14, 24
Life
  expectancy, 33, 34, 36, 37
  quality-enrichment, 32
Lifestyle
  diseases, 33, 236
  disorders, 22
  factors, 326, 327
Ligaments, 5
Linear development, 33
Lion posture, 151
Lipid profile, 163, 170, 171, 322
Literacy rate, 36, 272
Locust posture, 151

Low
density lipoprotein (LDL), 322, 324, 325
self-esteem, 28
Luxury, 31

M

Machine learning (ML), 81, 82, 87, 103, 104, 177, 181, 182, 186, 224, 244, 264
Mahābhūtas, 3, 4
Makarasana, 13, 165
Manas, 3, 5, 6, 14, 42, 190
Mandukasana, 13
Manomaya kosha, 5, 6
Mantra, 63, 64, 83, 137, 139, 140, 152, 165, 168, 187, 195, 229, 230, 235, 243, 246, 260–262, 267
yoga, 24, 63, 168
Marma, 1, 8, 9, 14
Martial posture, 151
Maslow's theory, 36
Mass, 5, 127, 260, 315, 320, 323, 326
Mathematical ability, 176, 195, 225
Matsyasana, 9, 318, 321
Matsyendrasna, 151
Matter-life engagement, 5
Maximization of
goal (MG), 124
strategy (MS), 124
Mean difference, 72–74, 280, 284
Medical care, 67, 275, 326, 327
Medicinal herbs, 180, 237, 255
Meditating, 25
Meditation, 1, 4, 16, 19, 28, 31, 41, 48, 50, 52, 61, 64, 65, 69, 70, 74–76, 79, 80, 82–84, 104, 107, 108, 113, 117, 119, 123, 135–137, 142, 144–148, 150–154, 159, 168, 175, 179, 181, 233, 235, 245, 246, 249, 260–262, 271, 274, 297, 304, 315, 317
techniques, 83, 145, 274
Memory
game, 232, 234, 250–253, 255, 257, 258, 265
assessment, 250–253, 255, 257, 258
power, 195, 225, 256
score, 256
tests, 248, 256, 258

Menstrual
blood, 5
cycles, 160, 163, 168, 170, 171
flow, 5
Menstruation, 9
Mental
afflictions, 32
alertness, 136
clarity, 136
component summary (MCS), 89, 90, 99–104, 111
fitness, 79, 80, 144, 243
health, 19–21, 27, 28, 65, 67, 69, 80, 84, 86, 102, 103, 135, 136, 150, 153, 163, 171, 176, 181, 185, 186, 188–193, 195, 209, 212, 223–225, 236, 237, 239, 242, 243, 247, 256, 275, 289, 291, 299, 300, 305, 307–309
illnesses, 29, 33, 67, 190, 191
modifications, 20, 25, 32, 62
pressure, 29, 234
serenity, 163
trauma, 176, 178, 226
turbulence, 21
Methodology, 32, 70, 81, 84, 88, 189, 192–194, 196, 234, 239, 247
Mild cognitive impairment (MCI), 271, 273–276, 279, 285, 286, 288, 290, 291
Mind
body
healing, 169
practices, 55
culturation, 57
Mindful
attention awareness scale (MAAS), 114, 118–120, 122, 124
based interventions, 116, 127
breathing, 304
Mindfulness, 28, 29, 83, 85, 107, 113–116, 118, 119, 122, 124–127, 152, 168, 169, 261, 280, 297, 298, 305–310
based intervention (MBI), 114, 115, 307
practice, 115, 298, 308, 309
techniques, 152, 306
Mini-Mental State Examination (MMSE), 271, 276, 277, 279, 285, 288

Ministry of Statistics and PI (MoS-PI), 175, 194, 195, 233
Mockery, 20
Monoamine oxidase (MAO), 191
Mood disorders, 13, 115
Moral
　disciplines, 48
　values, 20, 21
Muḍha, 44
Mudra, 136–144, 149, 151–154
Muscle endurance, 278
Muscular strength, 27, 29, 166
Mystical
　levels, 29
　sounds, 24

N

Naḍis, 1, 7, 9, 16
Nasti yogaatparam balam, 16
Nāth yogis, 46
Natural language processing (NLP), 87
Negative affect, 34, 113, 114, 117, 119, 120, 122, 124–126, 271, 272, 276–278, 285, 287–289, 291
Nerve, 3, 9, 190, 318
　impulse, 3
Nervous system, 13, 69, 148, 152, 168, 178, 179, 187, 239, 318
Neurodegenerative disease, 291
Neuroplasticity, 38, 52
Niruddha, 44
Nirvāna prakaraṇa, 46
Niyama, 4, 27, 32, 48, 49, 64
Non-insulin-dependent diabetes, 321
Nutrition, 46, 66, 107, 261, 273, 289, 326

O

Obesity, 160–163, 165, 168, 176, 178, 187, 224, 226, 243
Obey norms, 21
Om chanting, 280
Orchestrator, 3
Organizational framework, 7
Organs, 12, 13, 43, 52, 69, 135, 136, 144, 151, 164, 165, 317, 318
　function, 13

P

Padmasana, 13, 151, 165
Paired
　sample T-test, 119, 196, 199, 205, 208, 211, 212, 215, 219, 221, 234, 251, 252, 255
　T-test, 205, 208, 211, 214, 217, 219, 222, 252
Panas, 114, 117, 119, 120, 122, 127, 276–279, 286–290
Pancha mahavrata, 23
Paradox, 37, 38
Paraspinal muscles, 13
Parasympathetic nervous system, 69
Particulate matter (PM), 242, 263
Patanjali, 1–3, 12, 20, 23, 29, 44, 62, 63, 76, 136, 304, 318
　yoga sutra, 20, 23
Paves, 4, 177
Pedagogy interventions, 113, 127
Pessimism, 28
Philosophical ground, 46
Physical
　activity, 63, 165, 166, 169, 170, 178, 185, 188, 273, 274, 289, 290, 316, 317, 322
　ailment, 15
　body, 6, 46, 136, 151, 179, 266
　component summary (PCS), 90, 104, 111
　conditioning, 166
　evaluations, 5
　exercise, 41, 107, 167, 170
　fitness, 19, 107, 162, 166, 271, 272, 274–276, 278, 279, 285, 286, 288–291
　frailty, 278
　health, 26, 31, 33, 35, 67, 71, 80, 83, 84, 86, 144, 167, 176, 178, 179, 191, 224, 298–300, 305, 307–309
　　benefits, 305
　power, 26
　quality of life index (PQLI), 36
　strength, 29
　world, 14
Physiology, 9, 185
Physique, 25, 26

Placenta, 5
Pollution, 189, 229, 242, 243, 264
Polycystic ovarian syndrome (PCOS), 159–161, 163, 165–171
Positive
  activity model, 309
  affect negative affect scale, 34, 39, 114, 117, 119, 120, 122, 271, 278, 285, 287–291
  emotions, 34, 119, 237, 308, 309
  health, 297, 298, 305, 308–310
  psychology, 27, 28, 297, 298, 301, 302, 308–310
  thinking, 21
Post
  havan, 265
  performance, 250, 253
  test, 197, 203, 206, 209, 212, 215, 218, 221, 251, 253, 255, 275, 279, 280, 285, 287, 288
  scores, 251, 255, 287, 288
Posttraumatic stress disorder, 27
Posture, 4, 12, 13, 64, 82, 137, 144, 151, 161–163, 262, 317, 318, 320, 321
Prachodayat, 267
Pragmatism, 2
Prakriti, 3–7, 11–14
Prana, 3, 4, 7, 9, 13, 14, 50, 51
Pranayama, 4, 5, 23, 25, 29, 65, 137, 145, 148, 151–154, 163–165, 168, 170, 179, 195, 235, 240, 241, 245, 246, 274, 280, 318
  kosha, 5
Pranic
  energy, 255, 261
  healing, 261
Pratibhā, 40
Predispositions, 4, 9
Predominant
  definitions, 32
  goal, 33
Pre-havan, 265
Preservatory processes, 7
Pre-test, 275, 278, 285, 287
  scores, 285
Prevent dementia, 272
Psychiatric disorders, 27

Psychological, 6, 14, 20, 25–27, 35, 38, 45, 56, 61, 66, 67, 71–73, 75, 76, 83, 114–117, 164, 165, 176, 178, 180, 188, 239, 261, 288, 297, 302–309, 315, 316, 319–322, 325, 326
  disorders, 6, 25, 176, 188, 239, 306, 309
  health, 66, 67, 71, 164
  outcomes, 315, 321
  residues, 32
  well-being, 61, 76, 116
Psychology today, 21
Psychosomatic
  disorders, 25
  issues, 6
Public health and air pollution in Asia (PAPA), 229
Purgatory action, 9
Purusha, 3, 11, 12, 14

Q

Qualities
Quality of, 3–5, 7, 12, 15, 54, 71, 187, 190, 301
  digital well-being, 37
  in life-threatening illness patient (QOLLTI-P), 85
  life (QoL), 25–27, 29, 31–39, 45, 53, 55–57, 61, 65–76, 79, 80, 82, 85–90, 103, 104, 107, 135, 136, 142, 144, 150, 153, 154, 170, 184–186, 289, 305, 307, 308, 325
  benchmarks, 33
  indicators, 36
  levels and indicators, 36
Questionnaire, 71–74, 79–81, 85, 89, 104, 113, 117, 188, 275, 276, 321
Quiescent dispositions, 44

R

Rāga, 44
Raj yoga, 24, 29, 25, 62
Rajas, 3, 5, 11
Rational thinking, 14
Rehabilitation, 1, 27, 29
Relaxation techniques, 167
Remedy, 22, 192

Rhythm, 20, 85
Righteous behavior, 15
Rig-Veda, 23
Rishi, 23, 82, 236
Rituals, 23
Routine customary, 23

S

Saccidānanda, 32
Sage
  Maharshi Patanjali, 23
  Vyasa, 23
Salabhasan, 151
Salivary amylase activity, 189
Samadhi, 2–4, 24, 27, 49, 62, 65, 153
  Pada, 2
Sāmānya diseases, 46
Sama-veda, 23
Samidha, 267, 268
Samkhya karika, 15
Sample
  dataset, 108–110, 231, 232, 265
  size, 61, 75, 191, 199, 205, 208, 211,
    214, 217, 217, 219, 222, 224, 252,
    255–257, 326
Samskāras, 32, 43–45
Samvida, 267
Śaṅkarācārya, 39
Sanskrit, 7, 23, 62, 83, 230, 261, 262, 274
Saraswati Panchak, 176, 180, 190, 195,
  196, 226, 235, 237, 244–246, 256, 257
  havan, 235, 246, 257
  herbs, 256
  samagri, 245, 256, 257
Sarvangasana, 9, 151, 318, 320
Satavari, 195
Satisfaction theories, 35
Sattva, 3, 5, 11, 54, 190
Sattvik, 11, 15
Satvik ahara, 304
Savitur, 267
Self
  actualization, 36
  discrepancy theory, 36
  improvement, 28
  knowledge, 24

Seniors with mild cognitive impairment
  (SWMCI), 271, 275, 290
Sense organs, 6, 12, 27, 43, 51, 52, 239
Sensor, 182–184, 264
Serial learning, 289
Shankhpushpi, 195
Shavasana, 165
Short
  form-36 (SF-36), 79–81, 89, 104
  term memory, 276, 289
Siddhasna, 151
Simhasana, 13, 151
Simhasana, 151
Sinha's comprehensive anxiety test
  (SCAT), 242
Sleep quality, 315, 327
Slums, 27
Smart cities, 79, 84, 104
Social
  animal, 21
  behavior, 27, 29
  health, 71, 76, 307
  inactivity, 22
  interventions, 289
  life, 19–22, 29, 185
  philosophy, 21
  reforms, 29
  rehabilitation, 27
  relationship, 26
  support, 34
  wellbeing, 20
Somatic
  stress, 163
  symptoms, 308, 310
South Asian tradition, 23
Species, 13, 14
Sphaeranthus indicus, 195
Spinal cord, 25, 147, 148, 317
Spine agile, 13
Spiritual
  existence, 7
  focus, 27
  health, 305
  practices, 46, 107, 108, 179, 194
  reforms, 29
  wellbeing, 20, 55, 164, 193, 305, 165
Spirituality, 19, 136, 147, 150, 230, 303
Squatting posture, 151

Stagnation, 3
Standard deviation, 119, 199, 205, 208, 211, 214, 215, 219, 221, 251, 252, 254, 255
State trait anxiety inventory (STAI), 28, 29, 189
Statistical analysis, 72, 234, 249, 250, 252
Stress
  management, 164, 316
  reduction, 66, 144, 166, 306
Subjective well-being, 164, 237, 271, 277, 289–291
Sukshma kriya, 280
Surya namaskar, 23, 159, 161–165, 167, 168, 170, 171
Sushruta Samhita, 262
Sushumna
  breathing, 152
  Nadi, 147, 148
Suspended particulate matter (SPM), 263
Sustainable development (SDG), 34, 37, 104, 187, 298
Sutras, 2, 3
Suvah, 266
Svastikasana, 151
Sweating, 9
Swift-acting system, 14
Symbolic representations, 7
Sympathetic response, 189

T

Talahridaya Marma, 9
Tamas, 3, 5, 11, 44
Tamasic, 11
Tamasik, 15
Tantric customs, 23
Tapas, 24, 48, 64
Tat, 267
Temper, 9, 178
Terawatt/hour (TWh), 263
Terrorism, 19
Test
  scores, 198, 203, 204, 206, 207, 209, 210, 212, 213, 215, 216, 218, 219, 221, 222, 246, 249, 251, 253–255, 258, 269, 270, 285, 287, 288
  statistic, 199, 205, 208, 211, 214, 217, 220, 223, 251, 254, 272

Theoretical foundations, 32
Therapeutic measure, 170, 171, 237
Three-forked path, 2
Total cholesterol, 315, 322, 324
Traditional healing, 148
Tragic crop, 20
Tranquil, 42
Transcend, 2, 62–64
Transformation, 3, 4, 6, 7, 57, 68, 135, 225
  mechanisms, 7
Transtheoretical model, 309
Tree posture, 151
Tributaries, 9
Trimarga, 2
T-test, 61, 72–74, 76, 119, 196, 199, 205, 208, 211–212, 214, 215, 217, 219–222, 234, 251, 252, 255, 258, 272

U

Udana Vayu, 9
  vitiation, 9
Ultimate soul, 25
Unconditional
  happiness, 57
  love, 47
Understanding quality of life, 33
Unfavorable consequences, 6
Unfulfillment, 38
Unification, 2
Uninspiring, 4
Uninterrupted, 24, 52, 153
Union, 13, 20, 24, 62, 83, 304
Unique, 3, 7, 13, 56, 81, 137, 237, 264, 305, 309
  combination, 3, 237
  identifiers (UIDs), 264
United Nations (UN), 37, 62, 298, 304
Universal consciousness, 3
Universe, 3, 83, 161, 186, 237, 303
Unpleasant, 10, 114, 278
Unwinding, 50
Upanishadic legacy, 23
Upa-veda, 5
Urgent, 20
Urinary incontinence, 9
Urination, 9

Urvi marma, 9
Uterus, 9, 191
Utkatasana, 151

V

Vach, 195
Vairagya, 15
Vaishnavas, 23
Vareñyam, 267
Vayu, 1, 4, 7–9, 16, 138, 139
Vedas, 23, 161, 179, 187, 262
Vedic, 23, 24, 27, 64, 80, 137, 139,
  176–181, 189, 223–225, 230, 235,
  238–242, 260–262
  period, 23, 262
  protocols, 225
  times, 23
  yoga, 23, 24
Vein, 9, 322
Vernacular, 2
Vibhransha, 14
Vibration, 24
Victory, 25, 150
Vijñanamaya kosha, 5
Vikrutis, 6
Vikṣipta, 44
Violent, 20
Virasana, 151
Vital organs, 13
Vitiation, 9, 14
Volitional practice, 51
Vrkshasana, 151
Vṛtti, 32, 43, 47, 49, 55
Vyāsa Bhāṣya, 45

W

Weaker, 7, 235, 244, 245
Weight loss, 163, 165, 166, 170
Welfare, 21, 154
  formula, 154
  questionnaire, 321
Well-being questionnaire, 321
Willingness, 14, 271, 276
Wisdom, 5–7, 14, 15, 23, 39, 40, 56, 84, 177,
  185, 186, 197, 220–223, 231, 267, 298
Withdrawal, 27, 116

Witness, 3, 4, 6, 9, 12, 146
Work competition, 26
Workplace, 25, 136, 150, 307
World
  Happiness Report, 33, 34, 37, 38
  Health Organization (WHO), 20, 26, 35,
    61, 65, 71, 74, 86, 107, 108, 190, 230,
    272, 298, 299, 308, 316, 321
  War II, 33, 301

Y

Yagya therapy, 193, 194, 233, 235, 237,
  241, 243, 247, 255, 257
Yagyopathy, 187, 233–241, 244, 246, 247,
  249, 256, 258
  Research and Development Association
    (YRDA), 244
Yajna, 176, 177, 179–181, 186–188, 195,
  196, 224–226, 229–231, 243, 261, 267,
  268
Yajur-Veda, 23
Yama, 4, 2732, 42, 48, 49, 64
  niyama, 42
Yashasvati nadi, 9
Year fixed effects, 34
Yearning spawn, 4
Yoga, 1–4, 6, 7, 10, 11, 13, 16, 19, 20,
  22–29, 31, 32, 39–57, 61–65, 68–76, 79,
  80, 82–84, 103, 104, 107, 108, 113, 114,
  116–121, 123–127, 135–137, 142, 144,
  145, 151–154, 159, 161, 163–170, 175,
  176, 179, 181, 189, 195, 224, 226, 233,
  235, 245–247, 249, 271, 272, 274, 275,
  279–281, 283, 285, 288–291, 297, 298,
  304, 305, 308–310, 315–321, 323–327
  asanas, 245, 246, 320
  Darshan, 20
  Description, 23
  dynamics, 4
  effects, 26
  eight limbs, 2
  exercises, 68, 166, 168, 280
  gesture posture, 151
  group, 26
  intervention, 113, 170, 272, 279, 280,
    289, 291, 315, 320, 323

literature, 20
meditation, 28, 61, 69, 70, 74, 75, 82,
    84, 104, 135, 136, 142, 144, 152, 181
module, 271, 291
mudra, 151
needs, 25
origin, 2, 22
philosophy, 136
postures, 68, 280
practices, 23, 24, 27, 69, 144
practitioner, 74, 75, 168, 280, 290
purpose, 1
sadhana, 23
science, 23
sutras, 1–3, 23, 136, 304
therapy, 316
training, 113, 114, 116, 117, 119, 121,
    126, 127, 168, 271, 275, 279–281,
    283, 285, 288–291
    programs, 127
types, 24

Yogaś citta vṛitti nirodhaḥ, 2
Yogasutra, 3, 32, 42–45, 51, 62, 64
Yogi, 3, 4, 6, 12, 23, 153
Yogic
    asanas, 9
    breathing Pranayama and meditation
        techniques (YBMT), 145
    experience, 16
    formulations, 2
    history, 23
    level, 29
    life, 1
    paradigms, 32, 48, 56
    path, 14
    practice, 9, 22, 23, 25, 63, 163, 168, 305
    process, 1, 2, 4, 9
    system, 11
    techniques, 48, 57
    way, 16
Young generation, 19
Youth, 22, 29, 154